TEXTBOOK OF PSYCHI

Shazia.

Dedication

To Linford Rees, who taught us to understand psychosomatic relationships.

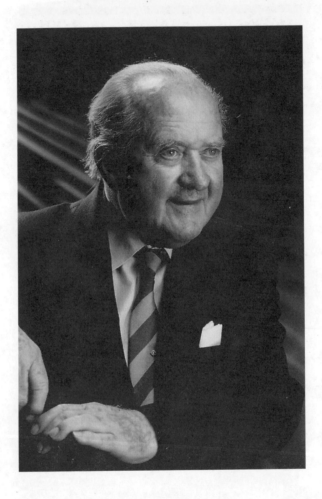

TEXTBOOK OF PSYCHIATRY

Edited by

Linford Rees

CBE, DSc, MD, FRCP, FRCPsych(Hon), LID(Hon), DPM

Emeritus Professor of Psychiatry, University of London; Past President of the British Medical Association; Past President of the Royal College of Psychiatrists

Maurice Lipsedge

MPhil, FRCP, FRCPsych

Consultant Psychiatrist, Lewisham and Guy's Mental Health Trust; Senior Lecturer, United Medical and Dental Schools, Division of Psychiatry and Psychology, Guy's Hospital, London

Chris Ball

MRCPsych

Consultant in Old Age Psychiatry, Lewisham and Guy's Mental Health Trust; Senior Lecturer in Old Age Psychiatry, United Medical and Dental Schools, Division of Psychiatry and Psychology, Guy's Hospital, London

A member of the Hodder Headline Group
LONDON
Co-published in the USA by Oxford University Press, Inc., New York

First edition published in Great Britain in 1997 by Arnold,
a member of the Hodder Headline Group,
338 Euston Road, London NW1 3BH

Co-published in the United States of America by
Oxford University Press, Inc.,
198 Madison Avenue, New York, NY10016
Oxford is a registered trademark of Oxford University Press

Whilst the advice and information in this book is believed to be true and
accurate at the date of going to press, neither the authors nor the publisher
can accept any legal responsibility or liability for any errors or omissions
that may be made.

British Library Cataloguing in Publication Data
A catalogue record for this book is available from the British Library

Library of Congress Cataloging-in-Publication Data
A catalog record for this book is available from the Library of Congress

ISBN 0 340 57195 0

2 3 4 5 6 7 8 9 10

Typeset in 9/11pt Palatino by Scribe Design, Gillingham, Kent, UK
Printed and bound in Great Britain by Alden Press

CONTENTS

LIST OF CONTRIBUTORS

Dr A.P. Boardman
Head of Department
Department of Psychiatry
Keele University
School of Postgraduate Medicine
Stoke-on-Trent

Dr Peter K. Carpenter
Consultant Psychiatrist in Learning Disability
Phoenix NHS Trust
and Honorary Clinical Lecturer
University of Bristol
Bristol

Dr David A. Collier
Senior Lecturer in Molecular Genetics
Head of Section
Institute of Psychiatry
London

Dr Anthony C.D. James
Consultant in Adolescent Psychiatry
Warneford Hospital
Oxford

Professor James P. Watson
Professor of Psychiatry
United Medical and Dental Schools
Division of Psychiatry
Guy's Hospital
London

PREFACE

Linford Rees' *Short Textbook of Psychiatry* went into five editions and was translated into seven languages between 1967 and 1988. However, three recent reports, namely the General Medical Council's *Recommendations on Undergraduate Medical Education* (1993), the British Medical Association's *Report of the Working Party on Medical Education* (1995) and the Conference of Medical Royal Colleges' *Arrangements for General Professional/Basic Specialist Training* (1995), have redefined the agenda for the teachers of future generations of doctors. The emphasis has moved away from detailed academic knowledge to a wider view that stresses skills, understanding and attitudes. It is with these changes in mind that we have approached the preparation of this new textbook.

The culture in which we practise is increasingly multi-cultural, ageing, community-orientated and focused on primary care, moving away from a medico-centric to a more multi-disciplinary approach. How to communicate in this complex domain and translating this dialogue into clinical concepts have been of great importance to us. Developing an appreciation of the influence of social, psychological, cultural, environmental and ethical influences, as well as biological factors, on the expression and experience of mental health problems has been our prime concern.

The book has been arranged in topics, with the emphasis being placed upon what it is important for the student to know. To this end we have shown how to describe a mental state, but have avoided the otiose scholasticism of detailed phenomenology. Similarly, although there is guidance on the management of violence and antisocial behaviour arising as a result of severe mental health problems, there is no account of the detailed work of the forensic psychiatric services. However, the legal and ethical considerations commonly encountered by doctors are addressed.

Finally, whilst the book is primarily directed at medical undergraduates, it will also be of value to those from other disciplines who are working in the mental health field, and to doctors passing through the period of general professional/basic training.

Linford Rees
Maurice Lipsedge
Chris Ball
Sidcup, Kent
1996

Recommendations on Undergraduate Medical Education. Education Committee, General Medical Council, December 1993.

Arrangements for General Professional/Basic Specialist Training. Conference of Medical Royal Colleges and their Faculties in the UK, June 1995.

Report of the Working Party on Medical Education. British Medical Association, August 1995.

FIFTY YEARS OF PSYCHIATRY: AN INTERVIEW WITH PROFESSOR LINFORD REES

Professor Linford Rees was formerly professor of psychiatry at St Bartholomew's Hospital in London. His career spans 50 years and encompasses the major developments in psychiatry during this time. Originally from the south of Wales, he acquired an interest in psychiatry early in his medical training. Subsequently he worked at the Maudsley Hospital and developed the psychiatric services in his home country of Wales. His interests range widely, and have included psychopharmacology, psychosomatic illnesses and the teaching of psychiatry. The following conversation between Chris Ball (CB) and Professor Rees (LR) explores the developments that have taken place over his long and distinguished career.

CB: Professor Rees, I would like to start by asking you a little bit about your background. I was wondering whether you came from a medical family?

LR: No, I come from a family of teachers. My father was a teacher, my grandfather was a teacher, and my aunts and uncles were teachers or headmasters, or directors of education, and all the boys in my class at the grammar school were going to become teachers, so I said 'well that's going to be difficult to get a job if I am going to be a teacher,' so I looked for alternatives. I went into medicine to avoid becoming a teacher, but I ended up as a teacher just the same!

CB: So from grammar school you went to the Welsh National School of Medicine in Cardiff. Was psychiatry part of the curriculum?

LR: It was a 3-month course of lectures and demonstrations, but I did 7 months as a resident clinical assistant at Whitchurch Hospital, and that gave me intensive in-patient as well as out-patient experience. I looked after the female side, did a morning round and an evening round, and then we had to do all the social histories for the out-patients at the Cardiff Royal Infirmary when the social worker was away – this was good experience for me. Similarly, we had to do the dispensing when the dispensers were away, and then even the post-mortems. It was a very varied experience. It was stimulating because Whitchurch had a very well-known and distinguished research scientist called Quaster. He had a team of biochemists who did research into psychiatric illness. I remember taking part in one of his investigations, as he wanted to study whether the liver of schizophrenics effectively detoxifies benzoic acid. My colleague and I were the so-called 'normal' controls. He was a very brilliant and stimulating person, so my interest in psychiatry emerged from that experience. I also went with the Superintendent to the teaching hospital where we did out-patients and treated patients ourselves.

CB: It seems you were exposed fairly early on to an organically based notion of mental illness. It also sounds as if taking social histories made a big impression on you early in your career.

LR: Exactly. The social histories were extremely detailed and took many pages of writing to get the full account.

CB: How was the teaching organized at that time?

LR: It was mainly a series of systematic lectures. They were given by Dr Henry, who was a good teacher and expressed difficult concepts with clarity. It was all didactic, clear and concise. There were the usual demonstrations of typical chronic, severe cases. This, of course, is not the best way of teaching or demonstrating psychiatry. It tends to put people off.

CB: Yes, I think some people find it uncomfortable to come in and to watch that kind of teaching. Was that something that influenced your later teaching style?

LR: Yes. I avoided that completely.

CB: I have heard stories of the very distinctive and memorable teaching style you perfected. Usually in small groups, and sometimes in the open air?

LR: Yes, that's right.

CB: When developing psychiatry as part of the undergraduate curriculum, were there any major problems to overcome?

LR: In Barts I was lucky – I had the support of the Professor of Medicine, Professor Eric Scowen, and Sir Aubrey Lewis, who was my mentor at the Maudsley. Professor Scowen was on the Committee of Management at the Institute of Psychiatry, so he was very keen. Initially I went to Barts only one afternoon a week to the out-patient department – there was no in-patient work. When I took over I succeeded in getting 3 months full-time for psychiatry. The students loved this and greatly appreciated it. In the first clinical term I gave a series of introductory lectures on the psychological aspects of clinical medicine. They then had 3 months full-time, and then in the final year they could do 2 weeks of elective psychiatry and used to go away to various hospitals. It gave them the choice of either child psychiatry, adult psychiatry or psychotherapy, or whatever. So having 3 months full-time was a tremendous bonus because it gave us plenty of time with the students. Teaching was done in small groups. Two or three students were allocated to a particular consultant, and that made it an intimate, close method of teaching, almost like an apprenticeship. There were regular case conferences, case presentations, talks and lectures. But it was all done on an informal, small-group basis.

CB: That sounded like a fairly major step forward that you introduced.

LR: It was a leap forward because there was no other medical school in London with that amount of time and availability of teaching throughout the 3 years of medical training.

CB: It is quite remarkable that psychiatry was so neglected until that time, given how important it was. You said earlier that you had the support of the Professor of Medicine. Was that a very important element?

LR: Oh yes, very important, because of the senior registrars in psychiatry. The first one to have

an appointment was with the Professor of Medicine. He welcomed it. Senior registrars would go on rounds with him and they discussed social and psychological aspects of every patient, whatever the illness was. It was the job of the senior registrar to discuss this not only with the Professor, but also with all the students and the junior staff. Later I was able to place senior registrars with many medical departments. I had an interesting experience. I once arrived about 5 minutes late for a lecture, and when I came to address the students, there sitting in the front row was Sir James Patterson Ross, Professor of Surgery. He liked the lecture, quoted it extensively, and came to a few more lectures. I'm sure that was a great boost.

CB: This kind of breaking down of barriers between the medical specialties and psychiatry seems to me to be something about reshaping the relationship between the physical and psychological parts of disease.

LR: The most important thing I found was that, if physicians and surgeons asked you to see one of their patients and you helped them to get better, this was the most powerful influence in gaining their support and recognition. That's a hard way to do it, but it's the only way in a teaching hospital like Barts in which psychiatry was relatively new.

CB: I would guess that the prevailing paradigm was very much a psychoanalytical one in the psychological causation of physical problems, but that was something you went beyond and took forward in a much more positive way, both at Barts and more widely.

LR: I had done a considerable amount of research in Wales on the relationship between psychological issues and physical problems – asthma, urticaria, vasomotor rhinitis, vagotomy and miner's nystagmus. So when I came back to London, half a dozen of us were interested in the holistic approach to disease. We were physicians, paediatricians, students, health officers, GPs and anthropologists. We all got together and decided to establish a Society for Psychosomatic Research. That took off and became quite successful. This was followed by the International College of Psychosomatic Medicine which involved people all over the world.

CB: One of the most important developments you have seen was the introduction of drugs particularly targeted at psychiatric disorders rather than non-specifically sedating patients. Could you say something about what kind of impact these drugs had?

LR: The impact was tremendous, really. Chlorpromazine was the first, and it had a tremendous impact on psychiatry because of its wide-ranging effects. At the first international meeting held in Paris in 1956 there were people from various parts of the world, all with impressionistic viewpoints. I was the only person who described results based on double-blind controlled trials. Professor Pierre Pichot, who was the chairman, was impressed by the elegance of the trial.

CB: Had the reputation of chlorpromazine come before it?

LR: Oh yes, absolutely, but I think sceptical scientists needed the randomized double-blind controlled trial method of assessing the drug before they would accept its validity or usefulness.

CB: I can imagine its arrival in the pharmacy was an exciting day.

LR: Oh yes, it was very exciting because here was something new which helped not only by calming severely disturbed patients, but also by specifically targeting hallucinations and delusions. Nothing like it had been available before, so it was very exciting.

CB: Do you think chlorpromazine actually lived up to its promise?

LR: Yes it did, but the promise, probably, was greater than was justified in the beginning because it had not been subjected to proper controlled studies.

CB: Have you seen other major changes that have been as important with psychotropic medications?

LR: A variety of other tranquillizers emerged, but chlorpromazine remained the measure, the standard of comparison. Then came the butyrophenones which proved helpful in mania. Brian Davies and I did the original study of haloperidol in mania at the Bethlem. The next big advance was the antidepressants. The monoamine oxidase inhibitors were introduced by the discovery of the serendipitous use of iproniazide in tuberculosis. Iproniazide often made patients overactive, excitable and elated, so Klein and Nathan tried it in depressives and got good results. I was not the first to use imipramine, but I was one of the first to carry out double-blind control trials with it. Maurice Lipsedge and I did the first controlled trial of dothiepin, which had been discovered in Czechoslovakia.

CB: Before these drugs were introduced, what was the likely career of a severely ill person?

LR: Well, there was ECT for the more severe cases, and that produced good results for withdrawn, depressed patients. Continuous baths were used, but that was of limited value. In fact there was very little then. Amphetamines were used, but these were of practically no value at all. So for severe depression ECT was the only choice.

CB: Was there much hope for someone developing a schizophrenic illness prior to this?

LR: Cardizol injections were used to induce therapeutic convulsions before ECT became widespread. I remember one very chronic patient at Worcester who showed significant improvement after intravenous injections. It was not pleasant for the patients because, prior to losing consciousness, they used to get very anxious.

CB: For most patients would it have meant a long term as an in-patient if they developed schizophrenia?

LR: Some recovered spontaneously, but the majority had quite prolonged illnesses. About 6 months before the inception of the National Health Service I was appointed to survey the Mental Health Services of Wales and plan the future services. When I completed that survey, I had a lot of spare time so I studied schizophrenia, comparing insulin coma therapy, electronarcosis and electroconvulsive therapy which identified all the prognostic features. People got quite excited about this method of evaluating different treatments, but electronarcosis did not prove to be of any value.

CB: I was wondering how you see the future, having been involved in many of the most important developments over the last 50 years.

LR: I see a promising future in the biological aspects of psychiatry. Genetics is a thriving science, and important discoveries have been made in this area. Genetic factors affect biochemistry by influencing enzymes, so I see tremendous advances in the development of new forms of treatment. This applies to Huntington's chorea, identifying the genetic basis and specific DNA profile not only for the patient, but for the relatives. All of these will help in the prevention of the transmission of Huntingdon's chorea. I see a bright prospect for the development of more specific psychotropic drugs. We will see a whole range of 5HT reuptake inhibitors, and new ones are coming out with improvements on the previous ones. Functional imaging of the brain will teach us a great deal about the biological basis of mental illness.

CB: I am wondering how you feel we can keep these developments in a proper perspective, while dealing with the social and psychological problems as well.

LR: I always taught my students that every illness, whatever it is, even if it's what appears to be exclusively a physical illness, always has a psychological aspect. Now the interesting thing is that I think psychological methods of treatment are going to advance, both behavioural therapy in its various forms and cognitive therapy, as well as short-term psychodynamic therapy.

CB: During your time in Cardiff you had an inspirational teacher, Dr Quaster, and you mentioned Sir Aubrey Lewis, who profoundly influenced more than one generation of British psychiatrists, including yourself.

LR: Sir Aubrey Lewis taught the most rigorous standards for research and clinical practice. His high intellect was inspiring.

CB: What is it that makes a good teacher, do you think?

LR: I think the first thing is that you must be able to communicate with clarity, but an equally important thing is that you must be enthusiastic and able to evoke emotional responses in an audience – to excite them and make them interested. I think that when people ask what are the most memorable lectures you can remember, and when you analyze that, they all have one common factor; an inspiring lecture, whatever its form or content, achieves an emotional response.

In Wales, some preachers evoke the 'hwyl', which is when they get the congregation to respond to what they say. It is an interaction that excites them. You get a lot of conversions happening when you get that emotional arousal. In other words, I think good lecturers have the ability to convey not only the academic content of the lecture but also, by the way it is presented, its capacity to evoke a reaction and in turn to stimulate interest, activity and endeavour on the part of the students.

One very stimulating lecturer was Sir Reginald Watson Jones. He spoke about fractures, but he spoke about it in such an interesting and enthusiastic way that we were all carried away and all wanted to become orthopaedic surgeons. I do not know whether he learnt that or whether it was part of his make-up. I think a lot of it does depend on the personality of the lecturer.

CB: If there is one message that you would like medical students to take away from this book, what would that be?

LR: There's something I feel very strongly about. I would like them to take on board the principles of aetiology. There has been a lot of debate about the Gulf War syndrome and somebody on television said 'we could not find a single cause and we could not find a single disorder, therefore it does not exist'. They overlooked the fact that all illnesses have a multifactorial origin – the social, psychological, biochemical, genetic, physical and environmental aspects. All of these things potentially play some part, and their effect on the organism is not necessarily a single discrete entity. What I would like to see is the student learn how to assess the patient and, having done that, to say what the predisposing factors are and which were the initiating or precipitating factors, which were the factors which make the illness continue and which factors determine the outcome. I feel very strongly that physicians and students should use this clear concept of what determines the cause and course of an illness.

CB: Professor Rees, thank you very much.

PART

1

APPROACHING MENTAL
HEALTH PROBLEMS

1 TALKING AND LISTENING TO PEOPLE

Interviewing in the psychiatric context can be a daunting prospect when looked at from the outside. Your introductory lecturers will have given you a detailed and complex schema for taking histories and burdened you with a thesaurus of words, some familiar but used in unfamiliar ways, and some unfamiliar and used for strange and unimaginable things (*Gedankenlautwerden*: hearing one's thoughts spoken out loud). A whole new concept, THE MENTAL STATE EXAMINATION, will have been introduced in hushed and reverent tones. Initiation into this world can only come after trials of fire, water and air. The other major problem concerns what you actually do or say in the interview.

- What do I do if they cry?
- What do I do if they get violent?
- What happens if it's funny and I want to laugh?
- How do I manage if they talk about things which I can't talk about?
- What if they say nothing?
- I can't ask things like that.

In the end there is only one way to get over this problem and that is to jump in and see some people. It may help to sit in with a person who is being interviewed, but in the end you have to do it yourself.

Issues in the interview

- developing the relationship
- current problems
- why are they presenting now?
- how did they get to this point?
- what sort of person are they?
- what has made them this type of person?
- hypothesis testing
- diagnosis
- shared understanding of the problems
- shared plan of action for the future

However, a little preparation can go a long way towards making this a rewarding and enriching experience.

Before seeing the person ask yourself the question, 'Why am I seeing this person?' 'Because I have to for the ward round' is probably the reason, but a number of other possibilities should be borne in mind.

Reasons for seeing people with mental health problems

TO ESTABLISH A RELATIONSHIP

Unless you establish a reasonably positive relationship with the person at the outset of the interview, then you might as well go home and not bother. Without some initial intimation that you will be a sympathetic and warm listener then it is unlikely that you will achieve any of the objectives of the interview.

This starts before you even meet the person to be interviewed. In most settings appropriate dress is required that demonstrates a certain respect if not extremes of formality.

The person needs to be warmly welcomed and invited into the room that is to be used for your interview. In people's homes it is even more important to be aware of the appropriate social behaviour as a guest. Ensure that you introduce yourself clearly to the person and that they are comfortable.

UNDERSTAND THE REASONS WHY THE PERSON IS SEEING YOU

For example, they may be seeking help in sorting out their marital relationships, or they may be seeing you because the police won't help them remove the neighbours who are beaming radio waves at them, or because they feel that life is not worth living.

Getting a verbatim account from the person of the problems that currently beset them is the first stage of the process.

UNDERSTAND HOW THIS PERSON CAME TO BE IN THIS SITUATION AT THIS PARTICULAR TIME

What is the story behind the reason they are seeing you? How long has this situation been going on, how did it first start, and what have you done about it up until now? A vital question is: why now? Why not several weeks ago? What has changed? What is different? If a person is coming of their own free will you are likely to get on much better than if they have been coerced into coming to see you ('Get help now or I am leaving you'.)

UNDERSTAND WHAT SORT OF A PERSON IS IN THIS SITUATION

What is their life story? What are their early influences and their responses to stress in the past? The biography and personality of the person will profoundly influence their responses to stress and their ability to work in particular psychological ways. It may also influence their compliance with medication.

UNDERSTAND THE PERSON'S IDEAS, CONCERNS AND EXPECTATIONS OF THE INTERVIEW

The idea of seeing a psychiatrist is a complete anathema not only to those who are psychotic and do not define their problems as psychological, but also for many others who worry they will be labelled as 'mad or crazy' as a result of the consultation, or that they will be locked up. It is also important to understand what the person hopes to derive from the interview. If it is a recommendation for rehousing and you offer 16 sessions of non-directive counselling the chances of success will be slim.

HOW TO GO ABOUT IT

Exploring these questions with people can be difficult in some cases, but most people are happy to talk about and explore these issues with you. A number of simple techniques can be used to make this part of the interview flow.

Venue

Choose somewhere quiet and private to talk. In practice this can be difficult, especially on medical wards where all your intimate business from details of your bowel resection to your visitors' problems in parking are common knowledge. A place where people are constantly coming in and out is no good, nor where the phone is ringing all the time.

The arrangement of furniture needs to be conducive to a relaxed interview (I rearrange my out-patient clinic each week from its medical layout to a more intimate one. I do not like conducting my interviews across a metre of beech veneer).

The venue must also feel safe for you. It should be near to other people and be fitted with a violence alarm. Try to sit nearer the door than the person if you suspect that there is any possible problem of violence (I was caught out in this way as an inexperienced junior and learnt the lesson the hard way). Conduct the interview with someone else present if you are at all concerned.

Time

Interviews that are conducted in a hurried way are not productive. Even if very stressed, a relaxed approach to the consultation will help the person to feel sufficiently at ease to unfurl their story at a comfortable pace. As time is often relatively limited it is perhaps best to make this clear at the beginning in order to avoid cutting people off just as they have got started.

We have 40 minutes today to look at some of the problems that took you to your doctor and to get some background information about you.

Non-verbal communication

Large amounts of information can be obtained by doing nothing in the right kind of way. If you spend the whole interview with your head down taking notes the person will not feel encouraged to talk and you will not notice any of the person's non-verbal behaviour (moving about more in the chair when discussing relationships, averting their eyes when describing painful events, etc.).

Silence is vital to enable people to search for the right words or to collect themselves. It is difficult to be silent.

Hold on and wait, something will happen.

Maintaining eye contact shows continuing interest in the person, unlike staring out of the window. Encouraging nods and hand gestures will help the person through parts of their tale, but fiddling with your tie, pen or personal organizer will not.

Verbal behaviour

The aim of any interview is to encourage the person being interviewed to tell you what they think is important and what you need to know in their own words. A person's verbatim account freely given might be as follows:

> Do you have any distressing experiences?
> I hear them laughing and talking about me. They say horrible things. They say I killed those children. I didn't, but they say they will tell the police.

This is more informative than an affirmative answer to a closed question:

> Do you hear people talking about you that you cannot see?
> Yes.
> Do they say horrible things about you?
> Yes.

By asking open questions in this way (How are you? What has been troubling you? Can you tell me more?), rather than closed questions (Did your mother hit you? Did the tablets help you?) where only yes or no answers are appropriate, the person is encouraged to talk. However, you may need this type of question in order to clarify details.

Make empathic remarks which show that you understand the feelings that the person is experiencing.

> That must have made you feel very sad
> I can imagine that being frightening
> How awful.

Try not to interrupt and cut across what the person is saying and allow the interview to grow organically rather than sticking rigidly to a single format ('We have talked about your children. Perhaps you could tell me about your own childhood'). If you do need to change tack it is perhaps best to acknowledge this so that the person does not feel cut off in their stride.

> Thank you for telling me this. I wonder if I could change tack completely and ask you about your first admission to hospital because it will help me to understand more about the current situation.

How to conduct the interview

- take your time
- find the right place
- ensure clear introductions are made
- ask open questions
- use non-verbal behaviour to encourage the person, e.g. eye contact, hand gestures, posture, etc.
- keep the flow of the interview as organic as possiblet
- make empathic remarks

'HMMM. I SEE, SO.......... '

Making hypotheses is an activity we are all involved in when seeing people. Is this mania? Is this because she experienced sexual abuse as a child? Is this because of changes in the medication?

These ideas tend to be formed very early in the interview and then need testing. If a person tells you he or she is influenced by a death ray gun manned by Nazi war criminals then one quickly switches into schizophrenia interview mode, asking appropriate questions to confirm your hypotheses.

> Do you hear them talking too?
> Oh, about you. To each other?
> Hmm. I see, so....do they influence you in other ways?

These narrow pathways are usually kept to. Keep listening! Unexpected cues can throw you on to other scents:

> It only happens after I have this strange sense of something about to happen and butterflies in my stomach which sort of come up towards my chin.

Such a statement will lead to a rapid switch to questions on temporal lobe epilepsy.

MAKING A DIAGNOSIS

Making a formal diagnosis by testing your hypotheses is important, and the mechanisms for doing this will be explored in the chapter on diagnosis and classification.

ACHIEVING A SHARED UNDERSTANDING OF THE PROBLEMS WITH THE PERSON

Defining and providing feedback of your understanding of the person's problems is vital. It allows you to give the person some information about the issues as you see them, and also enables them to re-evaluate their problems in the light of this. It also gives the person a chance to put right any misconceptions that you have developed during the interview. At this stage, agreement on the areas on which it is important to find a way forward is vital. It is unlikely that your therapeutic manoeuvres are going to succeed if they are totally at odds with the person's views about where the problem lies. It may be that with some people no agreement can be reached. After a time you will find areas within which you can agree to work, even if they are not what you define initially as the primary problem.

A severely psychotic man and I agreed not to discuss issues relating to the activities of the police, as neither he nor I could do much about them and had different views about the nature of these activities. We worked together over issues of housing, work and social life which we agreed were important and we could approach together.

AGREEING A PLAN TO TACKLE THE PROBLEMS

Having agreed what the problems are and how they came about, agreeing a further management strategy is the next step. This might only be a question of agreeing to meet again in order to extend your understanding of the problem or do some physical, psychological or social investigations before the next meeting, when you would go through the problems and your understanding of them again before agreeing how to tackle them.

The amount that the person can do for himself or herself may well be much greater than the amount that the doctor is able to do for them, but only with support and encouragement is this likely to take place. The learning of anxiety control depends largely on practice, which the person can only do for themselves.

DOING A MENTAL STATE EXAMINATION

Could I see you do a mental state?
I only had time to do a mental state...

'Doing' a mental state is one of the most alien things that you come across when starting psychiatry. It looks, when written down, rather like the physical examination. First you take a history, and then you examine the person. This is the classical teaching. If you have been attached to an Accident and Emergency department or to a busy medical firm you will have realized that the two activities usually go on simultaneously, and this is also the case with the mental state examination.

What are you doing when you do a mental state examination?

When 'doing' a mental state examination you are attempting to describe the person's behaviour and psychopathology at the time of your interview.

The examination involves not only describing the physical appearance of the person but also listening to what they say and how they say it. It is this last part that is difficult to grasp and takes some time to get comfortable with. Sometimes questions need to be asked about the way people are thinking, but mostly these will be part of your exploration of the person's story.

You may need to ask questions such as the following.

Have you had any unusual experiences?
Do people treat you well?
How have you been in your spirits?

If these issues have not come out in the general flow of the interview itself.

Learning to look and listen is the most important part of 'doing' the mental state examination.

VIOLENCE AND PSYCHIATRIC DISORDER

It was noted above that interviews should be conducted in a safe place. It is important to have some understanding of the relationship between violence and psychiatric disorder.

Most violence and violent crimes are committed by people who are not suffering from a psychiatric disorder, and the majority of those with psychiatric disorders are not violent. Apart from acute abuse of alcohol or drugs the single psychiatric category most widely associated with violence is schizophrenia, and it is important to emphasize that most people suffering from this condition are not dangerous. On the contrary, it would be both inaccurate and unfair to add to the stigma of this diagnosis by assuming that people with schizophrenia are necessarily violent.

The potentially risky period in schizophrenia is when people are experiencing psychotic symptoms, especially persecutory delusions and passivity experiences. Once these are treated, the risk of violent behaviour decreases significantly.

TABLE 1.1 Factors predicting violence in psychiatric patients

Antecedents:	A previous history of violence
Diagnosis:	Schizophrenia Morbid jealousy and erotomania Illicit drug use or alcohol misuse or both
Social and domestic factors:	Loss of family support and deterioration in personal relationships Loss of accommodation
Clinical:	The person's declared intentions and attitudes to previous and potential victims Threats of violence Presence of active symptoms, especially delusions of poisoning and sexual matters, passivity experiences, command hallucinations, depression and angry outbursts
Management:	Loss of contact with mental health services Poor compliance with medication

Predictions about violent behaviour are difficult to make and the longer the forecast period, the greater the inaccuracy. When assessing a person's potential danger to the public you should pay attention to those elements in their life which are subject to change, including the following:

- compliance with psychotropic medication;
- exacerbation of symptoms;
- a radical disruption of personal relationships;
- an escalation of drug or alcohol abuse.

How to approach violent or alarming behaviour

A wide variety of behavioural problems can arise anywhere people are seen, be that in their own home, on the ward in Accident and Emergency, or in the General Practitioner's surgery. It is important to be aware of the possibility of difficult behaviour and to ensure that you are aware of how this can be dealt with. Ensure that people know where you are and when you will be back if you are making community visits. If there is any possibility of violence ensure that there are enough people about for the interview to be conducted safely. Familiarize yourself with the local security arrangements.

Problems that can arise include the following:

- verbally abusive and threatening behaviour;
- destructive behaviour;
- self-destructive behaviour;
- physical attacks on others;
- over-activity leading to exhaustion (in mania).

These problems can be prevented by keeping the person fully informed about what is happen-ing to them and why. It is important to address questions and complaints quickly.

Underlying causes include the following:

- fear rather than anger;
- organic confusional state;
- the effects of drugs or alcohol on perception, reasoning and self-control;
- threatening hallucinations or delusions;
- misinterpretation of your intentions;
- manic disinhibition;
- communication difficulties, including thought disorder or reduced linguistic fluency.

Your own behaviour can go a long way towards defusing the situation. Introduce yourself and anyone who is with you. It is helpful to give information about your professional role. Providing the person with information about the nature and purpose of the interaction will help them to orientate themselves. This enhances their sense of control, whereas a feeling of powerlessness increases the risk of aggression.

Your non-verbal behaviour (body language) is important. Adopt an unthreatening posture (with your hands by your sides) and an attentive facial expression, and avoid undue eye contact. Speak quietly and calmly, and move in a slow deliberate way. Sitting beside someone is much less confrontational than standing in front of them.

Use the person's name and attempt to elicit any grievance (by asking open-ended questions and not interrupting) and offer reassurance that it will be attended to and that no harm will come to them. Acknowledge the person's feelings and their account by showing interest and respect. It is best not to make threats or promises, avoiding challenge and confrontation. Give feedback on how you perceive the person's mental state (I sense you are very angry/anxious/frustrated, etc.). Finally, make suggestions offering choices rather than issuing orders.

Dealing with difficult behaviour

Non-verbal behaviour

- sit beside the person
- don't make undue eye contact
- move slowly and deliberately

Verbal behaviour

- give information about yourself and why you are there
- keep the person informed
- listen
- ask open-ended questions

- acknowledge the person's feelings
- give reassurance
- avoid threats and promises
- communicate interest and respect

If the situation cannot be defused in this way, physical means (restraint and medication) may need to be employed. This must be done with an adequate number of trained staff to ensure that it is an effective and safe procedure.

Further reading

Gunn, J. and Taylor, P. 1993: *Forensic psychiatry: clinical, legal and ethical issues.* Oxford: Butterworth-Heinemann.

Pendleton, D., Schofield, T., Tate, P. and Havelock, P. 1984: *The consultation: an approach to learning and teaching.* Oxford: Oxford University Press.

Trzepacz, P.T. and Baker, R.W. 1993: *The psychiatric mental status examination.* Oxford: Oxford University Press.

2 CLASSIFICATION AND DIAGNOSIS IN PSYCHIATRY

There are major difficulties in classification and diagnosis in psychiatry.

- What are psychiatrists talking about, i.e. what is a mental illness, and when is a mental state abnormal? How do you decide?
- Psychiatric symptoms and signs are non-specific.
- Delusions and hallucinations occur in schizophrenia, mania and severe depression.
- Depression can be the primary problem or part of another disorder, e.g. agoraphobia.
- There are no reliable biological markers.
- Psychiatrists change their minds and cannot agree.

There are differences between the two most commonly used classifications of the World Health Organization (WHO) (International Classification of Diseases (ICD)-10) and the American Psychiatric Association (Diagnostic and Statistical Manual (DSM)-IV).

Since everyone is unique, should we bother with labels at all, or should we take each person's distress on its own merits? What help can a label be?

WHAT ARE MENTAL DISORDERS?

This term, like so many in medicine, has no agreed definition but should include the following elements (derived from DSM-IV):

- a behavioural or psychological syndrome;
- associated with distress or disability;
- associated with a risk of incurring death, pain or disability;
- not culturally appropriate;
- the disorder is a manifestation of dysfunction in the individual;
- not merely a conflict between the individual and society.

As you can see, it is very difficult to put clear boundaries around the concept, and individual psychiatrists will vary greatly in their approach to those who are on the margins (see Chapter 19 on personality and its disorders). Deciding who fits into these categories is not usually a major problem, but sometimes only long contact with the person and detailed work with their families will clarify the situation.

MAKING YOUR DIAGNOSIS

In medicine diagnoses are made at a number of different levels:

- aetiological, e.g. syphilis;
- pathological, e.g. ulcerative colitis;
- deviance from a physiological norm, e.g. hypertension;
- clinical symptoms, e.g. migraine.

Mental disorders are also diagnosed at different levels:

- aetiological, e.g. general paralysis of the insane;
- pathological, e.g. Alzheimer's disease;
- clinical symptoms, e.g. schizophrenia.

Most diagnoses in psychiatry are made at the level of symptoms and signs as syndromes. Psychiatric symptoms are non-specific and only make sense when considered together as a pattern. Rather than detail each possible symptom and its possible significance, we have described the patterns for each of the syndromes within the relevant chapter, and accompanied these with other information about the syndromes.

Some major divisions

CATEGORICAL VS. DIMENSIONAL

In this book and for most areas of psychiatry a categorical approach to classification is taken (this is schizophrenia, that is obsessive-compulsive disorder, and so forth). This can lead to defining rather disparate symptoms and signs under the same rubric. There is a big difference between the person with schizophrenia who has lots of florid symptoms and the next person who has many negative symptoms (see Chapter 7 on schizophrenia), yet both would be recognized as having schizophrenia by a competent psychiatrist.

Where the categorical approach fails is in primary care. Here the person will often display a little anxiety, a little depression, and perhaps some phobic elements too, or else the disorder presents too early in its course to meet the criteria set by psychiatrists for an illness. Under these circumstances it may be more sensible to define the person's symptoms along a series of axes rather than in a categorical manner.

ORGANIC VS. FUNCTIONAL

There was great hope in the nineteenth century that the underlying brain pathology of all mental disorders would be worked out. This endeavour failed, and those clinically defined disorders for which no underlying neuropathology could be demonstrated became known as functional disorders (schizophrenia, manic-depression, anxiety disorders, etc.).

With sophisticated techniques of investigation, more of the biology of the functional disorders is now known (e.g. the neurochemistry of depression). As a result, the historical division between organic and functional has begun to appear unhelpful. However, it remains an important distinction, as some reversible causes can be found for symptom clusters resembling the classical functional disorders (see Chapter 6 on organic states).

PSYCHOTIC VS. NEUROTIC

This division has been one of the mainstays of practice for many years. Psychotic patients have delusions and hallucinations, and have lost the ability to test reality in the normal way. Neurotic patients recognize their states as abnormal and do not suffer from delusions or hallucinations.

The term neurotic has been omitted from the most recent major classifications. Particular problems surrounding the classification of depression and the anxiety disorders have led to its demise (a much lamented development in some quarters).

Current classifications

For many years it was not clear that psychiatrists were speaking to each other in the same language. One doctor's schizophrenia was another doctor's mania. Personal classifications abounded, and depending on where you were trained you diagnosed in a certain way.

Attempts to get around this problem began in the late 1960s with the development of standardized interviews, so that all individuals would be asked the same questions (e.g. the Present State Examination, 1st edition 1967).

From such interviews standardized diagnoses could be derived because the information collected about the individuals was elicited in the same way in each case.

Developing from this, the World Health Organization and the American Psychiatric Association have produced clarifications which operationally define mental disorders (ICD-10 and DSM-IV, respectively). In this book the DSM-IV has been used to a large extent, because it provides the clearest criteria for each disorder.

WHY MAKE DIAGNOSES?

If each person is unique, bringing their own personality, biography and social circumstances to the consultation, what is the point of making a diagnosis and reducing them to a label?

A diagnosis does not define a person; it defines the disorder that they have. We have tried to avoid terms like 'a depressive' or 'an alcoholic'.

Making a diagnosis is a useful shorthand way of communicating between professionals. It provides a frame of reference within which they can orientate themselves rapidly.

Making a diagnosis implies a whole range of knowledge which the professional can bring to bear upon the case in hand. Making a diagnosis of Alzheimer's disease tells you about the likely course of the disease (prognosis), what problems the person is likely to experience as time passes, and what amelioration is available to that person.

It allows you to talk to both the person with the disorder and their carers in an informative way, preparing them for the future and setting up support systems for them.

It also allows research to be done. Without diagnoses only single case studies can be reported. This is fine for very rare conditions, but not for common and disabling ones. No move forward can be made in the treatment and care of people with mental disorders if it is not possible to define the population you are dealing with.

Reasons for making a diagnosis

- for communicating with the sufferer and carers
- for communicating between professionals
- for prognosis
- for planning management

MAKING A DIAGNOSIS IN PSYCHIATRY

Making a diagnosis in psychiatry can be difficult. The lack of biological markers and the non-specific nature of the histories and symptoms means that it is not always entirely clear what the diagnosis is (this is part of the fun).

Whenever you are making a diagnosis you are placing a bet. Sometimes it is 99.9 per cent certain (the movement disorder is classic, the family history is of Huntington's chorea and gene studies have been done). At other times theere is less certainty and you have a series of differential diagnoses with different odds on each one.

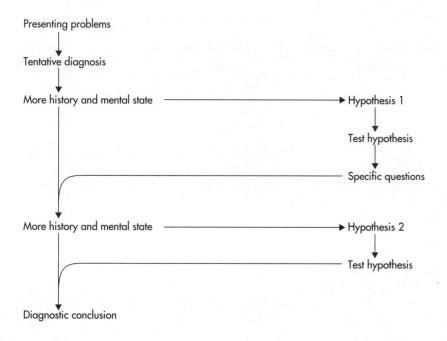

Presenting problems

Tentative diagnosis

More history and mental state ──────────────→ Hypothesis 1

Test hypothesis

Specific questions

More history and mental state ──────────────→ Hypothesis 2

Test hypothesis

Diagnostic conclusion

FIG 2.1 The diagnostic interview.

- 2:1 it is a cerebral vascular accident; 4:1 it is a cerebral tumour; 8:1 it is an abscess; 100:1 it is hysterical.

The classical route to a diagnosis is:

- take a history;
- do an examination;
- perform investigations.

Then and only then make a diagnosis.

However, in practice life is not like this. Early on in the interview clues will be given as to what the diagnosis might be. For example:

I feel so sad, I can't go on any more.
I can't face going out. My stomach churns, my head spins. I feel like I'm going to faint.
My mind can control the TV.

This will lead to you making hypotheses, which are then tested in the interview, being picked up and perhaps discarded as others are tested (Figure 2.1).

The diagnostic interview

The ultimate aim is to build up a pattern of the person's difficulties, signs and symptoms to see whether it fits with the pattern you know for each disorder. It is important to consider significant negatives. For example, if a person presents with poor concentration and impaired memory it is important to rule out depressive pseudodementia (see Chapter 21 on old age psychiatry) before making a diagnosis of dementia.

When you have taken the history and examined the mental state it is useful to provide a brief summary of the most salient features that point towards the diagnosis you have made.

When you think you have made the diagnosis it is important to construct an argument with pros and cons backing up your conclusions and why it has come about (aetiology).

Aetiology

A number of models exist for the generation of mental disorders. In most cases these are multifactorial and no single paradigm suffices.

BIOLOGICAL MODELS

There have been major advances in brain science over the last decade. More and more is known about the biology of mental disorders, but attempts to view them all as organic are pre-mature. Some mental disorders, e.g. Alzheimer's disease, clearly have a physical substrate, but even here the person's response to the organic deterioration of their brain is mediated through their personality, biography and social circumstances. Biological factors may include family history, drug use, physical illness, etc.

PSYCHOLOGICAL MODELS

The influence of psychodynamic explanations of illness has waned in recent years, but psychological factors in the causation of mental disorders are of major importance and should not be submerged under the current wave of interest in biological factors. Why does one person get clinically depressed following loss of his or her job, while another does not? There may be some biological predisposition, such as a family history, but it is more likely to be related to the person's ways of coping with stress and their previous experience of loss and rejection.

SOCIAL FACTORS

Social stressors such as poor housing, lack of a confidant, noise and poverty have all been associated with poor mental health. Continuing social problems make rehabilitation difficult and, unless they are resolved, make treatment of the mental disorder very difficult. Social factors may include job loss, poor housing, poor marital relationships, etc.

The bio-psycho-social model

Most psychiatrists employ a bio-psycho-social model. For each case the relative contribution made by each of the three elements is very different, even if the same disorder is present.

The aetiological factors can also be divided into the following categories.

Predisposing Those factors which made it likely that this person might experience a particular problem (e.g. a family history or disrupted childhood).

Precipitating Those factors which indicate why this problem has happened now (e.g. loss of job, physical illness, loss of a loved one).

Perpetuating Those factors which are likely to make resolution of the episode of illness less likely (e.g. poor housing, unstable relationship, chronic physical illness).

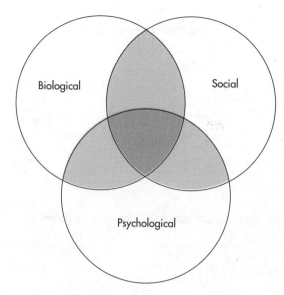

FIG 2.2 The bio-psycho-social model.

When you have made a provisional diagnosis and suggested the aetiology of the disorder, you need to state how you would like to proceed to confirm your diagnosis (i.e. by means of investigations).

SOCIAL INVESTIGATIONS

Collateral histories (you always want to know more!) may be obtained from people, case notes, social services, prison reports, etc. It is desirable to obtain the person's permission to make investigations in this way.

PSYCHOLOGICAL INVESTIGATIONS

Psychological investigations help to understand the psychological make-up of the person experiencing problems. Detailed neuropsychological testing can be used to help define a possible organic lesion.

BIOLOGICAL INVESTIGATIONS

These include physical examination, blood tests, urine screens, Computed Tomography (CT) and Magnetic Resonance Imaging (MRI), etc.

Only after these procedures have been carried out will a reasonably firm conclusion concerning the most likely diagnosis be made, and final plans for the management of the person be made. It is important to agree on this plan together with the person if it is to succeed (see Chapter 1 on talking and listening to people).

Further reading

American Psychiatric Association 1994: *Diagnostic and statistical manual of mental disorders.* 4th edn. Washington DC: American Psychiatric Association Press.
World Health Organization 1992: *The ICD-10 classification of mental and behavioural disorders 10.* Geneva: World Health Organization.

3 HISTORY, MENTAL STATE AND MANAGEMENT PLAN

In most cases you will not (and cannot) cover all the points outlined here in one session, either in out-patients or in an exam situation. Each interview needs to be tailored to the circumstances in which you find yourself (see Chapter 1 on talking and listening to people).

This schema outlines the major headings to cover. Details of the important features of each syndrome are outlined in the relevant chapter.

HISTORY

Orientating the listener

For example, 'John Hastings is a married 45-year-old unemployed bookbinder from Barchester who was referred to the clinic by his GP'. This helps to give the listener a picture of who the subsequent story is about.

Presenting problems or complaints

These are the reasons why the person is seeing you now. Get these in the person's own words if possible.

Note that the person may have no problems or complaints of their own beyond the fact that they are seeing a psychiatrist!

History of presenting problems

Why? How? When? (Tell me more... Then what happened?)
Try to include the history from someone else in addition to the interviewee at this time.

Family history

This includes parents, brothers, sisters, cousins and aunts. Did they have psychiatric or medical problems? What were relationships like between them?

Personal history

INFANCY AND CHILDHOOD

Did they have a normal birth? Did they walk and talk normally? Was their health fine?

EDUCATION

How much education did the person receive? How did they get on? Did they have a record of truancy? How did they do in examinations?

WORK

What sort of work have they done? Why did they move or change jobs? How often did this occur? What aspirations do they have?

RELATIONSHIPS AND SEX

How do they get on with people? Do they make strong relationships? What sort of sexual background did they have?
Are they or have they been married? Is the relationship a good one? Have they got children?

FORENSIC HISTORY

Does the person have any records of prison sentences, fines or other offences? The circumstances of these should also be noted.

DRUGS

What should they be taking? What are they taking (both legal and illegal drugs)? How much do they smoke and drink?

MEDICAL HISTORY

PAST PSYCHIATRIC HISTORY

This includes any previous consultations, admissions, treatments and outcomes.

PERSONALITY

What sort of a person is this? (See Chapter 19 on personality and its disorders.)

MENTAL STATE EXAMINATION

Appearance and behaviour

Describe as clearly as possible in plain language what is happening and how the person looks during your interview – whether you think their appearance is abnormal or not.

Speech

Keep this to the musical aspects of the speech. How much is there? Does it come unbidden? Is it loud, soft, fast or slow? Does it go up and down or is it monotonous?

Mood

SUBJECTIVE

Ask the person how they feel 'in themselves', 'in their spirits', in order to get a subjective view.

OBJECTIVE

Use this report together with your own observations of their behaviour and their thinking to get an objective view.

Note that sleep, appetite and diurnal variation are part of the history. They help to make a diagnosis of depressive illness, but say nothing about a person's mood.

Thought

Thought is reflected in the person's speech.

CONTENT

What are the main things that are preoccupying this person during the interview? Does the person have delusions or other abnormal beliefs?

FORM

Does the person express his or her ideas in a coherent way, or are they difficult to follow (thought disorder)? Are they fast or slow?

POSSESSION

Do the thoughts of the person belong to him or her alone, or are they interfered with in some way?

PERCEPTUAL DISORDERS

Does the person have strange experiences that he or she either cannot account for, or accounts for in a bizarre way? (People talking you can't see, funny smells, odd sensations in the body)

Cognitive function

ORIENTATION

Does the person know:

Who they are?
Where they are?
What the day, date and year are?

MEMORY

Short-term memory

Can the person repeat to you the names of three objects (a banana, a coat and a sledge) when these are said to them slowly?

If so, then ask them to repeat these words to you again after 5 minutes, during which time you will have been distracting them by doing something else.

Long-term memory

'What are the dates of the Second World War?'
'Who is on the throne?'
'Who is the president of the USA?'

CONCENTRATION

Ask the person to spell WORLD backwards.
Ask the person to subtract seven from 100, and then to subtract seven from that number, and so on (serial sevens).

VISUOSPATIAL ABILITY

Ask the person to copy simple drawings such as the following:

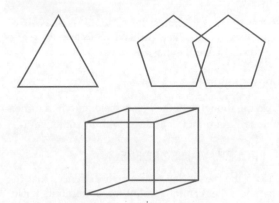

WRITING

'Please write a sentence for me.'

READING

'Could you read this sentence please?'

CALCULATION

Give the person several arithmetical problems of increasing complexity to solve.

LANGUAGE

Expressive dysphasia

Repeat after me 'No ifs, ands or buts'.

Nominal dysphasia

Name two objects (e.g. a watch and a pen).

Receptive dysphasia

Ask the person to carry out a command.

INSIGHT

'Why do you think you are in the situation that you are currently in? Are you ill? What do you feel about the treatment you have been receiving?'

SUMMARY

If the history outlined above was written by Proust, then this part should be written by Chekhov. It should be pared down to the bare necessities to show the wood from the trees.

DIFFERENTIAL DIAGNOSIS

- The most likely one and why
- Why this one is less likely, etc.

It is always best to include the possibility of an underlying organic disorder, as the symptoms are often the same as those of functional disorders (see Chapter 6 on organic states).

PROBLEMS

These are areas which you and the person identify as presenting difficulties which could be worked upon.

Having schizophrenia is not a problem, but hearing voices that tell you to kill yourself is.

AETIOLOGY

The biological, social and psychological factors that have brought about the mental disorder in this person can be divided into those that *predisposed* the person to a mental disorder and those that *precipitated* it at the present time.

FURTHER INVESTIGATIONS
Biological

Physical examinations, blood tests, etc.

Social

More information, collateral histories. Reports about work, living conditions, etc.

Psychological

Detailed cognitive testing or further exploration of the issues involved and the person's response to them.

MANAGEMENT

Acute

This may involve getting a seriously suicidal patient into hospital.

Longer term

The aim here is to ensure that the person improves, and that he or she maintains this improvement over a period of time.

BIOLOGICAL

Correcting biological abnormalities, e.g. treating a urinary tract infection.

Medication

Which medication and at what dose?

SOCIAL

Manipulation of social conditions, e.g. attendance at a day-centre in order to reduce isolation, provision of a home help, receiving benefits.

PSYCHOLOGICAL

Formal or informal treatments to work through issues and to develop new approaches to problems.

Prognosis

What is the likely long-term response of this person to your best therapeutic endeavours, and what factors make this likely?

Further reading

Hamilton, M. (ed.) 1985: *Fish's clinical psychopathology*. Bristol: Wright.

Sims, A. 1988: *Symptoms in mind*. London: Bailliere Tindall.

4 SOME WORDS PSYCHIATRISTS USE

Psychiatrists speak in a strange language. Some terms are completely incomprehensible, whilst others that you thought you understood no longer seem to have the same meaning. The signifier is nowhere more slippery and elusive than in the psychiatrist's hand.

In order to clarify some of the terms you will commonly meet, they are presented here as a glossary. Other terms crop up in the book and are explained at the appropriate point in the text.

Appearance and behaviour

AGITATION

Purposeless motor activity. The person wrings their hands, cannot sit still and walks about.

AKATHISIA (LITERALLY 'INABILITY TO SIT STILL')

This is an experience of the need to keep moving, usually as a side-effect of neuroleptic medication. It is often inferred from the person's movements, but there are many reasons for moving from foot to foot.

CATATONIA

The bizarre movements seen in schizophrenia. The person may adopt strange and uncomfortable postures, and the limbs can be moved and have a curious tone (known as waxy flexibility). These movements may alternate with periods of excitement (catatonic excitement).

ECHOPRAXIA

Repeating the interviewer's actions.

Speech

COPROLALIA

Compulsive and explosive exclamations of obscenities.

DYSARTHRIA

Speech that is difficult to understand because of lesions to the apparatus that produces the sound of speech, i.e. the lips, tongue, larynx or their innervation.

DYSPHASIA

An inability to use language as a result of damage to the brain, making it difficult to comprehend language (receptive dysphasia) or to express oneself coherently (expressive dysphasia).

ECHOLALIA

Repeating the interviewer's words.

PRESSURE OF SPEECH

The rapid speech seen in mania.

WORD SALAD

A complete mishmash of words that you cannot follow.

Emotion

AFFECT

A short-lived mood state.

ALEXITHYMIA

A person's inability to express their mood state in words. 'You know how it is...it's sort of...y'know'. Alexithymia is a source of great frustration to psychiatrists.

ANHEDONIA

The inability to derive pleasure from anything.

ANXIETY

An internal sense of apprehension and fear. It is a common symptom of many disorders.

DEPRESSION

This term has many lay uses and it is important to find out what it means for the person using it. It is a symptom associated with lack of pleasure and a feeling of misery. For it to be used as a syndrome, depression must be the primary symptom and other features, e.g. diurnal variation, must be present.

EUPHORIA

This is the normal end of a continuum of elevated mood which extends from euphoria via elation to ecstasy (seen in mania).

EUTHYMIA

Neither elated nor depressed. Normal mood.

FLATTENING OF AFFECT

A lack of emotional warmth.

INCONGRUITY OF AFFECT

This occurs when the emotion displayed is not in keeping with the subject under discussion, e.g. laughing when discussing distressing events.

LABILE AFFECT

Rapid changes in mood.

MOOD

A more persistent emotional state than an affect.

The experience of self and the world

DEPERSONALIZATION

The sense that you are unreal and not your usual self, unable to feel and respond in a normal way. The world is felt to be dull, flat and unreal (derealization). The feeling is intensely unpleasant.

Thought

DELUSIONS

A belief that is held with utter conviction despite evidence to the contrary, and that cannot be explained by the educational, social or cultural background of the person who holds the belief. It is the result of pathological thought processes.

DELUSIONAL PERCEPTION

Following a normal experience a delusion arises. 'I saw the vase and knew I was the Queen's son'.

FLIGHT OF IDEAS

A tenuously connected series of ideas which soar away from their intended goal. It is seen in mania.

OBSESSIONS

Recurrent thoughts that intrude into the person's mind unbidden. They are usually resisted and are recognized as arising from within the person's own mind. Compulsions are motor acts with similar properties and they often accompany obsessions.

OVERVALUED IDEA

Either a delusion-like idea held with some doubt (I think someone is following me everywhere, but I'm not absolutely sure), or an idea which influences the person's life unduly or which they pursue over-vigorously (e.g. a person who consistently engages in vendettas or litigation).

PASSIVITY PHENOMENA

The experience of having your thoughts removed or inserted into the mind by an external agency. Other people may experience their movements as being controlled by an external agency.

PHOBIAS

Fears that are out of proportion to the object or situation that causes them, leading to avoidance of the object or situation. The person recognizes that the fear is irrational.

THOUGHT BROADCASTING

The experience of having one's thoughts known by others, usually by telepathy or through the radio, television or Internet.

THOUGHT DISORDER

It is assumed that we think in straight lines. When these clear paths become disrupted or diverted then it becomes difficult to follow the person's line of reasoning. This may be subtle (loosening of associations) or abrupt (knight's move). Try to record it verbatim, as one man's thought disorder is another's learned discourse.

Perception

FORMICATION

The sensation of insects crawling under the skin.

HALLUCINATIONS

Perception in the absence of an external stimulus. Hallucinations can occur in any modality.

ILLUSIONS

Misinterpretations of external stimuli.

INSIGHT

The description of the person's view of why they are in their current situation. Is it because they are mentally ill, or do they have other explanations?

Further reading

Hamilton, M. (ed.) 1985: *Fish's clinical psychopathology*. Bristol: Wright.
Sims, A. 1988: *Symptoms in mind*. London: Bailliere Tindall.

5 PSYCHIATRY AND PRIMARY CARE

CASE 5.1

A 33-year-old married woman with three children presented to her General Practitioner (GP) requesting an urgent home visit as she had breathing difficulties and felt she was going to die. The previous night she had gone to the emergency department by ambulance with the same symptoms. She had also called out the GP night locum service the previous week and had been given a salbutamol inhaler. Subsequent consultations revealed that she had experienced autonomic symptoms of anxiety since her last child had been diagnosed as having pyloric stenosis. This had been corrected by surgery and the child had made a complete recovery. She came to her GP at that time with nausea and a churning sensation in her stomach. These symptoms had worsened and she now had episodes of overwhelming anxiety with palpitations, tingling in her fingers and difficulty getting her breath, especially at times when she was feeding her child. Between these episodes she was tense, restless and had tension headaches. Her sleep was intermittently disturbed. She believed that her child's illness had been due to breast-feeding. Her other two children had been bottle-fed.

She was referred to an anxiety management group at the health centre and attended most of the sessions. She showed some improvement, but still had intermittent panic attacks. Her youngest child had no more problems, but she had a continuing poor relationship with her husband who was not supportive and in whom she could not confide.

If you had an emotional problem who would you turn to?

It is unlikely that you would first visit your local psychiatrist. You would probably seek assistance from your friends, partner or other relatives. You may ask others in your community, such as neighbours or religious leaders. However, if you sought medical help you would be most likely to visit your GP who, in many countries, is the first port of call for those with emotional, psychological or psychiatric problems.

There are approximately 33 000 GPs working in the National Health Service (NHS). There are more hospital doctors, about 55 000, of whom 20 000 are consultants and 35 000 are 'junior hospital doctors'.

PRIMARY CARE

What is primary health care?

This is health care that begins at the time of the first encounter between a person and a provider of health care. In many parts of the world this may be a paramedic or a 'barefoot doctor'. In the UK primary care is synonymous with general practice. Other countries have similar systems to the UK, e.g. the Netherlands and Canada. In the USA, primary care is provided by both family practitioners and specialists.

Secondary care is provided by hospitals and specialists, although some primary care is given at this level (e.g. Accident and Emergency departments). Sometimes the term 'tertiary care' is used to denote super-specialist services such as renal transplant and cardiac surgery (Figure 5.1). The

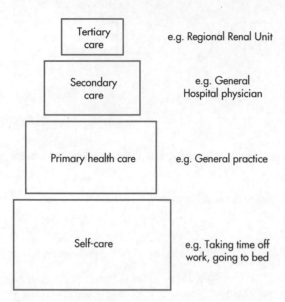

FIG 5.1 Levels of care.

World Health Organization (1984) definition of primary care is rather broader and emphasizes the importance of non-medical personnel and prevention.

The primary health care team

GPs now often work as part of a primary health care team which usually consists of a practice manager, receptionists, secretaries and a practice nurse. Other professionals, such as district nurses, health visitors and community midwives, are often attached to the team. Others may be employed or attached to the practice, e.g. dispensers, physiotherapists, psychologists, social workers, counsellors and community psychiatric nurses. Some practices have employed complementary therapists such as acupuncturists and aroma therapists.

How many patients do GPs see?

Ninety-eight per cent of the population are registered with general practitioners. The average number of people registered with each GP, the 'practice list', is around 1900 and has fallen in number since 1950.

In any given year 70 per cent of all people and 90 per cent of families on a GP's list will consult their

GP at least once. Over a 5-year period the GP will treat more than 90 per cent of his or her patients.

Of course, many people will only be seen once or twice by their GP in the course of a year, but some will be seen on many occasions. The average number of times that a person will consult their GP during a year (the annual consultation rate per person) is between three and four. An average GP will thus do between 6000 and 8000 consultations per year. Most of these consultations take place in the GP's surgery, but about 10 per cent will occur in the patient's home. GPs are available 24 hours a day (on a rota) and will make about 1 night visit per week each.

Some groups of people attend their GP more often than others, e.g. the young, the elderly and women aged 18–45 years. GPs spend an average of 8–9 minutes with each person.

Important features of general practice

- National system – 98 per cent of people are registered with a GP
- Single route of entry into NHS (except, for example, accidents and emergencies, sexually transmitted diseases)
- First contact care – diagnosis, assessment and management
- No financial barrier – free at the time of use
- Availability – direct access, 24 hours a day (for registered patients)
- Gatekeeping – selective referral to hospitals and other agencies
- Personal care – emphasis on this in NHS regulations. The GP is a personal physician
- Family care – many families and couples register together
- Long-term and continuing care – about 40 per cent of people have at least 20 years of continuous registration with their GP
- Local care – care is provided for a known small practice population, often by the same GP, for many years
- Home visits – flexible, especially for the elderly.

The particular strengths of general practice are as follows:

- it provides whole population care;
- it reduces stigma;
- it is acceptable to patients (less dissatisfaction is reported about attending a GP than is reported by hospital out-patients).

Features of illness in primary medical practice

Professor McWhinney, a Canadian family physician, has outlined these as follows.

- The patterns of illness approximate to the pattern of illness in the community, i.e. there is:

  a high incidence of transient illness;
  a high prevalence of chronic illness; and
  a high incidence of emotional illness.

- The illness is undifferentiated, i.e. it has not been previously assessed by any other physician.
- Illnesses are frequently a complex mixture of physical, emotional and social elements.
- Disease is seen at an early stage, before the full clinical picture has developed.
- The relationship with the individual is a continuous one and transcends individual episodes of illness.

From what has been outlined so far, it should be clear why primary care is an important source of health care for the population, and why you would be likely to visit your family doctor, rather than a psychiatrist, with your emotional problem. It may also have occurred to you that, overall, the types of illnesses seen in general practice will cover a broader spectrum and be seen at an earlier stage than those seen in the hospital, and that primary care may act as a filter or gateway to secondary care. With these points in mind, let us turn to look at psychiatric disorders in primary care.

THE PATHWAY TO PSYCHIATRIC CARE

If the general practitioner is the first port of call for people living in the community, then it follows that most individuals with psychiatric disorders should visit their GP before being referred to the psychiatric services. Goldberg and Huxley have described the path that people with psychiatric disorders take on their way to see a psychiatrist

Level 1	**The community** 250–315/1000/year	
		First filter Illness behaviour
Level 2	**Attenders in primary care** Total psychiatric morbidity 230/1000/year	
		Second filter Ability to detect disorder
Level 3	**Mental disorders identified by doctors** 'conspicuous psychiatric morbidity' 101.5/1000/year	
		Third filter Referral to psychiatric services
Level 4	**Psychiatric services – total morbidity** 20.8–23.5/1000/year	
		Fourth filter Admission to psychiatric beds
Level 5	**Psychiatric in-patients** 3.4–5.71/1000/year	

FIG 5.2 Pathway to psychiatric care.

(Figure 5.2). The five levels each correspond to a stage on the pathway to psychiatric care. Between each level is a filter which selects certain individuals at each stage. For example, whilst more women suffer from mental illnesses than men, a man is more likely to be an in-patient in a psychiatric ward than a woman.

You should examine the rates of psychiatric disorder at each level, and from this you will see that the rates of disorder seen by the psychiatric services are about 10 per cent of those general practice attenders who are identified as having psychiatric illness. It would seem that the majority of people with psychiatric disorders remain within primary care and are not sent on to secondary care.

Before we go on to examine the levels and filters in detail, two issues deserve consideration.

First, should we speak of 'psychiatric disorders' in primary care? After all, if these disorders do not reach the psychiatric services, then can they truly be called 'psychiatric'? Some may wish to call them 'emotional disorders' or 'psychological problems'. However, this is of less importance than being clear about the nature of these disorders and how they are defined and measured, a topic that we will return to later.

Second, do all persons with psychiatric disorders follow this pathway? No – the model will require modification depending on the national health care system you are considering and the way in which the individual presents. In some countries, e.g. the USA, the psychiatrist may act as the primary care physician. Some acute disorders may present to the secondary services via the accident and emergency department (e.g. after an overdose), the criminal justice system (e.g. after arrest, or on Section 136), or via Social Services.

Psychiatric disorder in the community (Level 1)

- mental ill health affects one in four of the UK adult population at any point in time
- one in two women and one in four men will experience an episode of depression of such a degree that medical care is indicated at least once in their lives

How do we know these facts?

They come from the study of the occurrence of diseases in populations, which is known as epidemiology.

WHAT IS EPIDEMIOLOGY?

It is a scientific discipline which is concerned with the following:

- populations (from the Greek *demos* meaning the 'populace'), *not* individuals;
- the number of cases of a particular disease in a population;
- how these diseases are distributed among groups of people (according to age, sex, social class, etc.);
- factors that are associated with these diseases.

Epidemiology was traditionally concerned with infectious diseases, i.e. epidemics, but is now concerned with the modern epidemics of cancer, heart disease, AIDS and mental illness.

The functions of epidemiology

- to describe disease in a population
- to explain causes of disease by discovering factors that put the population at risk, and thus to predict occurrences and prevent them

In addition, epidemiology provides data that is essential for the planning of health services.

The precise measurement of disease in a population is difficult for several reasons, but mainly because matters do not remain stable for long enough. This is because people move about, and also because people fall ill and may then recover, stay the same, deteriorate or die. This latter aspect is illustrated by the difference between *incidence* and *prevalence*.

$$\text{Incidence} = \frac{\text{number of events that occur during a period of time}}{\begin{array}{c}\text{sum for each individual in}\\\text{population of length of time}\\\text{at risk of incurring this event}\end{array}}$$

$$\text{Prevalence} = \frac{\begin{array}{c}\text{number of individuals with a}\\\text{condition at a specified time}\end{array}}{\begin{array}{c}\text{number of individuals in a}\\\text{population at that point in time}\end{array}}$$

Prevalence = incidence × duration of disorder

It is also important to define precisely what is meant by a 'case' of disease. This may be difficult in psychiatry, where there are no tests that can be readily applied and where disorders may be considered to be on a continuum from the normal.

This is not unique to psychiatry (try defining a 'case' of chronic bronchitis or of hypertension).

Psychiatric epidemiology has generally approached this problem by using semi-structured interviews in which the interviewer is directed to ask the subject a number of questions which are designed to elicit the presence of a symptom that is defined in an associated manual. The ratings from the interview are usually then linked to a definition of the disorder which is of interest (e.g. depression), and which is usually defined in terms of the number and type of symptoms and the time period for which they have been experienced. This allows cases to be reliably identified, and means that the occurrence of the disorder can be compared between different populations, countries, time periods, etc.

How many people suffer from psychiatric disorders in the community?

The answer to this question will depend on a number of factors which are outlined below.

Possible explanations of the variation in rates of morbidity

- the populations used could vary, e.g. with regard to age, sex or class. Morbidity levels may vary between different countries
- the sampling procedure used could vary, e.g. including institutions or not
- different methods of measurement of morbidity, e.g. the use of questionnaires as opposed to interviews
- diagnostic classification – definition of cases
- use of estimates, e.g. using admission rates as a measure of morbidity
- recording procedure, e.g. does this miss individuals or encourage non-response?
- rates reported, e.g. prevalence, incidence
- time period considered, e.g. life-time, year, point
- analysis of data, e.g. correctly done, taking account of non-responders
- characteristics of the recording clinician, e.g. different clinicians may use different thresholds for recording symptoms

The above are all sources of error. It could be that differences in rates of morbidity (e.g. between populations, or over time) could represent true differences in rates.

Measurement of the number of people with mental illnesses in the population at large is relatively recent, and most of our knowledge comes from studies carried out since the 1940s.

Studies conducted in the USA and Canada during the 1950s suggested that 60 to 70 per cent of the population had symptoms of mental ill health. These were symptoms such as worry, tiredness and sleepless nights, which were often experienced in isolation and did not amount to psychiatric disorder. The experience of such subjective feelings is common. People often report physical symptoms, but this does not necessarily mean that they have physical diseases. However, the same studies did suggest that between 20 and 30 per cent of people had mental disorders.

A recent study of a representative national sample of adults conducted in the USA (the National Comorbidity Survey) found that:

- nearly 50 per cent of all respondents reported a lifetime history of at least one DSM-III-R disorder;
- 30 per cent of respondents had reported at least one DSM-III-R disorder in the previous year;
- major depression was the most common single psychiatric disorder reported, with an overall lifetime prevalence of 17.1 per cent and a 12-month prevalence of 10.3 per cent.

Importantly, in this study *less than 50 per cent* of the respondents who reported a lifetime DSM-III-R disorder had obtained any treatment for it.

Few national studies have been carried out in the UK. A recent survey (the National Survey of Psychiatric Morbidity in Great Britain) was carried out as part of the *Health of the Nation* action plan. This showed that:

- one in every seven adults had some form of neurotic health problem in the week before they were interviewed;
- the most prevalent neurotic disorders were mixed anxiety/depressive disorder (7.1 per cent) and generalized anxiety disorder (3.0 per cent).

The most consistent finding in epidemiological studies of psychiatric disorders worldwide is that they are more common in women than in men.

Consultation – going to the doctor (Filter 1)

Not all people who suffer from symptoms will consult their GP. For example, 12 per cent of men and 14 per cent of women reported episodes of acute sickness leading to reduced activity over a 14-day period, but only 41 per cent of these individuals consulted their GP. Furthermore, 8 per cent of people with no illnesses consulted their GP.

However, it has been shown that:

■ having a mental illness increases the likelihood of a person going to his or her GP;

■ a person suffering from a psychiatric disorder is twice as likely to consult their GP within a given time period than someone who does not have a psychiatric disorder;

■ about 25 per cent of probable cases of psychiatric disorder who live in the community will consult a GP over a 2-week period;

■ almost 25 per cent of a GP's consultations can be regarded as attributable to psychiatric morbidity;

■ people with psychiatric disorders attend more frequently than other patients, and are often among those who most frequently attend their GP.

Psychiatric disorders in general practice (Level 2)

CASE 5.2

A 45-year-old man, divorced but now living with a new partner, came to see his GP with indigestion, which was treated symptomatically with no benefit. Subsequent consultations revealed that he had been feeling low in mood and increasingly irritable since being made redundant. His low mood was variable from day to day, he had lost his appetite and he had difficulty in getting to sleep. He would repeatedly wake in the night, and when he woke in the morning he did not feel like getting up. He experienced loss of interest and pleasure in addition to loss of libido. He had a pessimistic view of the future and at times believed that life was not worth living and that he would be better off dead. However, he had made no suicidal plans and rejected the idea of killing himself. He experienced periodic autonomic symptoms of anxiety when he thought about the future and often felt tense. His concentration and energy were reduced.

There was no previous record of emotional problems and he was not known to be a frequent attender at the surgery. He had previously been married, but the marriage had never been satisfactory and he finally divorced his wife. He was now living with a new partner, and as a result of this his family had rejected him. He had never experienced depressive episodes in the past, but had been unhappy in his first marriage and had then drunk heavily, although he now drank infrequently. As a result of his job loss he had financial difficulties which had necessitated selling his house and moving to a council property.

He was given antidepressants and support from a CPN who attended the practice.

Much of the information about psychiatric disorders in general practice has been unearthed since the 1940s. During the 1960s, researchers at the Maudsley Hospital in London, led by Michael Shepherd, conducted the first large-scale study of psychiatric disorder in general practice. This was conducted in 46 practices in the London area, and it was found that, according to the GPs' reports, 14 per cent of patients consulting them had some form of psychiatric disorder.

However, as we shall see later, GPs tend to underestimate the number of patients with psychiatric disorders. Shepherd's study also found that, when a questionnaire was used, an estimated 25 per cent of the attenders had a psychiatric disorder.

Several types of study have been carried out in general practice in order to examine psychiatric disorders.

■ *GP-reported rates of disorder in individual practices* Many of these were carried out in the 1950s and 1960s and pointed to the large numbers of psychiatric disorders in general practice. As a measure of prevalence these rates are of limited value, as they used GP estimates and it is difficult to generalize from single practices to general practice as a whole.

■ *Multi-practice studies using GP-reported rates* These still only provide estimates of prevalence; the study by Professor Shepherd found a ninefold variation in reported rates across the practices.

■ *National Morbidity Surveys* Four of these have been conducted in England and Wales between 1955/56 and 1991/92 using a selection of general practitioners. They again used GP-reported rates of disorder, and gave rates for all disorders that the GPs saw, not just psychiatric disorders.

■ *Questionnaire studies, e.g. using the General Health Questionnaire to estimate morbidity* These may give more 'objective' measures, but they may also overestimate the number of psychiatric disorders.

■ *Interview studies, e.g. using the Present State Examination* These give the best estimates, but are time-consuming to carry out.

These different studies indicate the following.

■ The results obtained from the multi-practice and National Morbidity surveys provide an estimate that between 14 and 34 per cent of attenders in general practice suffer from psychiatric disorders.
■ The questionnaire studies show that 30 to 40 per cent of people are suffering from psychiatric disorders.
■ Interview studies have shown that about one third of people are suffering from a psychiatric disorder.
■ As in the general population, emotional symptoms are common and are present in people who do not have a psychiatric disorder, e.g. almost 30 per cent of people with no psychiatric disorder suffer from fatigue and 12 per cent suffer from depressed mood.
■ Disorders of the respiratory system represent the largest proportion of a GP's workload, comprising over 20 per cent of total consultations. Mental illness comes in either second or third place, representing about 20 per cent of all consultations.
■ The majority of people with psychiatric disorders present to their GP with physical symptoms.
■ Disorders such as schizophrenia are relatively rare.
■ The most common disorders are those of anxiety and depression, sometimes known as the 'neuroses'.
■ There is a large overlap between anxiety and depression, e.g. over 40 per cent of people have mixed anxiety/depressive disorders.
■ About 10 per cent of people will be suffering from depression – probably about half of these will be severe enough to require antidepressants.
■ Many of the mood disorders are short-lived problems of adjustment to stress in people's lives – the adjustment disorders.
■ Psychiatric disorders are more common in women than in men.

Classification of psychiatric disorder in general practice

The classifications outlined in the other chapters of this book (ICD-10, DSM-IV) can be used in primary care, but are generally considered to be too complicated for use in general medical settings.

The World Health Organization has produced a new classification for use in primary care – ICD-10 (PHC) – which outlines 24 common conditions. This has not yet been fully tested out or agreed upon.

The Mental Disorders section of ICD-10 for use in primary care

■ F0 Organic disorders
   F00   Dementia
   F05   Delirium
■ F1 Psychoactive substance abuse
   F10   Alcohol use disorder
   F11   Drug use disorder
   F17.1 Tobacco use
■ F3 Psychotic disorders
   F20   Chronic psychotic disorder
   F23   Acute psychotic disorder
   F31   Bipolar disorder
■ F4 Mood, stress-related and anxiety disorders
   F32   Depression
   F40   Phobic disorders
   F41.0 Panic disorder
   F41.1 Generalized anxiety
   F41.2 Mixed anxiety and depression
   F43   Adjustment disorder
   F44   Dissociative disorder
   F45   Unexplained somatic complaints
   F48   Neurasthenia
■ F5 Physiological disorders
   F50   Eating disorders
   F51   Sleep problems
   F52   Sexual disorders
■ F7 Developmental disorders
   F70   Mental retardation
■ F9 Disorders of childhood
   F90   Hyperkinetic disorder
   F91   Conduct disorder
   F98   Enuresis

Specific disorders
DEPRESSION AND ANXIETY

CASE 5.3

Mrs JW, a 40-year-old married woman with two daughters, came to the surgery on several occasions over the past year accompanying her 16-year-old daughter when she consulted her GP for dysmenorrhoea and problems with the contraceptive pill. On one of these occasions she broke down in tears when explaining her daughters' problems. She had had problems in coping with her job as a receptionist over the past year and had experienced periods of low mood and poor sleep lasting for about a week at a time. These episodes had begun after she was called to see the headmistress at her daughter's school, who told her that her daughter had been found smoking cannabis. Her daughter was expelled from school as a result, and then said that she had been having sex with an older boy and that she might be pregnant. This later proved not to be the case. This daughter had always been cherished by her mother, since she had been born prematurely and overprotected in her early years. Mrs JW had found it hard to believe that she would take drugs, and was not aware of her relationships with boys.

Mrs JW also experienced tension headaches on most days, and autonomic symptoms of anxiety when at work or when she dropped her younger daughter, aged 12 years, off at school. This daughter had just started her menstrual periods. She had always been a robust girl who had challenged her mother's authority, and Mrs JW was concerned lest she should get into trouble at school. Her husband was a reticent man who often worked away from home and did not like to speak to his wife about the children. She felt unable to confide in him, and often spoke to a workmate about her difficulties.

Mrs JW had not felt able to come to the GP about her problems for fear of being perceived as a poor mother. She did not want to take antidepressants and after several consultations with the GP on her own she was referred to the practice counsellor. Her confidence increased, her symptoms declined and her fears about her daughters never materialized. However, her relationship with her husband deteriorated and they subsequently divorced.

We have already noted that symptoms of depression and anxiety are common in people visiting their general practitioners, and that such symptoms occur in people without psychiatric disorder.

Severe depression, e.g. manic depression (bipolar affective disorder) or major depression (DSM-IV), is much less common than less severe forms and adjustment disorders (see Table 5.1). Anxiety disorders (phobias, panic disorders and generalized anxiety disorder) are also common,

TABLE 5.1 Psychiatric disorder in general practice (Blacker and Clare, 1988)

Diagnostic category	Percentage of consulting patients
Overall psychiatric disorder	35.3
Stress/adjustment disorder	17.9
RDC minor depressive disorder	5.7
RDC major depressive disorder	4.3
Anxiety neurosis (including panic and phobic disorder)	3.2
Alcoholism	2.6
Personality disorder	2.6
Schizophrenia and related psychotic disorders	1.0
Drug dependence	1.2
Bipolar affective disorder	0.9

but may overlap with depressive disorders or depressive symptoms.

The cost of depression is high.

To the individual:

■ psychological suffering;
■ somatic discomfort;
■ social consequences, e.g. loss of earnings, loss of job;
■ increased rate of accidents and self-harm;
■ increased rate of alcohol abuse;
■ increased mortality.

To the family:

■ psychological distress;
■ social consequences, e.g. financial, marital break-up;
■ forensic problems, e.g. shop-lifting;
■ long-term psychological effects on children, e.g. children of mothers with postnatal depression.

To society:

■ high health and social services costs; and
■ loss of productivity.

It is difficult to put precise monetary figures on the costs of depression and other psychiatric disorders, but the following estimates have been made.

■ In the USA, the costs of depression are thought to be in excess of $16 billion each year.

■ The costs of psychiatric disorders in general practice in the UK have been estimated to be:

Direct costs (e.g. consultation, treatment) £120 million

Indirect costs (e.g. loss of earnings, social security) £255 million

Total £375 million

However, these UK costs are very conservative estimates, and the figure may be closer to £5 billion each year.

SCHIZOPHRENIA

This disorder is much less commonly seen by general practitioners than depression and anxiety. The number of new cases occurring in a population each year is about 20 per 100 000, but as it is a chronic disorder its prevalence is between 140 and 420 per 100 000 members of the population.

Whilst the majority of people with schizophrenia will be in contact with psychiatric services, it is estimated that about 25 per cent of people with schizophrenia who are discharged from psychiatric facilities are managed only by their family doctor.

People with schizophrenia attend GP surgeries up to three times more often than the average attender, and physical problems are more common among people with schizophrenia. The GP has an important role to play in the shared case (with psychiatric services) of patients with schizophrenia, especially in dealing with their physical problems.

ALCOHOL ABUSE

CASE 5.4

A 27-year-old single man living at home with his parents went to see to his GP because of tiredness and loss of energy which had developed over the past year. He worked as a clerical assistant in a large firm of solicitors, a job which he normally enjoyed, but he had recently found the increasing workload difficult. The GP could find no abnormalities on examination, but did notice a faint smell of alcohol on the man's breath at the time of the evening surgery. Blood tests showed a raised gamma GT and MCV, but there were no other abnormal liver function tests. When asked about his alcohol consumption he admitted to drinking 3 or 4 pints of beer at lunchtime and the same on his way home from work in the evenings. He would drink up to 12 pints each day at weekends with his friends. He drank to relieve the tensions that he felt at the end of the day, and because his workmates spent each lunchtime and evening in the pub. He felt that drinking increased his sociability, especially with women, with whom he found relationships difficult. Discussion about his drinking habits and education about the effects of alcohol encouraged him to cut down his alcohol consumption and alter his lifestyle.

Up to 20 per cent of adults seen in general practice are consuming harmful amounts of alcohol. At one end of the spectrum are low users of alcohol who show no signs of harm; at the other end are highly dependent drinkers with multiple medical and social problems. Most alcohol problems seen in general practice are among moderate drinkers, i.e. men who drink between 21 and 50 units per week and women who drink between 15 and 35 units per week.

GPs themselves have been noted to have a high risk of dying from excessive alcohol consumption, but this trend has decreased in recent years. However, even now one in five GPs still drinks too much.

As with the psychiatric problems we have discussed, severe alcohol problems (e.g. the 'skid-row' alcoholic) are uncommon, and less severe although damaging forms are the rule. However, the view of the extreme stereotype has been common amongst GPs, who generally dislike dealing with 'alcoholic' patients, although the GP is in an ideal position to intervene at an early stage in cases of alcohol abuse. Studies carried out in the UK have demonstrated that 10 to 15 minutes of GP advice results in a 15 per cent reduction in alcohol consumption and a 20 per cent reduction in the proportion of excessive drinkers.

DRUG ABUSE

The patterns of drug abuse have changed greatly in the past 15 years in terms of prevalence, types of drugs misused, and age and social background of the users. GPs, particularly those in inner cities, are often confronted by drug abusers.

GPs see the entire range of drug misusers:

■ intermittent experimentation with drugs;
■ regular involvement in illicit drug-taking with its associated lifestyle and social problems;
■ stable dependent use of pharmaceutical or controlled drugs, usually obtained by prescription.

They also see the range of drugs abused, e.g. opiates, cocaine (including crack), amphetamines, LSD, Ecstasy (MDMA), solvents and benzodiazepines.

Benzodiazepine dependency has been highlighted as a particular problem in general practice – often because the GP is the source of the prescribed drug. A single GP with a list size of 2000 patients will have 60 who are long-term users of benzodiazepines, of whom 45 individuals will be over the age of 60 years; the majority will be women, and 50 per cent will have been taking the medication for more than 5 years.

Benzodiazepine use in general practice

- each GP has a list of about 2000 people
- 60 people are long-term users (50 per cent for over 5 years)
- 45 are over the age of 65 years
- the majority of users are women

SUICIDE

The rate of suicide in England and Wales is about 11 per 100 000 members of the population. A GP with a list size of 2000 patients should see one suicide in a 4-year period. Whilst for an individual GP this is an uncommon although tragic and disturbing occurrence, the significance for GPs lies in the fact that patients who commit suicide are likely to be in contact with their GP shortly before they kill themselves.

- two thirds of people who commit suicide will have seen their GP in the previous month
- forty per cent will have seen their GP in the previous week

More recently a rise in suicides by young men has been noted, and these same men are less likely to have been seen by their GP in the weeks leading up to their successful suicide. High rates of suicide have also been noted in young Asian women in the UK.

SOMATIZATION

CASE 5.5

A 47-year-old divorced woman who lived with her elderly father had experienced low-grade abdominal pain since her divorce 8 years previously. She also experienced episodes of more intense pain, piercing in nature, which was localized to her lower abdomen, and she complained of intermittent diarrhoea and heavy periods. She had been sent for a range of investigations by her previous GP, and had seen two hospital surgeons, a physician and a gynaecologist. Apart from an abnormal cervical smear, no abnormalities had ever been found. Her cervical smear was under review by the GP and local gynaecologist. She had requested a hysterectomy but this had been refused her as no pathology was found except for the abnormal smear. She had had an emergency appendicectomy 3 years previously, but no abnormality was found in the appendix. Her previous GP had finally removed her from his list as she had repeatedly called him or his partners out to see her in the night. She had been allocated to the present practice by the Family Health Service Authority (FHSA).

During her first year in the new practice she presented almost weekly to any of the five partners, demanding analgesia. She would often storm out of consultations saying that the doctors did not care about her. One of the practice GPs managed to form a therapeutic relationship with her and saw her for the majority of her consultations. It emerged that her abdominal pain appeared to increase at times when she was depressed, as indicated by low mood, tearfulness, irritability, poor sleep and low self-esteem. She attributed her abdominal pain to a retroverted uterus which she believed was stuck to her bowel, and to the fact that she had never had children. She often complained that she could not cope with her 78-year-old father who was a difficult man and had poor mobility secondary to osteoarthritis, and she expressed feelings of intense hatred towards him. He had been a heavy drinker during her childhood, and had often been absent from the family home. She recalled him returning home when drunk and having fights with her mother. She had supported her mother, who had diabetes, until she was 27 years old, when her mother died. Following this she had married a businessman and had moved out of the parental home. She had initially had a good marriage, until her husband began to drink and was finally made bankrupt. He eventually left her for another woman, and she was forced to return to her father's home.

She was persuaded to take an antidepressant, and arrangements were made for her father to be seen by a district nurse and some day care was arranged for him through social services. Her analgesia was reduced and her consultations were mainly prearranged. She made no further requests to be seen at the hospital, but continued to see the gynaecologist for review. She continued to experience low-grade abdominal pain and did not accept that there was a link between her depressive symptoms and her abdominal pain, although she did accept that she was coping better with both of them.

We have already noted that the majority of people with psychiatric disorders consult their GP with physical symptoms. There may be several explanations for this:

- the person has coexisting physical and psychiatric disorders which are essentially independent, e.g. heart disease in a person with depression;
- the person has a physical disorder which is distressing to them, e.g. a newly discovered breast lump;
- the person has an emotional problem, but presents with physical symptoms as they believe the doctor will find these acceptable, i.e. the physical symptoms are used as a 'ticket' to see the GP;
- the person presents with physical symptoms of their psychiatric disorder, e.g. palpitations in anxiety disorders.
- the person believes that he or she has a physical disorder, although there is no medical evidence for this.

The last two explanations are examples of somatization. Four conditions describe a case of somatization:

- they must be seeking help for somatic symptoms
- the person must attribute these symptoms to some physical disorder
- a specific psychiatric disorder must be present
- the somatic symptoms are not due to physical disease, but can be thought of as being part of the mental disorder

Between 50 and 60 per cent of new psychiatric disorders presenting to a GP are cases of somatization. The majority of these people will have anxiety and/or depressive disorders.

About 50 per cent of these somatizers will be adamant that they are suffering from a physical disorder rather than an emotional one. The remainder will admit on closer questioning that their physical symptoms are the result of stress or psychological problems.

What happens to people with psychiatric disorders in general practice?

This question could also be phrased as follows. What is the outcome for people with psychiatric disorders who are seen by general practitioners?

One problem in giving an answer to this question is that, as we have seen, there is a range of different disorders. However, if psychotic disorders are excluded, then, for new disorders presenting to GPs:

- about 25 per cent will remain psychiatrically ill after 3 years;
- 75 per cent will thus have recovered. The majority of these will have recovered after 1 year, and many by 3 months after presenting to the GP.

Many of the disorders are therefore short-lived. However, for those people who have disorders which last for 12 months or more (these are usually then called 'chronic' disorders) the outcome is poor, with about 10 per cent of cases showing recovery in the next year. Of those who do recover, about 50 per cent will show a variable course.

Factors affecting the outcome of psychiatric disorders in general practice

- *initial severity of the disorder* – more severe disorders are associated with poor outcome
- *early improvement* – people showing improvement over the first few weeks show a better outcome overall
- *age* – older age is associated with variable or chronic cause
- *physical illness* – the presence of physical illness is associated with poor outcome. Such cases sometimes improve more slowly than non-somatizers
- *life events* – major life events are associated with a poorer outcome. Life events which represent an important change and give new hope ('fresh start events') are associated with a better outcome. Support at the time of crisis is associated with a better outcome
- *social factors* – continuing social, family and marital problems are associated with poor outcome
- *personality* – external 'locus of control' is associated with a poorer outcome
- *detection by GP* – being recognized as being psychiatrically ill by one's GP results in a better outcome

Detection of psychiatric disorder by general practitioners (Filter 2)

It should be apparent from the above discussion that not all people who go to see their GP with a psychiatric disorder will be identified by their doctor. In fact, GPs vary enormously in their ability to detect psychiatric disorder and, on average, identify about 60 per cent of those cases that consult them.

What then determines whether a person's psychiatric problems will be detected or missed? The answer to this lies in both the person and the doctor.

PATIENT FACTORS RELATING TO THE DETECTION OF DISORDER

CASE 5.6

A 41-year-old married, employed man presented to his GP complaining of indigestion, the experience of regurgitation of food and feelings of food sticking in the lower end of his gullet. He had suffered an episode of depression 5 years previously, and three members of his family had died from cancer during the previous 10 years. He was preoccupied with his symptoms and believed that he might have cancer. He was a poor communicator, was brooding over his problem and was sleeping poorly. A gastroscopy was arranged which revealed no abnormality and the consultant gastroenterologist suggested prescribing an H2 blocker.

He did not consult his GP again until a year later when he came after encouragement from his wife, having become increasingly withdrawn, irritable and low in mood. He had encountered problems at work and had been suspended because of drinking problems. He was brooding over feelings of failure and hopelessness about the future and he experienced autonomic symptoms of anxiety, including sweating, palpitations and churning in the stomach. He had lost interest in his usual activities and derived little pleasure from these. His sleep was poor and his appetite was reduced, although he had lost no weight. He had experienced suicidal thoughts, had attempted to harm himself with a knife, and had been found by his wife standing on a motorway bridge contemplating suicide.

In retrospect, his current presentation could be seen as identical to that 5 years previously. He was started on antidepressants which initially produced little change until they were changed to an alternative preparation. He eventually made a full recovery after referral to psychiatric services.

The people whose problems are detected are usually those with more obvious features of psychiatric disorder. Those patients in whom the psychological distress is not identified, the 'hidden psychiatric morbidity' group, give out less obvious signals of disorder.

- GPs rarely miss those people who present directly with psychological complaints
- people who present with physical symptoms are more likely to be missed
- people who have coexisting physical and psychiatric disorders are likely to have their psychiatric disorder missed

The characteristics of those people who are missed

- they describe fewer symptoms of emotional distress (emotional 'cues') during the consultation
- they are less likely to have a past history of psychological disturbance which is known to the GP
- they have had fewer recent consultations

Some people may hold attitudes and beliefs which encourage them to present to their doctor in a particular way. A person may fail to disclose distress because he or she believes the following:

- doctors do not deal with psychiatric problems
- doctors do not have the time or inclination to help
- the somatic problems that the person experiences are not caused by a psychological problem
- doctors do not need to know about the person's emotional problems
- doctors will reject or dismiss their emotional difficulties

Patient factors relating to the detection of psychiatric disorder by general practitioners are as follows:

- presentation – physical or psychological
  – psychiatric disorder with or without physical disorder
- severity of disorder
- cues given out in consultation
- disclosure of distress to doctor
- past psychiatric history known to GP
- number of recent consultations with GP

PRACTITIONER FACTORS RELATING TO THE DETECTION OF PSYCHIATRIC DISORDER

Those general practitioners with an accurate concept of the type of disorder that presents in primary care, and who hold the view that psychological factors play an important role in illness, are better at case detection. They also express an interest in psychiatric problems and tend to have a more 'liberal' personality.

Some doctors may believe that psychiatric disorder is not an important, legitimate problem that is treatable. Others may be repelled by or anxious about psychiatric patients, or may think that the patient will be offended, angered or stigmatized by a psychiatric label.

Doctors generally show a physical bias in their assessments. Although many problems in primary care present with a mixture of physical, psychological and social pathology, emphasis will frequently be placed on somatic features. In medical school we are often taught an either/or approach to diagnosis, and this may encourage us to view psychological problems as simple alternatives to physical ones, which may cause coexisting problems to be overlooked.

The behaviours of GPs that are related to an increased likelihood that a person's psychological problems will be detected are generally those that seek to clarify and tease out these problems and difficulties. That is not to say, however, that these doctors should neglect the physical symptoms or illnesses – it is important that these are taken seriously. Some of these interview behaviours are associated, in individual doctors, with a clear concept of what constitutes psychiatric morbidity in primary care. In other words, those doctors who know what they are looking for will find it, especially if they have efficient interview techniques.

In addition, the interview skills associated with detection are those that put the person at their ease, make them feel that they are being taken

Practitioner factors relating to the detection of psychiatric disorder by general practitioners

- attitudes: roles of psychological factors in illness; interest in psychiatric problems; attitudes towards psychiatric patients; confidence/expertise in dealing with psychiatric problems
- personality – 'liberal' or 'conservative'
- bias in assessment – psychological/physical
- interview skills

GPs who are better at detecting psychiatric disorder

- make early eye contact with the patient
- clarify the person's presenting complaint
- show empathy
- are sensitive to emotional cues
- are less authoritarian in their interviewing style
- use appropriate psychiatric questions and probes
- ask questions that invite the person to give details about a particular topic (clarification)
- make supportive comments
- are good at dealing with interruptions and garrulous people
- spend less time talking, and interrupt the person less, but are more effective when they do and appear to be less rushed
- give less information during the first 3 minutes of the consultation

GPs who are poor at detecting psychiatric disorder

- bury themselves in their notes and do not look at the patient much
- over-use technical jargon
- carry out rushed interviews using questions based on their theoretical knowledge rather than on the person's comments
- appear to be less interested and make fewer empathic comments
- interrupt people
- give information before their problems are fully elicited

seriously and increase the chances that the doctor can observe features of distress in the person. When people present to doctors who have better interview techniques they give out more signals of psychological distress. This is because the doctor's techniques promote this behaviour; it also means that the doctors are less likely to miss the person's distress.

Does detection of psychiatric disorder by GPs matter?

Give this matter some careful consideration – it could be that missing some psychological distress does not matter. After all, many people recover without help from doctors.

Consider first why the GP should bother to detect psychiatric disorder. Central to this question is a concern over the effects of psychological disturbance on the individual, his or her family, and the health services.

- failure to detect a psychiatric disorder, e.g. depression, denies the person potentially effective treatment
- psychological distress undermines the person's family and social network, and ill-advised life decisions may be made at these times (e.g. leaving a job, partner or home)
- people may be sent for costly, potentially harmful and inappropriate diagnostic procedures to try to find an explanation for their physical symptoms

The real test is whether detection of psychiatric disorder has an effect on the outcome of the person. There is some evidence for this.

- detection of psychiatric disorder reduces the number of subsequent consultations with the GP
- people with psychiatric disorder who are not detected have longer episodes of psychological distress than those who are detected
- being recognized as psychiatrically ill by the GP results in a fourfold greater likelihood of symptomatic improvement and a threefold greater likelihood of social improvement than not being recognized

One intriguing finding in a Dutch study was that improvement after detection was not just related to the treatment given. This suggests that there is something important in itself about recognizing a person's distress.

Improving detection of psychiatric disorder

Can the detection of psychiatric disorders by GPs be improved, or is it the case that once doctors are in practice their habits are set for the rest of their career?

Several projects have been initiated in the UK, involving a variety of GPs of varying ages and experience, which have attempted to change the doctors' interviewing styles. These projects have used video-taped feedback of real consultations and have been shown to:

- improve the detection of psychiatric disorder;
- change the doctors' interviewing style – especially those skills and behaviours that are related to better detection. These changes are maintained over time;
- be regarded with enthusiasm by GPs.

There is also evidence that training in interview techniques and increasing GPs' awareness of psychological problems can:

- influence outcome for people – particularly in people with mixed anxiety/depression;
- produce more satisfied people;
- reduce anxiety in people;
- make people feel more understood.

Conspicuous psychiatric morbidity (Level 3)

This term refers to the psychiatric disorders that GPs detect, as opposed to those psychiatric disorders that are not recognized (the 'hidden psychiatric morbidity'). As we have seen, GPs are very variable in their reporting of psychiatric problems, and the figures for such disorders can be obtained from the studies using GP-reported rates which we discussed above.

The amount of psychological problems seen in primary care and the community makes them a cause of considerable concern for the health of a community and a major public health challenge.

In view of the major public health implications of mental illness, the government has included it as one of its key areas in the *Health of the Nation* document.

The targets for mental illness are as follows:

- to improve significantly the health and social functioning of mentally ill people;
- to reduce the overall suicide rate by at least 15 per cent by the year 2000;
- to reduce the suicide rate of severely mentally ill people by at least 33 per cent by the year 2000.

Primary care has a part to play in helping to meet these targets.

One successful initiative has taken place in Gotland, Sweden. Gotland is a small island off the coast of Sweden, and has 56 000 inhabitants and 18 GPs. An educational programme covering psychiatric topics was given to all the GPs, and this was found to:

- lead to improved treatment of psychiatric problems by GPs and less use of psychiatric services;
- reduce the suicide rate on Gotland.

Unfortunately, the effects of this programme were not maintained, and there is a need for constant updating of education.

In the UK, public and media awareness has probably been partly responsible for the decrease in the number of benzodiazepines prescribed.

The international perspective

We have mainly concerned ourselves with psychiatric disorders in general practice in the UK. However, much of the above discussion can be applied to primary care settings across the world.

In 1993, the World Bank published a report on health and the burden of disease. For mental disorders they found that:

- for non-communicable disease in women in the developing world, neuropsychiatric disease (15 per cent of the total) created the second largest burden of disease after cardiovascular disease;
- depressive disorders account for 24 to 31 per cent of the total burden of disease in women caused by the neuropsychiatric disorders;
- the main burden is in younger age groups (15–44 years old).

The World Health Organization (WHO) has repeatedly emphasized the importance of primary care and its role in the management of people with psychiatric disorders. In its 1973 report the WHO

stated that 'the primary medical care team is the cornerstone of community psychiatry'.

Worldwide, depression and anxiety are among the most commonly presenting problems in primary care. In a large study conducted by the WHO in several countries, 20 per cent of primary care people were found to be suffering from depression or anxiety. A further 10 per cent of people were suffering from mixed anxiety/depression, brief recurrent depression and mild depression.

Studies carried out in Australia, Greece, the Netherlands and the USA also show that primary care doctors miss 30 to 40 per cent of the mental illness presenting in their surgeries.

Referral to psychiatric services (Filter 3)

Only 5 to 10 per cent of people with psychiatric disorders are referred to psychiatric services. This means that the majority of people with emotional problems are cared for in general practice.

As with detection, GPs are very variable in their referral habits, and to some extent the likelihood of a person being referred may be regarded as something of a lottery.

Several factors have been shown to affect referral by GPs of people with psychiatric problems to specialist psychiatric services.

Factors influencing referral by GPs to secondary care

- male gender
- younger age group
- severity of disorder
- experience of separation from parents in early life
- associated alcohol/drug abuse
- suicide attempt or suicidal ideation
- social problems
- inappropriate responses to medical attention

Whilst the more severe disorders have an increased chance of referral (e.g. it is likely that all people with schizophrenia are referred), there is not necessarily a linear relationship between the severity of a disorder (e.g. depression) and referral. Some people with a moderate to severe depressive disorder may be referred, whilst others may not.

When thinking about referral it is worth asking:

- why this person?
- why now?
- why by this GP?

That is, the decision to refer will represent an inter-action of the following:

- factors in the person, e.g. how distressed they are, how they are acting;
- factors in the GP , e.g. how confident they are, their past experience;
- the circumstances, e.g. the availability of psychi-atric services, time of day.

Psychiatric services

Psychiatric services tend to see the more severely ill people with disorders such as schizophrenia and bipolar affective disorders. The majority are seen as out-patients.

Psychiatric services have undergone considerable change, especially since the 1940s. The biggest change has been the reduction in size of the large mental hospitals (formerly known as asylums) and the development of services outside psychiatric hospitals – so-called 'Community Psychiatry' or 'Community Mental Health Services'. Out-patient clinics and day hospitals have developed since 1948.

Since the 1950s a series of government policies has put forward plans for the closure of the large hospitals and the development of alternative services. These began with two government White Papers in 1962 and 1963, produced at the time when Enoch Powell was Minister for Health. A quote from Enoch Powell sums up the view of the asylums:

> There they stand, isolated, majestic, imperious, brooded over by the gigantic water tower and chimney combined, rising unmistakable and daunting out of the countryside....It is out of duty to err on the side of ruthlessness. For the great majority of these establishments there is no appropriate use.
>
> Enoch Powell (1961)

Management of psychiatric disorders in primary care

General practitioners have four options open to them concerning the treatment of psychiatric disorders:

- to give no specific treatment;
- to employ psychotherapeutic techniques them-selves;
- to prescribe psychotropic drug treatment;
- to refer the person to other professionals.

NO SPECIFIC TREATMENT OPTION

As a proportion of psychiatric disorders in people are not detected, then some individuals will not receive direct treatment for their psychiatric problems. Detection and acknowledgement of distress by the GP is probably all that a proportion of patients require. Knowing that someone has taken the time to listen and to take their problems seriously is sufficient for one category of people.

PSYCHOTHERAPY BY GPS

As the GP spends on average less than 9 minutes with each person there is insufficient time to engage in structured psychotherapy. However, many of the GPs who are good at detecting psychi-atric problems are also better at managing these disorders.

Good detectors tend:

- to explain the reasons for treatment
- to negotiate treatment
- to check that advice and treatment are understood by all people
- to give psychosocial information, advice and treatment to their emotionally distressed patients

Poor detectors tend:

- not to provide educational information
- not to check that advice and treatment were understood by the person
- not to tell people what was presented or what the main effect of medication was supposed to be

GPs are not psychotherapists. However, they can and do use psychotherapeutic and counselling techniques in their consultations for the benefit of patients. One study has shown GPs' use of brief structured counselling to be as effective as anxiolytics (e.g. diazepam) in the treatment of anxiety disorders.

PSYCHOTROPIC DRUG TREATMENT

Most treatments for psychological disorders in general practice are pharmacological, principally involving the benzodiazepines and antidepressants. In the UK, most psychotropic drugs are prescribed by GPs, amounting to about one in six prescriptions.

The prescribing of such drugs increased during the 1960s and continued to do so, at a slower pace, during the 1970s. Prescriptions for benzodiazepines decreased in the 1980s, mainly due to uncertainty about the long-term use of these drugs, reports of dependence, public distrust and threats of litigation. GPs have often been criticized for prescribing inadequate doses of antidepressants for too short a period.

REFERRAL TO OTHER PROFESSIONALS

As we have seen, only a small proportion of people seen in general practice are referred to psychiatric services. However, in recent years there has been an increase in the number of mental health professionals providing services to GPs in the GP's own surgery. Around 50 per cent of general practices now have a mental health professional of some kind working with them.

Counsellors/psychotherapists

About one third of practices in England and Wales have a counsellor of some kind working with them. Some of these are community psychiatric nurses or clinical psychologists, but one third are individuals without a specific professional background in the psychiatric services who are employed as practice counsellors.

The use of psychological therapists in primary care has been advocated for a wide range of problems, including anxiety, phobias, depression and relationship difficulties, as well as smoking, obesity, alcohol abuse, postnatal depression, benzodiazepine dependency and high-risk sexual behaviour.

Approaches have included the following:

■ non-directive (Rogerian) counselling;
■ behavioural and cognitive therapies;
■ anxiety management;
■ marital and family therapy.

Some general practitioners have established their own psychotherapy/psychoanalytical seminars and discussion groups, known as 'Balint groups' after the psychoanalyst Michael Balint who developed such groups in general practice during the 1960s.

Community psychiatric nurses (CPNs)

Community psychiatric nursing services were first established in the 1950s, and began to expand in the 1960s. They have increased in numbers faster than any other category of mental health professional, and in 1990 there were almost 5000 CPNs in the UK. Traditionally CPNs were employed to assist in the follow-up of people who had been discharged from psychiatric hospitals, but during the 1980s they began to work more in general practices, taking referrals directly from GPs.

Some people argue that CPNs should work mainly with those people with severe mental illness (e.g. schizophrenia). Others maintain that they have an important role in providing therapy for those with psychological problems in primary care.

CPNs have been shown to be as effective as psychiatrists in dealing with chronic neurosis. However, they may not be any more effective than GPs in dealing with acute neurotic problems.

Some nurses – known as nurse behaviour therapists – are specifically trained in behavioural therapy and often work in primary care. These nurses are few in number but are effective in treating patients with, for example, phobias and obsessive-compulsive disorder.

Social workers

Some social workers are attached to general practices, but this situation varies in different local authorities. Social workers are known to have a useful role in managing patients with chronic depression.

Clinical psychologists

GPs often refer patients directly to clinical psychologists, some of whom may be based in their practices. Clinical psychologists give opinions, assessments and advice to GPs, and have skills in behavioural, cognitive and other psychotherapies.

Liaison between GPs and psychiatrists

Psychiatry and general practice have traditionally come into contact with each other through a semi-formal system of referral and consultation.

In the UK, the following are traditional contact points between the GP and the psychiatrist:

■ psychiatric out-patient clinics;
■ domiciliary visits – the GP can request any hospital specialist to visit the person at home –

the specialties of geriatrics and psychiatry are the ones most frequently used;
- admission to hospital (including Mental Health Act assessment for compulsory admission).

The following schemes have also been set up:

- emergency clinics;
- crisis intervention teams;
- walk-in services.

Psychiatric services are now increasingly organized to serve local populations of 30 000 to 70 000 people. Some of these local services are based in 'Community Mental Health Centres' which often offer an early opportunity for referral by GPs. These local community services frequently employ multidisciplinary teams consisting of psychiatrists, mental health nurses, occupational therapists, clinical psychologists and social workers.

There are three main models of collaboration between GPs and psychiatric teams.

- *The replacement model* The psychiatrist or team becomes the primary care agent. This model has applied mainly to the USA. However, some secondary psychiatric services in the UK allow people to refer themselves and thus bypass the GP.
- *The increased throughput model* This allows for increased referral by GPs to psychiatric services. Some Community Mental Health Centres do allow for this, but the GP remains the main gatekeeper to secondary services.
- *The liaison/attachment model* Psychiatrists and teams move out of the hospital into general practice surgeries.

In practice, in the UK many services are a mixture of traditional services with elements of the last two models. These are supplemented to a greater or lesser extent by the attachment of other mental health professionals in primary care.

About 20 per cent of psychiatrists in England and Wales and 50 to 60 per cent of psychiatrists in Scotland spend some time in general practice. Three main methods of working are used:

- *shifted out-patients* – conducting out-patient clinics in general practice premises;
- *consultation* – the psychiatrist carries out the assessment of the person and the referring doctor carries out the treatment plan;
- *liaison-attachment* – the psychiatrist provides a supervisory and consultatory role after setting up working and training links with other allied professionals.

Letters between psychiatrists and general practitioners

The letter and discharge summary are the main written channels of communication between GPs and psychiatrists. However, they are the source of much complaint, contention and debate.

REFERRAL LETTERS FROM GENERAL PRACTITIONERS

The often seen 'Please see and do...' referral letter is a poor way to start the referral process. The initial letter is of vital importance, as it is the first impression of the patient that the psychiatrist receives. There are no set rules regarding the content of the letter, but it should contain:

- the person's name, address and demographic details
- reason for referral (include the degree of urgency, what the GP wants, e.g. advice, treatment)
- main symptoms or problems (and any relevant life events and difficulties)
- medication prescribed so far (including non-psychotropic medication) and any other treatment given
- past psychiatric history and treatment
- any family history

A suggested format is a one-page letter with the above headings.

LETTERS AND DISCHARGE SUMMARIES FROM PSYCHIATRISTS TO GPS

Remember that these are written for two reasons: to communicate information to the GP, and to provide a clear and permanent record in the hospital notes.
The initial letter should contain:

- the person's name, address and demographic details
- current problems
- present circumstances
- the person's background
- mental state
- diagnosis and reasons for diagnosis
- any suicide risk
- prognosis
- treatment plan and any follow-up arrangements

More information may be included to give a complete history of the case. However, it is useful to write a summary at the end of the letter, to which the GP can easily refer.

Follow-up letters should contain information about the person's current state, any changes to the treatment plan, current medication and the immediate plan.

Discharge summaries should contain full details of the admission, and should contain the headings that you normally use when taking a history and recording the mental state. Again it is useful for the GP to have a brief summary to which he or she can refer, and this should include the details suggested for the letters above. It is now often customary to send the GP a brief summary of the person's admission, which is issued on the day of discharge, acknowledges that the person has been in hospital, and gives details of their medication on discharge and the immediate follow-up plan.

Remember that good communication between GPs and hospital services is fundamental to good patient care. Letters are only one way of communicating, but they are especially important because they provide a permanent record. However, never hesitate to pick up the telephone or talk to your colleagues face to face. Faxes and E-mail links can also be used.

Training for general practitioners

GPs gain specific training in psychiatry in four settings:

- as medical students;
- as a psychiatric SHO in a vocational training scheme;
- during the 1-year trainee appointment;
- as an experienced GP – as part of their continuing medical education or as a clinical assistant in psychiatry.

Since 1982 all new GPs in the UK have had to undergo a compulsory 3-year vocational training in which they hold a series of hospital posts (one of which may be in psychiatry) and spend a year as a trainee in a practice with a recognized GP trainer.

SUMMARY

- Primary health care is the point of first contact between a person and a provider of health care.
- In the UK, primary health care is synonymous with general practice.
- A series of selective filters operates between the community and psychiatric services, and involves primary health care.
- Worldwide, psychiatric disorders are common in primary health care, and relatively few of the psychiatric disorders seen are referred to secondary care.
- Emotional symptoms and distress are common in the community and primary care, but not all of this distress amounts to psychiatric disorders.
- Psychiatric disorders account for 20 to 30 per cent of disorders seen in primary care.
- Psychiatric disorders represent a large proportion of the GP's workload.
- Most psychiatric disorders in primary care are short-lived affective disorders (depression and anxiety), but 25 per cent are chronic 'neurotic' disorders.
- GPs vary enormously in their ability to detect psychiatric disorders.
- The treatment of psychiatric disorders in primary care has not been widely researched, but the use of a range of professionals in primary care to treat these disorders is becoming more common.

Further reading

Goldberg, D. and Huxley, P. 1980: *Mental illness in the community. The pathway to psychiatric care*. London: Tavistock Publications.

Goldberg, D. and Huxley, P. 1992: *Common mental disorders. A bio-social model*. London: Tavistock/Routledge.

Pullen, I., Wilkinson, G., Wright, W. and Gray, D.P. 1994: *Psychiatry and general practice today*. London: Royal College of Psychiatrists and Royal College of General Practitioners.

Shepherd, M., Cooper, B., Brown, A.C. and Kalton, G. 1981: *Psychiatric illness in general practice*, 2nd edn. Oxford: Oxford University Press.

PART

2

CLINICAL SYNDROMES

6 ORGANIC STATES

ref. Neurology.

INTRODUCTION

In recent years the increasing sophistication of neurobiological and neuro-imaging techniques (Figure 6.1) has provided major insights into the underlying neurological substrate of the so-called 'functional' disorders. There remain, however, a number of psychiatric syndromes which occur as a result of processes such as physical disease, degeneration, infection or trauma, the underlying cause of which can be sought through medical investigation, and these are known as 'organic states'. Sleep disorders are traditionally included with the organic disorders.

These have been classified in a number of ways:

- acute (delirium) vs. chronic (dementia);
- local vs. general;
- disorders of specific psychological domains, e.g. language, memory;
- disorders associated with specific medical disorders, e.g. thyroid dysfunction.

Clinically the most important division is into acute and chronic states.

DELIRIUM (ACUTE CONFUSIONAL STATE)

FIG 6.1 Coronal MRI scan of a normal 67-year-old man.

Features of delerium

- acute onset
- decreased awareness of the surroundings and self (fluctuations in consciousness)
- poor attention
- memory impairment
- illusions and hallucinations
- fragmentary delusions
- worsening at night
- fluctuating course

A 74-year-old woman was admitted to hospital for a routine operation on her inguinal hernia. She became increasingly disturbed during the night following her operation, believing that she could hear children being tortured and that she was being prevented from helping them by 'soldiers'. A small dose of haloperidol settled her for the night and she had no recollection of the incident in the morning.

Delirium is a common disorder in hospital practice, particularly affecting the elderly and children. The importance of making the correct diagnosis lies in the possibility of treating the underlying physical cause of the delirium, leading to a rapid resolution of the symptoms. The important features are outlined above. The importance of getting a good history of acute onset and fluctuations in severity cannot be too highly stressed. The management of delirium involves skilled supportive nursing and the treatment of the underlying cause (see below). The psychiatric symptoms may take longer to resolve than the medical disorder. In some cases (as in Case 6.1) there may be a need for the symptoms to be treated in their own right.

Management of delirium

- identify and treat the underlying cause
- nurse in a constant and well-lit environment
- use small consistent teams of nursing staff
- reduce the possibilities of misinterpretations
- maintain fluid balance
- administer medication only in cases of extreme disturbance

Common causes of delirium

- infections (urinary, chest)
- postoperative causes
- drugs (anticholinergics, sedatives, digoxin, cimetidine, steroids)
- alcohol and drug withdrawal
- myocardial infarction
- strokes, transient ischaemic attacks
- metabolic disorders
- epilepsy
- trauma

If medication is required, haloperidol, 0.5–2 mg in the elderly and up to 10 mg in younger patients, may be given orally or intramuscularly each 3 to 4 hours.

DEMENTIA (CHRONIC ORGANIC BRAIN SYNDROME)

A 76-year-old woman was found wandering the streets in the early hours of the morning wearing her nightclothes covered by a light coat. She was unable to say where she lived or where she was going. She believed it was early afternoon and wanted to get her shopping done before her father got home from work. Her sister reported that she had been increasingly forgetful over the last 2 years, losing her keys and pension book, not locking her door, and leaving saucepans on the stove. Formal testing showed her to be disorientated in place and time, and to have problems with both short- and long-term memory. Although she was able to talk about her school-days without problems. She had word-finding difficulties and problems copying three-dimensional figures.

Features of dementia

- long history of gradual decline
- memory impairment – inability to learn new information and recall once known information
- disorientation with regard to year, month, date and day of the week is common
- disorientation with regard to place usually occurs in unfamiliar settings, e.g. in hospital
- apraxias and agnosias
- impairment of judgement and reasoning
- delusions and hallucinations
- personality change

Dementia is a chronic, acquired and usually progressive impairment of a wide range of cognitive areas sufficient to interfere with the day-to-day life of the sufferer. The major features are outlined above. The commonest problem is the failure of new learning and forgetting information that was once known. CT or MRI scans show dilation of the ventricles and atrophy of the cortex.

Dementia is seen in approximately 5 per cent of those aged 65 to 70 years, rising to 20 per cent in the 80+ age group. With the increasingly ageing population the number of cases of dementia is going to rise over the next 20 years.

Early studies suggested that 50 per cent of cases of dementia had Alzheimer's disease, 20 per cent were multi-infarct cases and 15 per cent were a mixture of the two, the remainder being a mixture of the unusual forms. Recent advances in microscopy have revealed that Lewy Bodies, the characteristic finding in Parkinson's disease, are much more common in the cortex than was previously believed. It is suggested that Senile Dementia of the Lewy body type (SDLT) represents 20 per cent of cases, making it a common cause of dementia. The associated clinical syndrome is outlined below. (For more details on the presentation and management of dementia, see Chapter 21 on old age psychiatry.)

Classification of the dementias

- Degenerative – Alzheimer's disease, Diffuse Lewy Body disease, Pick's disease
- Vascular – multi-infarct, sub-arachnoid haemorrhage, subdural haematoma
- Infection – HIV, syphilis, Creutzfeldt-Jacob disease
- Demyelinating disorders – multiple sclerosis
- Endocrine disorders – hypothyroidism
- Movement disorders – Huntington's chorea, Parkinson's disease.

Alzheimer's disease

Alzheimer's disease is the commonest form of dementia both in those under 65 years (pre-senile) and in those over 65 years of age (senile). The onset is gradual with relentless progression. It has a characteristic neuropathology of plaques and tangles (see Chapter 21 on old age psychiatry for more details).

Multi-infarct dementia

The characteristic history is one of a stepwise deterioration in the illness, with stable plateaus between. There are often focal neurological signs and a history of hypertension and/or stroke.

Senile dementia of the Lewy body type (SDLT)

The main features are as follows:

- dementia;
- fluctuating course with lucid and confused periods;
- hallucinations (often visual);
- Parkinsonian features;
- falls;
- sensitivity to neuroleptics.

The clinical picture of SDLT is outlined above. This group of people do very badly when exposed to neuroleptics.

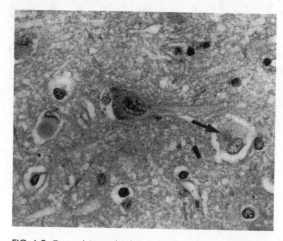

FIG 6.2 Cortical Lewy bodies.

Reversible dementias

Most forms of dementia are chronic conditions for which no treatments are available. However, a small but important group of conditions cause a dementia-like picture which may be reversed or at least halted by intervention at the right time.

Causes of 'reversible' dementia

- normal-pressure hydrocephalus (dementia, gait disturbance, incontinence, CT findings of ventricular dilation without cortical atrophy)
- hypothyroidism
- syphilis
- nicotinic acid deficiency (dementia, dermatitis, diarrhoea)
- Vitamin B_{12} deficiency

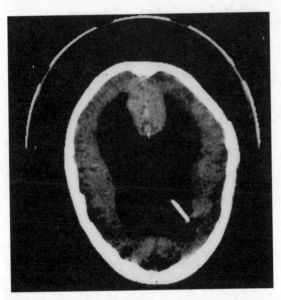

FIG 6.3 CT scan showing the hugely dilated ventricles of normal-pressure hydrocephalus with a shunt to divert cerebrospinal fluid to the peritoneum.

Pseudo-dementia

The withdrawal, apathy, agitation, inability to complete tasks and poor concentration (leading to memory problems) of a depressive illness may appear to be the result of a dementing illness. Making the correct diagnosis is important, as the depressive illness is treatable.

The features of pseudo-dementia
■ depressed mood and cognitions
■ short history
■ past history of depression
■ poor concentration
■ no confabulation
■ 'Don't know' or approximate answers
■ no neurological signs

DISORDERS OF SPECIFIC PSYCHOLOGICAL DOMAINS

Memory disorders

Memory disorders may be divided into those which are transient (delirium, head injury, etc.)

and those which are persistent (amnestic syndrome, dementia). In the Amnestic Syndrome the memory alone is affected, whereas in the dementias all domains of cognition are affected (see above).

Memory disorders	
Transient	**Persistent**
delirium	dementia (global)
epilepsy	amnesic syndrome
transient global	■ thiamine deficiency
amnesia	(alcohol abuse)
	■ head injury
hypoglycaemia	■ anoxia
	■ vascular lesions
	■ 3rd ventricle tumour
	■ TB meningitis

AMNESTIC SYNDROME (KORSAKOFF'S SYNDROME)

The features and causes of the amnestic syndrome are outlined below. The major feature of amnestic syndrome is a disorder of recent memory and time sense in the absence of generalized cognitive decline. The patient's remote memory remains intact. Gaps in the memory are filled by confabulating (giving an account of actions and events which are found to be false).

Alcohol abuse (thiamine deficiency) is the commonest cause of this problem (see Chapter 20 on addiction). Similar problems can be caused by anoxia, trauma (e.g. head injury), vascular lesions, third ventricle tumours and TB meningitis. Transient amnestic syndrome may be caused by delirium, epilepsy, transient global amnesia and hypoglycaemia.

Features of Amnestic Syndrome
■ normal registration of information
■ failure of recent memory
■ clear consciousness
■ confabulation
■ no other cognitive abnormalities

TABLE 6.1 Differential diagnosis of memory disorders

	Delirium	Amnestic syndrome	Dementia
Immediate memory	Poor	Normal	Moderate
5-minute memory	Poor	Poor	Poor
3-month memory	Fair	Poor	Poor
Consciousness	Impaired	Normal	Normal
History	< 2 weeks	> 1 month	> 6 months
Course	Fluctuating	Stable	Slow decline
Language	Variable	Good	Impaired
Praxis	Variable	Good	Impaired
Thinking	Disorganized	Normal	Poor
Hallucinations	Present	Absent	Rare
Sleep	Disturbed	Normal	Fragmented

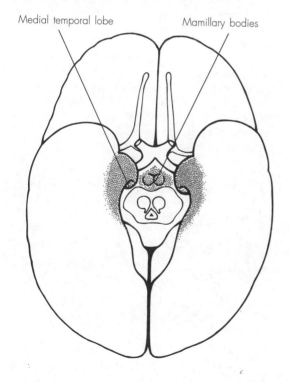

FIG 6.4 Areas of the brain associated with memory dysfunction.

Medial temporal lobe

Mamillary bodies

SYMPTOMS ASSOCIATED WITH SPECIFIC REGIONS OF THE BRAIN

The frontal lobe (Figure 6.5)

Symptoms of frontal lobe dysfunction include:

- decreased intellectual drive, and apathy;
- loss of awareness of social expectations;
- personality change;
- tactlessness;
- irritability;
- euphoria;
- concrete thinking, perseveration, poor sequencing.

CASE 6.3

A 64-year-old man presented with a 2-year history of increasing neglect of himself and his garden. Despite spending many hours there, it was becoming increasingly unkempt. He was irritable and threatening towards his wife and had become more sexually demanding. A colostomy which he had managed for many years became difficult and messy. Having made lewd comments and touching

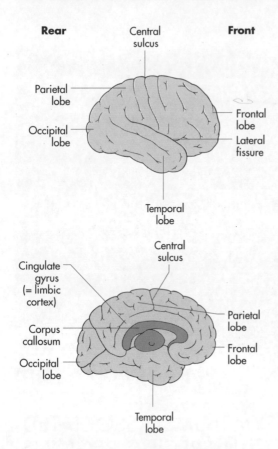

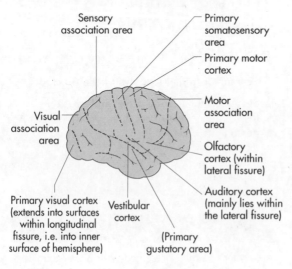

FIG 6.5 The lobes of the brain.

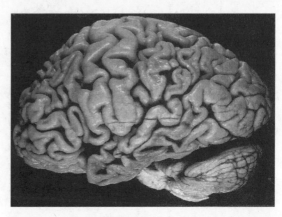

FIG 6.6 Frontal atrophy of the brain seen in Pick's disease.

the bottom of a girl on the street he was questioned by the police. He was unkempt, and his speech was sparse with word-finding difficulties. He was irritable and revealed a poverty of thought. His apathy made testing difficult, but his memory was intact. He gave concrete interpretations of proverbs and was perseverative in responses to problem-solving exercises. He had no insight into the changes in his personality. Neurological examination was unremarkable and a CT scan showed bilateral frontal atrophy. A diagnosis of Pick's disease (selective frontal lobe atrophy with the distinctive Pick body seen on microscopy) was made (Figure 6.6).

The major features of frontal lobe disease are well illustrated in this case history and outlined above. Changes in personality are predominant, with problems in concentration, memory and the planning of complex tasks. People become stuck in one area of thinking or activity and are unable to switch to another area (perseveration).

Causes of frontal lobe dysfunction

- Pick's disease
- trauma
- tumour
- syphilis

Tests of frontal lobe function

- verbal fluency
- sequencing tasks, e.g. hand, fist, palm test
- grasp reflex
- Wisconsin Card Sorting Test

The temporal lobe

Symptoms of temporal lobe dysfunction

- personality alteration
- dense amnesia if there is bilateral damage
- psychosis (secondary to epileptic foci)
- complex hallucinations
- depression
- visual field defect
- dominant hemisphere damage
  poor verbal memory
  sensory dysphasia (Wernicke's dysphasia)
- non-dominant hemisphere damage
  poor visual memory
  poor facial recognition (proposoagnosia)

Temporal lobe lesions are rarely silent, and produce more mental disturbance than lesions in any other area of the brain. The temporal lobes are involved in many of the highest abstract functions of the brain, but rarely produce neurological signs. As such, they are often diagnosed late in their course.

Tests of temporal lobe function

- tests of verbal and visual memory
- facial recognition tasks
- repetition of sentences

Causes of temporal lobe lesions

- tumours
- trauma
- infection
- thiamine deficiency

The occipital lobe

The features of occipital lobe lesions

- visual field disturbances
- complex visual hallucinations
- visual recognition disturbance (micropsia, macropsia, visual agnosias)
- cortical blindness

The symptoms of occipital lobe lesions are ill-defined. Visual field defects occur in the opposite visual field and, when extensive, can produce cortical blindness with preserved pupillary light reflexes. Complex visual recognition disturbances occur when the lesions spread to the borders of the parietal and temporal lobes. Hallucinations are often the result of cerebral vascular accidents producing epileptic foci.

The parietal lobe (Figure 6.7)

The features of parietal lobe lesions

- visuo-spatial abnormalities
- topographical disorientation
- dysphasia
- motor apraxia
- Gerstmann's syndrome (finger agnosia, dyscalculia, agraphia, left–right disorientation)
- disturbance of body image or neglect
- cortical sensory loss (loss of two-point discrimination, lack of object recognition by palpation, figures written on the palm of the hand not recognized)
- sensory Jacksonian march
- depression
- tactile hallucinosis

CASE 6.4

A 26-year-old man suffered from a classical depressive illness with biological features following the death of a member of his family. He had a strong family history of depression and previous episodes of mood disturbance. He was started on tricyclic antidepressants and began to recover. He developed episodes of paraesthesia occurring in one arm, which began at the fingers and travelled centrally. A CT scan revealed a dominant parietal tumour. Whilst the depression was unlikely to be related to the parietal lesion, the tricyclic medication reducing the epileptic threshold probably revealed the tumour at an earlier stage than might otherwise have been the case.

Lesions of the parietal lobe usually present with complex cognitive disorders. Depression is common, but bizarre hallucinatory experiences are rare (sensory Jacksonian march; see Case 6.4 above). Gerstmann's syndrome (see above) is rarely found in its pure form, but elements may be present. Motor apraxias in which there is difficulty in executing motor tasks despite having the power to do them are common. Non-dominant lesions produce unusual disturbances of body image with unilateral neglect or denial of abnormality. Cortical sensory loss involves the failure to recognize objects by palpation (astereognosis), failure to recognize numbers written on the palm of the hand (dysgraphaesthesia) and loss of two-point discrimination.

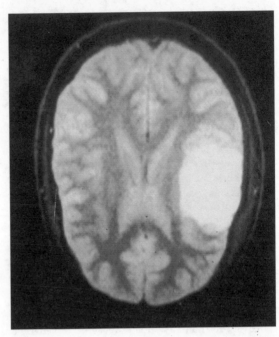

FIG 6.8 CT scan of Case 6.4 showing the parietal lobe tumour.

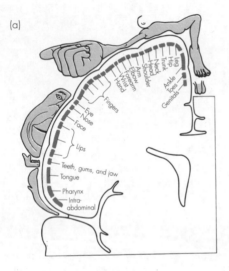

(a)

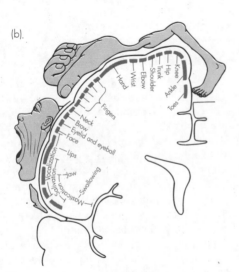

(b)

FIG 6.7 The somatosensory areas of the parietal lobes. (a) Somatosensory cortex, right hemisphere. (b) Motor cortex, right hemisphere.

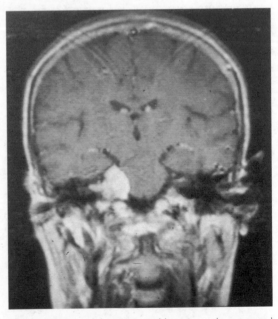

FIG 6.9 MRI scan of a 54-year-old woman who presented with paranoid delusion and hallucinations. The scan shows a petrous temporal meningioma distorting the brain stem.

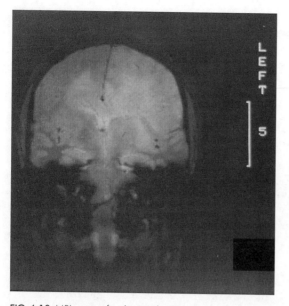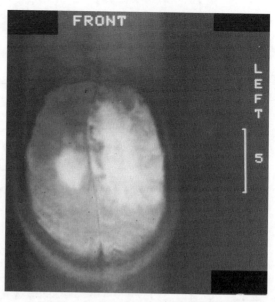

FIG 6.10 MRI scan of a large glioma crossing the corpus callosum in a young man presenting with an illness indistinguishable from schizophrenia.

Cerebral tumours

CASE 6.5

A 70-year-old woman was admitted to hospital with a 3-month history of increasing withdrawal, apathy and self-neglect. She had poor concentration and some slowness in thinking, but no other evidence of cognitive decline. There were no localizing neurological signs. She failed to respond to medication, and spent more and more time asleep. A CT scan revealed a large tumour of the dominant parietal lobe. She was not felt to be a suitable case for surgery and she died 2 months later (see also Figures 6.9 and 6.10).

There is no single picture that is representative of all cerebral tumours, although psychological symptoms are common. The factors involved in the generation of mental symptoms are outlined below. These factors interact in complex ways which vary from one tumour to another. There is no clear correlation between the degree of raised intracranial pressure and the production of mental symptoms.

Factors involved in the generation of mental symptoms in cerebral tumours

- tumour location and size
- speed of growth (fast-growing tumours produce more symptoms, and slow-growing tumours are more likely to present only with mental symptoms)
- histological type (gliomas are worse than meningiomas)
- malignant or benign
- raised intracranial pressure
- pre-morbid personality

EPILEPSY

Classification of epilepsy

- Partial (focal) seizures
  (a) Simple partial seizures (consciousness not impaired)
  (b) Complex partial seizures (consciousness impaired)
  (c) Partial seizures evolving to generalized seizures
- Generalized seizure
- Unclassified seizures

Revised Classification International League Against Epilepsy (ILAE) 1985

An 18-year-old man was admitted to hospital following a 2-week period of increasing disturbance. He was not sleeping and had become irritable with all those who stood in the way of his grandiose plans. He believed that he had been chosen by God for a special mission and was being persecuted as a result. He experienced third-person auditory hallucinations. There was no evidence of clouding of consciousness. The attack occurred after an increase in frequency of his grand mal seizures.

Psychiatric disorders and epilepsy

The psychiatric disturbances associated with epilepsy can be divided into those associated with the seizure itself (peri-ictal symptoms) and those which are unrelated to the seizure (inter-ictal symptoms).

Peri-ictal symptoms

- auras, churning of the stomach, *déjà vu, jamais vu*, hallucinations, lip-smacking, fear and anxiety;
- automatisms (complex motor activity with impaired consciousness occurring during seizure activity. Usually brief and purposeless, rarely prolonged with wandering (fugue));
- delusions and hallucinations.

Post-ictal symptoms include:

- malaise and sleep (usually);
- continuing psychotic symptoms (which may be long-lasting).

Partial seizures (i.e. with a focal origin) are most commonly associated with psychiatric disturbances, especially if the focus is within the temporal lobe. The seizure may be heralded by an 'aura'.

During the seizure itself consciousness is usually impaired but the person can undertake complex motor behaviour (automatism). Delusions and hallucinations often accompany the seizure and can be vivid and complex.

Post-ictally most people experience some malaise and will sleep, but people with temporal lobe epilepsy may undergo a prolonged period of disturbance when they are clearly confused but continue to experience psychotic symptoms.

The diagnosis of temporal lobe epilepsy is a clinical one in which the report of a witness is vital.

A negative electroencephalogram (EEG) does not preclude the diagnosis.

Inter-ictal disorders

PSYCHOSIS AND EPILEPSY

The relationship between psychosis and epilepsy has been difficult to unravel. In addition to the disturbances described above, which are clearly related to the seizure activity itself, some people display impairment of consciousness with hallucinations and paranoid delusions associated with abnormalities of electrical activity which do not amount to a seizure. A third group of people who experience epilepsy develop schizophrenia-like episodes between the seizures without any disturbance of consciousness. These may be chronic and occur more frequently than would be expected by chance for coincident diagnoses of schizophrenia and epilepsy.

Psychotic symptoms and epilepsy

- as part of an 'aura'
- as part of the seizure itself (with impaired consciousness)
- as a post-ictal phenomena (usually with impaired consciousness)
- between seizures, with EEG abnormalities not amounting to a seizure (with impairment of consciousness)
- between seizures with a normal EEG (consciousness not impaired)

DEPRESSION AND EPILEPSY

The diagnosis of epilepsy has profound effects on a person's life, which may leave them feeling miserable. In addition, a greater degree of depressive illness is suffered by those with epilepsy than by the general population, and is the commonest psychiatric problem associated with epilepsy. The problem is primarily associated with temporal lobe epilepsy, as is an increased suicide rate (five times higher than that of the general population).

DEMENTIA AND EPILEPSY

There is a long tradition of equating mental deterioration with epilepsy. However, more careful diagnosis (excluding degenerative disorders) and changes in treatment regimes have weakened the association. Problems in cognition are associated with early-onset seizures, frequency of seizures and the type of seizure, generalized seizures being worse. Temporal lobe epilepsy is associated with memory problems.

PSEUDO-SEIZURES

'Seizures' without an organic basis are frequently encountered in emergency departments, but differ from the 'true' seizure in a number of ways (see below). The person may have a documented history of 'true' epilepsy and become very sophisticated. Until a definitive diagnosis is made, the seizure should be regarded as 'organic' in origin and appropriate medical and nursing care given. A normal EEG during a fit is diagnostic.

The features of pseudo-seizures

- they follow a psychological trauma
- no aura
- no fall, tongue-biting or incontinence
- purposeful movements
- abdominal muscles not involved
- no post-ictal effects
- no EEG changes during the fit

HEAD INJURY

Acute consequences of head injury

Mild

The person loses consciousness only very briefly, if at all, and remains dazed for a short time but continues to function. He or she returns to normal within a few hours, with amnesia for the incident (a normal Saturday afternoon for most rugby players!).

Moderate

The person is unconscious for several hours and is disorientated and confused before returning to normal. There is amnesia for the period before (retrograde amnesia, RA) and after (post-traumatic amnesia, PTA) the accident.

Severe

Unconsciousness lasts for several hours to days. The period of confusion is prolonged, as is the RA and the PTA. If consciousness is not regained within 1 month 40 per cent of cases will die and only 20 per cent return to work.

Penetrating injuries and intracranial bleeding also worsen the prognosis.

Significance of post-traumatic amnesia (PTA)

PTA is defined as the time from the trauma to the establishment of normal continuous memory.

- PTA >1 hour. Return to work within 1 month
- PTA >1 day. Return to work within 2 months
- PTA >1 week. Return to work within 4 months

Chronic sequelae of head injury

Factors that influence the long-term outcome of head injury

- volume and severity of the damage
- location of the damage
- epilepsy (30 per cent with penetrating injuries and 5 per cent with closed injuries)
- pre-morbid personality
- personal and family psychiatric history
- the person's interpretation of the trauma
- continuing compensation

A complex mixture of personal, social and medical factors contributes to the long-term outcome of head injuries. In the most severe cases the volume and site of the damage are of major importance. In less severe cases the personality of the person and their ability to deal with stress become more important as does the 'meaning' of the injury for the individual. Ongoing compensation or legal action will complicate any picture.

Psychiatric sequelae of head injury

- post-concussional syndrome
- personality change
- cognitive impairment
- psychoses

POST-CONCUSSIONAL SYNDROME

Post-concussional syndrome is the commonest after-effect of head trauma, occurring in 10 to 20 per cent of severe cases. The initial symptoms of dizziness and headache usually resolve over a period of weeks, and may be related to subtle organic changes. Other symptoms, fatigue, depression, anxiety and phobia may take much longer to resolve, and are related to the personal factors outlined above.

PERSONALITY CHANGES

Personality changes occur in 5 to 15 per cent of people with severe injuries. These may occur as part of a dementing process or due to damage to the frontal lobes. Where there is no gross structural damage a coarsening of previous personality traits is seen.

COGNITIVE IMPAIRMENT

Trauma resulting in a persistent vegetative state, in which there is an absence of all discernible mental activity, represents the most extreme end of this spectrum. There is more likelihood of cognitive impairment if the injury has caused a prolonged PTA. Penetrating injuries, with haemorrhage and infection, increase the degree of cognitive impairment. Recovery of function may be very slow and may continue over many years.

PSYCHOSES

Both schizophreniform and affective psychoses have been described as a result of head injuries. Depressive illnesses are the commonest of these and are associated with frontal and non-dominant hemisphere damage, while schizophreniform illnesses are linked to temporal lobe damage.

Repeated head injury (punch drunk syndrome)

Features of punch drunk syndrome

- cerebellar symptoms
- extra-pyramidal and pyramidal motor disorder
- intellectual deterioration
- paranoid illness (rarely)

Repeated head trauma can lead to widespread neurological damage. Dysarthria, gait disturbance, lack of facial mobility and ataxia are common. Memory impairment is the commonest cognitive problem, but personality change with apathy, irritability and outbursts of temper is also seen. In those with intellectual deterioration, paranoid illnesses, including morbid jealousy, are seen.

INFECTIONS OF THE CNS

HIV infection

CASE 6.7

A 24-year-old man was visited at home 2 years after he had been found to be carrying the HIV virus. The house was in great disarray, with magazines, clothes and computer equipment strewn across the floor. He had been incontinent and the kitchen was filthy. He showed little concern about the state in which he was living. He was ataxic, and cognitive testing revealed global deficits. He had a chest infection and was admitted to the medical ward, where he died a few weeks later.

PSYCHOLOGICAL PROBLEMS RELATED TO HIV INFECTION

These may occur:

- in relation to diagnosis or progression of the infection
- as a result of direct infection of the brain
- as a result of secondary processes in the brain
- as a result of drug problems

At the time of diagnosis and at times of progression of the infection, levels of uncertainty and anxiety are high. The need for adequate pre-test and post-test counselling and for support throughout the subsequent phases of the infection cannot be stressed too strongly. At times these reactions may develop into frank psychiatric problems, such as depression, which require treatment in their own right.

PROBLEMS OF DIRECT INFECTION OF THE BRAIN

In most cases sero-conversion is accompanied by only a mild transient malaise. However, it may progress to encephalitis and require hospital treatment.

All forms of psychotic illness, paranoid states, schizophreniform illnesses, catatonia and affective disorders have been described and related to the presence of HIV in the brain. Clues to the diagnosis lie in a history of high-risk behaviours or the presence of cognitive defects when testing the mental state.

The presence of cognitive impairment has been a source of debate. It is rare for there to be cognitive impairment (HACC) without immunosuppression (i.e. CD4 count of below 400). The first changes are slowing of the mental processes and poor concentration (HMCD). In 10–15 per cent of cases there is progression to dementia with problems in all realms of cognition.

Secondary processes causing meningitis (e.g. cryptococcus) or space-occupying lesions (e.g. toxoplasma or lymphoma) may also cause abnormalities in mental functioning. Any change in the mental state of a person with HIV demands a full neurological assessment and appropriate neuroimaging. The issues surrounding drug use and HIV are beyond the scope of this chapter (see Chapter 20 on addiction for more details).

Problems of direct infection of brain

- encephalitis at sero-conversion
- apparently functional psychoses
- HIV-associated cognitive/motor complex (HACC). This includes HIV-associated minor cognitive/motor disorder (HMCD) and HIV dementia complex (HDC)

Syphilis

Approximately 10 per cent of those infected with *Treponema pallidum* develop some form of neurosyphilis.

Forms of neurosyphilis

- asymptomatic
- acute meningitis
- meningo-vascular, with insidious onset leading to dementia or episodes of delirium
- general paralysis of the insane (GPI)
  (a) simple dementing form
  (b) grandiose form
  (c) depressive form

Meningo-vascular syphilis can present with psychiatric symptoms, but General Paralysis of the Insane (GPI) has been a much more important although now increasingly rare form of the infection. The person is expansive and often euphoric and a belief that they are a very important person, sometimes from the past, can be held despite their living conditions. In the simple dementing form the cognitive impairment is to the fore without the grandiose front. A third important type is the depressive form in which all of the features of a functional depressive illness are mimicked. Clues to the underlying diagnosis may lie either in the history or in the physical examination, which reveals evidence of Tabes Dorsalis in 20 per cent of cases.

Tuberculous meningitis

Tuberculous meningitis has an insidious onset in which psychological symptoms predominate. Headache and photophobia may be absent, and the pyrexia is low grade. Apathy, irritability and personality change are the early signs. People go on to develop delirium and, if left untreated, die. Early intervention attenuates the course of the disease. There is a prolonged amnesic phase which slowly resolves, and with the return to a normal cerebral spinal fluid (CSF) most people have no residual symptomatology. If not treated at an early stage, elements of the personality change may remain despite the return of normal cognitive function.

Herpes simplex encephalitis

Herpes simplex encephalitis is the commonest cause of sporadic encephalitis in the UK. The onset is rapid, with a high fever. There is a delirious phase which can be very similar to delirium tremens, with vivid hallucinations. Coma and death often ensue. Following recovery of consciousness, the person may once again be very disturbed. The outcome is frequently fatal (70 per cent of cases), and the survivors are often very impaired. Dementia or amnestic syndromes are common, often with behaviour suggestive of temporal lobe damage. The reason for the florid presentation and the persistent sequelae is the tendency for the virus to cause necrosis and haemorrhage in the medial temporal lobes.

Encephalitis lethargica

This now rare infection caused great disabilities following epidemics between 1918 and 1920.

SOMNOLENT-OPHTHALMOPLEGIC FORM

This was the commonest variety, in which the person slept for prolonged periods and had paresis of the third and sixth cranial nerves. Sleep disturbances were experienced long after the neurological signs had gone.

PARKINSONIAN FORM

Rigidity and akinesis were the prominent features of this variety. Catatonic features were often present.

PSYCHOTIC FORM

This was an unusual presentation, but mistakes in diagnosis were made until neurological signs presented themselves.

LONG-TERM PROBLEMS

Many people developed long-term problems with severe Parkinsonism, often accompanied by repetitive activities or oculogyric crises and dementia. Personality change was also frequent, as were a variety of psychotic illnesses.

Forms of encephalitis lethargica
■ somnolent-ophthalmoplegic form ■ parkinsonian form ■ psychotic form ■ chronic form (combining the features of the above plus dementia)

Creutzfeldt-Jacob disease

Interest in this rare form of pre-senile dementia has grown in recent years. The agent responsible for the transmission is thought to be a prion (a glycoprotein without RNA or DNA) which causes a spongiform degeneration.

There is a prodromal period of lassitude and depression before the cognitive impairment and neurological symptoms (myoclonic jerks are the most characteristic) emerge. Finally, the person becomes rigid, adopting a decorticate posture. The CT scan may be normal, but the EEG shows characteristic triphasic sharp waves. Fifty per cent of people die within 9 months of diagnosis.

ENDOCRINE AND METABOLIC ABNORMALITIES

Thyroid dysfunction

HYPOTHYROIDISM

Features of hypothyroidism
■ fatigue ■ psychomotor retardation ■ apathy ■ depression ■ slowing of cognitive functions ■ delirium, dementia (especially in the elderly)

CASE 6.8

A 27-year-old woman presented with increasing lassitude, and failure to care for herself and her family. She took no interest in the world around her and wanted only to sleep. She was miserable and felt that life was not worth living. Her cognitive function was slow, with poor concentration. Physical examination was unremarkable, but an electrocardiogram (ECG) revealed low-voltage complexes. Thyroid function tests revealed low T_4 and T_3 levels with a greatly elevated thyroid stimulating hormone (TSH). Treatment with thyroxine restored her to her premorbid state.

The lack of thyroid hormone may mimic a functional depressive illness, but other features of myxoedema (e.g. cold intolerance, weight gain, coarsening of the skin) may give clues as to the diagnosis. People may need antidepressant treatment in addition to replacement therapy. The dementia resulting from hypothyroidism is not always reversible if present for 2 or more years. Occasionally, hypothyroidism may present as a paranoid state.

HYPERTHYROIDISM

Features of hyperthyroidism
■ restlessness ■ irritability ■ distractability ■ anxiety ■ functional psychosis

CASE 6.9

A 30-year-old woman found that she had developed greater energy, poor sleep and, despite an increased appetite, was losing weight. She was able to complete many small tasks, but became easily distracted and unable to concentrate on longer ones. Those working with her described her as irritable. Treatment with carbimazole effected a return to her normal mental state.

People with hyperthyroidism usually have psychological symptoms and, when severe, these can be difficult to differentiate from an anxiety neurosis. Measurement of serum T_4, T_3 and TSH levels is diagnostic. Acute organic reactions are now uncommon, as thyroid crises are rare. Functional psychoses of both schizophreniform and affective types are rare. An unusual variant, known as 'apathetic hyperthyroidism', may present as a depressive illness in the elderly.

Cushing's syndrome

Psychiatric effects of hypercortisolaemia

- depression
- acute anxiety
- paranoia
- euphoria (usually secondary to exogenous steroids)
- delirium (usually secondary to exogenous steroids)

CASE 6.10

An 86-year-old woman who had been started on steroids earlier in the day, having been diagnosed as suffering from polymyalgia rheumatica, dealt a doctor a severe blow to his right temple with his stethoscope. She believed that he had been sent to perform painful experiments on her in the early hours of the morning.

Depression is by far the most common psychiatric disorder reported in Cushing's disease, and it is often accompanied by paranoid features. Fluctuation in the severity of the mental features is a commonly noted characteristic. Cognitive dysfunction is common but mild. Treatment of the underlying disorder usually brings about a resolution of the symptoms. Exogenous steroids may cause elation of mood and delirium in the elderly (as in Case 6.10).

Addison's disease and the effects of hypocortisolaemia

Psychiatric effects of hypocortisolaemia

- depression
- apathy
- schizophreniform psychosis
- cognitive impairment

Psychiatric symptoms are ubiquitous in Addison's disease, depression being the most common. Schizophreniform psychoses occur, but are unusual. Cognitive impairment can present a dementia-like picture. In Addisonian crises the person may present with panic, delirium and eventually stupor.

Hypopituitarism (Simmond's disease)

Psychiatric effects of hypopituitarism

- depression
- apathy
- irritability
- cognitive impairment
- delirium, stupor, coma
- chronic paranoid psychoses

There is a high level of psychiatric disturbance in those with hypopituitarism, which is not due entirely to the concomitant metabolic disorder. The common causes of hypopituitarism include postpartum haemorrhage (Sheehan's syndrome), pituitary tumour or fractures involving the base of the skull. Often there is a long history prior to presentation. Depression is often very marked, and the metabolic disturbances may result in delirium. Occasionally a chronic paranoid psychosis develops.

Parathyroid abnormalities

HYPERPARATHYROIDISM

Psychiatric disturbances are common with hyperparathyroidism, depression being the most

Psychiatric features of hyperparathyroidism

- depression
- lethargy
- irritability
- cognitive impairment
- delirium

frequent presentation. Cognitive impairment is insidious, but hallucinations and paranoia can present acutely as part of the 'parathyroid crisis'. A small group of people present without clinical evidence of bone disease or kidney stones, but the diagnosis can be confirmed by a raised calcium and parathyroid hormone (PTH) assay.

HYPOPARATHYROIDISM

Psychiatric features of hyperparathyroidism

- delirium
- cognitive impairment
- emotional lability
- epilepsy
- pseudoneurosis

Psychiatric symptomatology is common in this group of people. Tingling in the hands, feet or around the mouth and muscular cramps need to be distinguished from similar symptoms resulting from an anxiety attack. Where the problem has developed insidiously, cognitive impairment and irritability come to the fore. 'Pseudoneurosis' can occur at any age, with adults becoming depressed and nervous, with fluctuations in their mental states.

Uraemia

Features of uraemia

- fatigue
- cognitive impairment
- depression
- delirium
- psychotic episodes
- drowsiness, stupor and coma

The psychiatric symptoms of uraemia are more likely to present to a psychiatrist if the develop-

ment of renal impairment has been slow. Nevertheless, symptoms are common in both acute and chronic renal impairment. These often fluctuate over time and in severity. Delirium is common in acute cases. The pre-morbid personality contributes to the rare cases where psychotic illnesses have developed.

Liver failure

Features of liver failure

- impairment of consciousness
- hypersomnia
- cognitive impairment
- hallucinations
- coma
- fluctuating course
- rarely functional psychoses
- neurological signs (flapping tremor, fluctuating motor signs)

The psychiatric features of liver failure may be present for many years, fluctuating markedly in their severity and form. Impairment of consciousness is usually present, with cognitive problems and hallucinations. Hypersomnia is seen early in the disorder. Neurological signs also fluctuate with the severity of the disorder. In its final stage, coma and death ensue.

Phaeochromocytoma

Features of phaeochromocytoma

- panic and fear
- flushing
- sweating
- tachycardia
- hypertension

Tumours of the adrenal gland secrete adrenaline and noradrenaline. As a result, the person has acute episodes of hypertension accompanied by palpitations and flushing. The accompanying mental symptoms are of intense fear and panic. The most important investigation is the measurement of the urinary catecholamine metabolite vanilomandelic acid (VMA). The symptoms mimic those of panic disorder, depression with marked anxiety, or even temporal lobe epilepsy.

Porphyria

- family history (autosomal dominant inheritance)
- precipitated by drugs
- abdominal pain
- peripheral neuritis
- epilepsy
- delirium
- schizophreniform psychosis

Porphyria presents with a wide variety of neurological and psychiatric problems precipitated by drugs (alcohol, sulphonamides, barbiturates and the contraceptive pill). It is an unusual cause of epilepsy, but can present either with a delirium or as a schizophreniform psychosis. Diagnosis is made by measuring urinary porphorbilinogen.

MULTIPLE SCLEROSIS

Psychiatric features associated with MS

- euphoria
    greater cerebral involvement
    more neurological signs
    poorer cognition
    relapsing course
    large ventricles
- depression
    less cognitive impairment
    unrelated to overall disease severity
- emotional lability
- memory dysfunction
- disturbance of higher cognitive functions
    abstraction
    concept formation
- personality change
- psychosis

The wide range of neurological symptoms which can herald an episode of multiple sclerosis (MS) and its erratic natural history make diagnosis difficult. The major psychiatric symptoms associated with MS are outlined below.

About 25 per cent of people experience euphoria, but fewer than 10 per cent do so consistently.

Depression occurs in about 25 per cent of cases, and appears to be unrelated to the overall severity of the disorder, but worsens during exacerbations. Memory dysfunction is the most consistent cognitive change in MS (occurring in about 50 per cent of cases). Language disturbances are rare, although dysarthria is common. Complex cognitive tasks such as concept formation and abstraction are disrupted. Personality changes and psychotic symptoms are also seen.

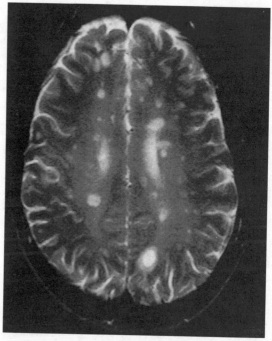

FIG 6.11 MRI scan of a patient with multiple sclerosis showing multiple plaques of demyelination.

MOVEMENT DISORDERS

The three D's of movement disorders are:

- Dyskinesia
- Depression
- Dementia

Parkinson's disease

CASE 6.11

A 76-year-old man had suffered from Parkinson's disease for 5 years. He had awoken at night on several occasions believing that he was in a hotel in Dublin (he had never been to Dublin) and had to find a particular person with some urgency, although he did not know who he was looking for. Examination revealed a slowing of mental processes, disorientation in time, and poor short- and long-term memory. Reducing his night-time dose of Sinemet alleviated his distress but made him stiffer in the morning.

Approximately 80 000 people in the UK suffer from Parkinson's disease. The classic features are rigidity, tremor and bradykinesia (slowing of movement).

DEPRESSION AND PARKINSON'S DISEASE

Depression may be difficult to diagnose in people with Parkinson's disease. The mask-like *facies*, slow movement, thinking (see below) and speech all make diagnosis difficult. About 40 per cent of people have depression, which is usually associated with anxiety features. The depression can be treated effectively by both tricyclic antidepressants and ECT.

Depression and Parkinson's disease

- diagnosis is difficult
- 40 per cent of people are affected
- marked anxiety
- more common in women
- early onset
- bradykinesia and gait disturbance
- responds to treatment

DEMENTIA IN PARKINSON'S DISEASE

Around 20 to 30 per cent of people suffer from cognitive impairment, which is a so-called subcortical dementia.

Dementia and Parkinson's Disease; subcortical dementia

- slowing of mental processes (bradyphrenia)
- poor short- and long-term memory
- language normal
- visuo-spatial skills impaired at an early stage
- concrete thinking

PSYCHOSIS IN PARKINSON'S DISEASE

In people with idiopathic Parkinson's disease the anticholinergic and dopaminergic agents can produce florid psychotic symptoms. It is often difficult to balance the benefits of treating Parkinson's disease with the disabilities caused by the psychosis. D2-selective neuroleptics (e.g. sulpiride) may be effective without causing exacerbations of the movement disorder. Clozapine (an atypical neuroleptic) can be beneficial under these circumstances, and may improve the symptoms of Parkinson's disease.

Huntington's chorea

Features of Huntington's chorea

- autosomal dominant inheritance (chromosome 4)
- age of onset 25–50 years
- progressive choreiform movements
- psychiatric symptoms often have an insidious onset
- personality change
- depression
- dementia
- schizophrenia-like episodes

Huntington's chorea is associated with a single autosomal dominant gene located on chromosome 4. It has almost complete penetrance. The onset of the movement disorder usually occurs between the ages of 25 and 50 years. The presentation of the illness is equally divided between the psychiatric and the neurological. The psychiatric presentations outlined above are insidious in onset. Depression occurs in 33 per cent of cases, and precedes the onset of the chorea in about two thirds of cases. Schizophrenia-like episodes also occur, and will respond to neuroleptics. Dementia is ubiquitous in those with marked chorea.

Diagnosis is usually made clinically, with emphasis on the family history. CT-scanning shows atrophy of the caudate nucleus, as well as generalized cortical atrophy and ventricular dilatation.

Hepatolenticular degeneration (Wilson's disease)

Abnormalities of copper metabolism, leading to its deposition in the liver and basal ganglia, usually present in late childhood. Forty per cent of cases present with liver problems, 40 per cent present with neurological problems and 20 per cent present with psychiatric problems.

Personality changes occur at an early stage, and dementia is present later in the disease. Schizophrenia-like syndromes have been described, usually of the paranoid type. Treatment is with penicillamine, but management of psychotic symptoms may be difficult with the abnormal liver function.

Basal ganglia calcification

Basal ganglia calcification is often secondary to abnormalities of calcium metabolism, but may be a primary abnormality, often associated with calcification in the cerebellum (Fahn's syndrome). Both schizophrenia-like and major affective disturbances are seen. Dysphoric mania (a simultaneous combination of depressive and manic symptoms) seems to be unusually common, and is very difficult to treat.

Dystonias

The dystonias represent a heterogeneous group of disorders characterized by sustained muscle contractions, which frequently cause twisting and repetitive movements or abnormal postures. They may be limited to one or two muscle groups (torticollis, blepharospasm, writer's cramp), or they may be more generalized. The change in severity as a result of emotional experiences and the lack of any clearly defined neurological cause for the dystonias has in the past led to them being regarded as hysterical in origin. Of major concern to the psychiatrist is the neuroleptic-induced tardive dyskinesia.

CEREBROVASCULAR DISORDERS

Cerebrovascular events are a common cause of disability and death worldwide. Lack of appreciation of the psychological effects of these events has been shown to hinder rehabilitation and return of the person to optimum functioning. The effects of infarction or haemorrhage depend primarily on the vessels involved.

Middle cerebral artery (Figure 6.12)

- contralateral hemiplegia
- cortical sensory loss
- dysphasia (dominant hemisphere)
- agnosia and body image disturbances (non-dominant hemisphere)
- delirium

Anterior cerebral artery

- contralateral hemiplegia (more marked in the leg)
- grasp reflex
- cortical sensory loss
- motor dysphasia
- dementia-like syndrome
- personality change of the frontal lobe type
- depression

Posterior cerebral artery

- contralateral hemiplegia
- visual hallucinations
- visual agnosia and disorientation
- alexia without agraphia
- thalamic syndrome
- cortical blindness with denial (Anton's syndrome)
- delirium
- memory disorders

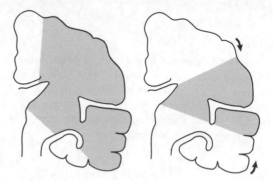

FIG 6.12 Areas of the brain supplied by the middle cerebral artery.

Cognitive function

The presence of cognitive dysfunction following a stroke is usually of a focal nature, unless the damage is very large. Problems of apraxias and agnosias hinder rehabilitation, as may the denial of disability or syndromes of neglect. Dementia is rare following a single stroke, but the repeated insults of small strokes can lead to a dementing picture (vascular dementia; see above).

Depression

The natural reaction to disability is one of misery and despair. However, the development of depressive illnesses following stroke is commoner than either in the general population or in populations matched for levels of disability but without cerebral damage. One third of people develop depression following a stroke. The effects of the stroke will depend upon a number of factors, including pre-morbid personality, past psychiatric history and family psychiatric history. Strokes which affect the non-dominant hemisphere are more frequently accompanied by depression, as are those closer to the frontal poles.

Untreated, depression represents a major barrier to rehabilitation, because of its associated lack of motivation and poor concentration. Depression may be difficult to diagnose in the presence of communication disorders.

Subarachnoid haemorrhage

The onset of symptoms following a subarachnoid haemorrhage is acute and often catastrophic. People may be confused and irritable, but a continuum from full consciousness to coma can be seen. Psychiatric problems are common in the survivors.

COGNITIVE CHANGES

Forty per cent of people experience some form of cognitive change, especially if there is a middle cerebral artery aneurysm. Some people are profoundly demented, whilst others show much milder defects. Memory difficulties represent the most prominent abnormality.

PERSONALITY CHANGE

One fifth of people experience personality change following a subarachnoid haemorrhage. This usually involves a loss of drive, interest and initiative. Such people become emotionally labile and prone to catastrophic reactions. Some people report feeling much better, less irritable and less anxious following the haemorrhage.

ANXIETY AND DEPRESSION

Anxiety is common and dependent to a large degree on the pre-morbid personality of the person. The major worry is often the possibility of recurrence of the bleed. Depression is equally related to the pre-morbid character of the sufferer, showing no clear relationship with the extent of brain damage.

Subdural haematoma

CASE 6.12

A 78-year-old woman was described by her husband as 'going from a Rolls-Royce to a Mini' over 6 weeks. She had previously been fit and running the household independently. There was a history of a fall, but no head trauma. She became ataxic, drowsy and confused. Unable to perform the simplest of daily tasks, she lay in bed and became incontinent. A CT scan showed bilateral subdural haematomas which were drained, and she subsequently made a complete recovery.

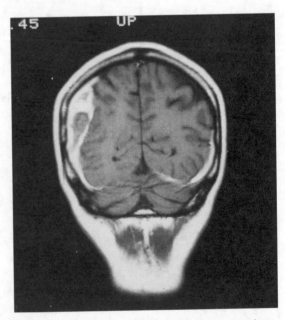

FIG 6.13 MRI scan of a 50-year-old man who was detoxified from alcohol but became increasingly unwell and developed unilateral neurological signs. The scan shows a subdural haematoma.

Subdural haematomas usually occur following head trauma, but such a history may be absent, classically in people with alcohol problems with no memory of their falls, in the elderly (see above), or in those with coagulation problems. The clinical picture is a fluctuating one with headaches, poor concentration and memory problems. Hemiparesis can be seen, but the neurological signs may be slight. As time progresses the person becomes more drowsy, and eventually lapses into a coma. A high index of suspicion is needed to make the diagnosis. Skull X-ray may show some shift of the midline structures, but a CT scan should be definitive (Figure 6.13).

Transient global amnesia

Transient global amnesia is characterized by a period of several hours during which the individual is unable to access recent memories or to learn anything new. Consciousness is not disturbed, and the person may be able to perform quite complex tasks, but is often bewildered and unable to comprehend the experience. The disorder occurs mainly in middle-aged men. The origin of the disturbance is thought to be vasospasm.

SLEEP DISORDERS

Sleep has two important phases: rapid eye movement (REM) sleep and non-REM sleep. Non-REM sleep consists of four stages, during which sleep becomes increasingly deep.

Classification of sleep disorders

Disorders of initiation and maintenance of sleep (DIMS)
- primary insomnia
- secondary insomnia (mental illness, physical illness or medication)

Disorders of excessive somnolence (DOES)
- primary hypersomnia
- secondary hypersomnia (mental illness, physical illness, medication, narcolepsy and sleep apnoea)

Parasomnias
- dream anxiety disorders (nightmares)
- sleep-walking
- night terrors

Disorders of initiation and maintenance of sleep (DIMS)

INSOMNIA

The definition of insomnia is essentially a subjective one in which the individual reports not getting enough sleep or experiencing poor-quality sleep. It is important to exclude causes such as pain, prostatism or medication (e.g. diuretics given at the wrong time of day), or a psychiatric disturbance (e.g. depression) which may be causing the disturbance of sleep.

If all of these possibilities have been excluded, then simple measures of 'sleep hygiene' can be advised.

Sleep hygiene

- develop a routine
- reduce caffeine (tea and coffee) intake prior to retiring, and keep fluid intake low
- reduce alcohol intake (none after 6pm)
- sleep in a warm, quiet, comfortable place
- exercise in the late afternoon or early evening, not just before bedtime
- only eat light snacks before bed

Many people become increasingly worried as bedtime approaches and need to develop relaxation strategies with a period of 'wind down' in the latter part of the evening, avoiding alerting activities such as reading and watching television when they go to bed. Relaxation techniques may be useful. Sleep will come when it is ready and the person is relaxed; forcing sleep is doomed to failure.

Disorders of excessive somnolence (DOES)

HYPERSOMNIA

It is important to exclude medical and psychiatric illness, as well as drugs, as the cause of hypersomnolence.

NARCOLEPSY

The hallmark of narcolepsy is that the individual goes to sleep under unusual circumstances, when they are assailed by an urge which they cannot resist. In addition, sleep paralysis occurs in about 25 per cent of cases. This can be profoundly distressing and may lead to the avoidance of sleep. Catalepsy, in which the person experiences a sudden loss of muscular tone and collapses to the floor, often in response to emotional stimuli, occurs in most cases but is less terrifying. The age of onset is between 10 and 20 years, and males are more frequently affected. Almost all cases are associated with HLA DR2. Schizophrenia-like episodes are more common in this group than would be expected by chance, but the reasons for this are unclear. The treatment available is not satisfactory. The person is advised to try to take frequent short sleeps. Tricyclic antidepressants have some effect on the frequency of catalepsy, and amphetamines are used to prolong wakefulness.

Features of narcolepsy
■ irresistible urges to sleep ■ catalepsy ■ sleep paralysis ■ HLA DR2 ■ schizophrenia-like episodes

SLEEP APNOEA (PICKWICKIAN SYNDROME)

Named after the 'Fat Boy' of Dickens' *Pickwick Papers*, this is a common cause of excessive daytime sleepiness and a sense of having had unrefreshing sleep. Most people snore loudly, get short of breath at night, and undergo periods when they stop breathing. The problem of daytime sleepiness can lead to major disruptions of work and relationships. Treatment involves alcohol avoidance, weight loss, stopping smoking, and sleeping on your side. For those in whom these measures fail, keeping the airway open with a positive-pressure nasal airway can be very effective.

KLINE-LEVINE SYNDROME

This is a rare syndrome in which the individual experiences hypersomnia accompanied by intense hunger. The episodes may be prolonged, lasting for days or weeks, and they may be separated by weeks or months of normal behaviour. During the attacks the person is irritable and can become aggressive when disturbed. He or she may be agitated at times and confused. Rarely hallucinations occur. The cause is benign and the attacks disappear over time.

PRIMARY HYPERSOMNIA

People with primary hypersomnia have longer daytime sleeps than those with narcolepsy and do not experience catalepsy or sleep paralysis. Such people also sleep deeply at night. The onset is between 10 and 20 years of age and the disorder tends to be a lifelong affliction. A wide range of neurotic disturbances have been described in these people. It is suggested that psychogenic factors are not important in the genesis of the syndrome, although the underlying organic substrate has not been clarified. Treatment is with amphetamines.

Parasomnias

NIGHTMARES (DREAM ANXIETY DISORDER)

Nightmares occur when there is a transition from REM sleep to full consciousness with detailed recall of a distressing dream. They are common in children, occurring most frequently between the ages of 5 and 6 years. They may be stimulated by external experiences such as a particular event, or they may occur at times of persistent anxiety.

NIGHT TERRORS

These occur much less frequently than nightmares. Usually they begin and end in childhood, but they may persist into young adulthood. Within a few hours of going to sleep the child will sit up and scream, appearing terrified. After some minutes the child then settles back into a calm sleep. These events occur during non-REM sleep and there is no recall of the event later on. Both benzodiazepines and imipramine have been shown to be effective in relieving these problems, but their prolonged use is not recommended.

SLEEP-WALKING

Sleep-walking occurs during non-REM sleep, usually in the early part of the night. It occurs between the ages of 5 and 12 years and 15 per cent of children will sleep-walk at least once. The automatism does not usually consist of walking, despite the name, but of sitting up in bed and making repetitive movements. The child's eyes are usually open and, if walking, they will avoid familiar objects in the room. Rousing the individual is difficult and they do not respond to questions. The episodes are usually of short duration, lasting for only a few minutes. Whilst walking, the person must be protected from harm, largely by predicting the places of danger and ensuring that there are stair gates, and that doors and windows are closed and any dangerous objects removed.

Benzodiazepines can be effective if the problem is severe.

Further reading

Lipowski, Z.B. 1990: *Delirium: acute confusional state.* Oxford: Oxford University Press.

Lishmann, W.A. 1987: *Organic psychiatry*, 2nd edn. Oxford: Blackwell Scientific Publications.

McKeith, I.G., Galasko, D., Wilcock, G.K. and Byrne, E.J. 1995: Lewy body dementia – diagnosis and treatment. *British Journal of Psychiatry* **167**, 709–17.

Piel, J. (ed.) 1992: Mind and brain. *Scientific American (Special Issue)* 267(3).

Trimble, M. 1989: *Biological psychiatry.* Chichester: John Wiley & Sons.

Schizophrenia has been at the centre of psychiatrists' interests for many years. Although the term was not coined until 1911, by Bleuler, reports of people suffering from symptoms that would suggest schizophrenia were recorded as far back as the second millennium BC. For many years a large number of the long-term occupants of asylums were suffering from this chronic relapsing condition. With the introduction of new models of care, more positive attitudes to the mentally ill and also more effective treatments, the number of people requiring long-term hospital care is far smaller. None the less, care in the community for those with this disabling illness is often fragmented and inadequate.

CASE 7.1

An 18-year-old man was seen at home following a request to his GP by his mother. A shy only child of a now-divorced couple, he left school at the age of 16 years and got a job with the local parks department. After being asked to go for a medical he stopped going to work and spent less and less time out of his bedroom. He kept the curtains drawn all day, cared little about his personal hygiene, and rarely ate. He could be heard at night pacing about and sometimes shouting.

When seen he was dishevelled and huddled in the corner of the room. He was reluctant to speak, but when he did so his voice was very quiet and it was often difficult to follow his story. It emerged that he believed that the people in the opposite house, at the request of the government, were looking at him through a telescope and in ways he could not understand they were able to hear all that he said and to understand all his thoughts. They would talk both to him and about him, saying what a terrible person he was and ordering him to do things he did not want to do. He wondered if they could control his thinking. He did not believe he was ill, nor did he understand why these people should pick on him in this way.

CLINICAL PRESENTATION

Prodromal phase

Schizophrenia can develop in any person of almost any age, but the most common time is during late adolescence or early adult life. The presentation is often insidious and hard to date. The person becomes more withdrawn, doing less, and losing their drive. This is reflected in reduced achievement at school or college, not holding down a job and making fewer contacts with the outside world. It may be only with hindsight that these changes are recognized as leading to a more acute phase of the illness. There may be no prodrome but an acutely stressful event which appears to start the process.

Acute phase

BEHAVIOUR

Behaviour during the acute phase is very varied and depends on the psychopathology of the person affected. Some become mute and withdrawn, and are entirely wrapped up in their abnormal experiences. Others may take action, sometimes violent, against those who they believe are persecuting them. The behaviour may seem very bizarre to onlookers. Some adopt strange postures which are maintained for long periods of time despite extreme discomfort (catatonia). These can alternate with episodes of overactivity which can be very destructive (catatonic excitement). They may be seen responding to their hallucinations, looking around the room for their source or answering back to them. Very often they will have neglected their personal hygiene.

AFFECT

People who are frightened by their experiences can be highly aroused, whereas others are bemused and bewildered as they try to make sense of their experiences. Frequently the affect shown by the person is at odds with the problem that they are describing (incongruent affect), or they do not appear to be experiencing or expressing any deep emotion (flattening or blunting of the affect).

SPEECH

The speech of a person with schizophrenia is assumed to echo their thought patterns. When a person develops thought disorder their speech can be difficult to understand. Stories which should be progressing in a particular direction undergo drifts away from the narrative line. They proceed in tortured loops away from the subject in hand. Abrupt changes in subject matter or sense take place (knight's-move thinking), and strange words (neologisms) are used (e.g. Twas brillig and the slivey toves did gire and gimble in the wabe) (Edward Lear). Words which sound the same are used, although out of meaningful context (clang associations), and speech may dissolve into complete incoherence (word salad). It is always best to record the person's speech verbatim. Thought disorder is difficult to define, and one man's thought disorder is another man's profound or poetic analysis of a situation.

THOUGHT

People with schizophrenia have delusions, i.e. firm, fixed beliefs that are not amenable to reason or evidence to the contrary which are arrived at by some abnormal thought process. These beliefs are incompatible with the affected person's cultural, religious and educational background.

They are frequently persecutory in nature, with a belief that the person is being followed, watched or hounded by people or organizations. The evidence for this frequently comes from the experience of hearing voices telling them that this is so. Once the possibility has been raised by the voice that this is happening, the world provides supporting evidence; people are watching them on the street and talking about them, news stories in papers and on television hold specific meanings just for them (delusions of reference). One man believed that the colour of each car that passed him in the street held a specific message for him, sent by his persecutors.

Occasionally a delusion may arise out of the blue with no precursors (primary delusion), or as a result of a normal perception (e.g. 'I saw the vase and knew I was the Queen's son') (delusional perception).

A number of other problems with thinking are important for diagnosis. The beliefs that your thoughts can be read, spoken out loud (echo de la pensée) or are available to others (thought broadcasting), or that they can be withdrawn (thought withdrawal) or alien thoughts inserted into one's mind (thought insertion) are often distressing.

Passivity phenomena are the beliefs that one's bodily feelings ('I have a burning all over me from the ray gun') (somatic passivity), actions ('the force moves my legs') and moods are not one's own but are imposed by an outside agency.

HALLUCINATIONS

Hallucinations may occur in all five sensory modalities, but auditory hallucinations are the most common. Often there are several voices which discuss the person amongst themselves (third-person auditory hallucinations). They will also directly address the person (second-person, auditory hallucinations), usually in an unpleasant and derogatory way. A running commentary on the person's actions may occur (e.g. 'He's going to read the next sentence now'). Bodily sensations can feel bizarre ('I have snakes in my belly') (somatic hallucinations). Visual hallucinations are less common and suggest an organic cause. Sensations of smell are usually noxious. A man with a history of schizophrenia reported being gassed by his neighbours. A home visit from hospital revealed a gas leak from his fire that required attention from the gas company! Beware of dismissing apparent hallucinations when they are in fact true perceptions being given a delusional interpretation by the person experiencing them.

INSIGHT

People with schizophrenia frequently do not agree that they are unwell ('I know what I tell you is not normal but it is true. I am not ill. The police should sort these people out'). This disparity between the medical perception of the person, society's perception and the person's own view of the situation may lead to conflict, and at times legal steps to ensure the well-being of the person and those in close contact with him or her need to be taken.

CASE 7.2

A 66-year-old woman vacated her room in a hostel 2 days before Christmas. She refused to return, despite subzero temperatures, becoming physically aggressive towards the staff. Her voices had explained that her estranged husband was coming to pick her up shortly, and MI5 had told her to wait. She was admitted under Section 2 of the Mental Health Act 1983.

The development of insight is a crucial factor in the future management of the person (see below). Some people have partial insight. This leads to unusual situations of complaining to a doctor about persecution when a more consistent action would be to go to the police.

DIAGNOSIS

The diagnosis of schizophrenia has in the past been an erratic affair. No pathognomonic signs exist for this heterogeneous syndrome. Diagnosis has been largely based on Kurt Schneider's 'First Rank Symptoms'. The presence of any one of these was said to be diagnostic, but it soon became clear that they occur in other disorders as well.

More recently, attempts have been made to diagnose the illness in a standardized manner, and operational criteria have been defined. One such is the *Diagnostic and Statistical Manual* (4th edition) (DSM-IV) of the American Psychiatric Association.

Schneider's first rank symptoms of schizophrenia

- third person auditory hallucinations
- a running commentary on the person's actions
- voices repeating the person's thoughts aloud
- thought insertion or withdrawal
- thought broadcasting
- delusional perception
- somatic passivity
- outside agencies causing the person's feelings or actions
- primary delusions (sudden delusional ideas coming to the person without preceding events, e.g. hallucinations or changes in mood)

DSM-IV diagnostic criteria for schizophrenia

1. At least two of the following for 1 month
   a. delusions
   b. hallucinations
   c. disorganised speech
   d. grossly disorganized or catatonic behaviour
   e. negative symptoms
2. Social/occupational dysfunction
3. Duration of at least 6 months' disturbance of social/occupational functioning, including 1 month of symptoms from 1
4. Both schizo-affective disorder and psychotic depression have been excluded
5. The disorder is not due to substance abuse or a general medical condition

SUBTYPES OF SCHIZOPHRENIA

Paranoid type

This is the commonest form of schizophrenia (see Case 7.1 above), in which the person is preoccupied with particular delusions or hallucinations but does not show a major disturbance of speech or behaviour (e.g. catatonia).

Disorganized type

Disorganized speech and behaviour and inappropriate affect are all common in this type of schizophrenia.

An 18-year-old woman on an acute psychiatric ward would frequently interrupt meetings, remove her clothes and give long accounts of exotic adventures and tortures she was experiencing. Despite the seriousness of what she described she would frequently laugh and rarely engaged in sustained discussion.

Catatonic type

In this type of schizophrenia there are disturbances of motor activity. The person will maintain bizarre postures despite extreme discomfort, and this immobility can amount to stupor. The examiner is able to shape these postures, the limbs having a characteristic tone (waxy flexibility) when moved. These periods of immobility may alternate with episodes of extreme over-activity, which are often repetitious and purposeless. The person may repeat what the examiner says to them (echolalia) or what the examiner does (echopraxia), or they may do the opposite of what the examiner requests (negativism).

A 30-year-old man was admitted following a frenzy of activity during which he had destroyed the contents of his flat and broken several windows. He described voices and influences coming from the television. In the ward he adopted a stooped posture and would allow his arms to be moved into uncomfortable positions, in which they would remain.

Catatonia is less commonly seen nowadays, and its frequency in the past might have reflected the unstimulating social milieu of the large asylums.

DIFFERENTIAL DIAGNOSIS

A number of major syndromes may mimic schizophrenia.

Brief psychotic reaction

Symptoms develop and subside rapidly in this disorder, usually following a stressful event (see below).

Schizophreniform disorder

This is essentially the same as schizophrenia, but has not been going on for the requisite 6 months (see below).

Depression

The major distinction from schizophrenia is that the individual has a depressed mood and this came prior to the psychotic symptoms, which will have a depressive flavour. Voices experienced by the person are much more likely to be second rather than third person in nature.

Mania

Once again the mood disturbance is primary, and the content of the delusions follows this. First rank symptoms can be seen in 15 to 20 per cent of manics.

Schizoaffective and delusional disorders

See below.

Drug intoxication

Especially amphetamines and LSD but also cocaine.

Medical disorders

See Chapter 6 on organic states for details.

Schizophrenia-like symptoms may be part of many organic conditions, e.g. temporal lobe epilepsy, Huntington's chorea, Wilson's disease and cerebral tumours.

Differential diagnosis of schizophrenia

- brief reactive psychosis
- schizophreniform disorder
- affective disorder (depression or mania)
- schizo-affective disorder
- drug-induced psychosis
- medical disorders

MANAGEMENT OF THE ACUTE PHASE

CASE 7.5

A 26-year-old man, who had recently moved from Scotland to London and was living alone, was admitted to casualty following a self-inflicted knife wound to his abdomen. This was performed on the instruction of the 'Great Spider' who spoke to him through his radio. The instructions continued during a brief stay in the surgical unit and he was transferred to the acute psychiatry ward.

An initial assessment of the person's ability to care for themselves, their danger to themself or others, and the strengths of their support network is needed to determine whether admission to hospital is required, if necessary under a section of the Mental Health Act (1983).

The psychological approach to a person with disturbing or violent behaviour is described earlier (see Chapter 1 on talking and listening to people).

Should these techniques fail to defuse the situation, then drugs can be used. For these to be safely and effectively administered, enough people trained in control and restraint techniques must be present.

If the person will accept oral medication, lorazepam (2–4 mg) is effective.

If this is not accepted, then intramuscular medication should be considered: lorazepam 2–4 mg every 4 hours in combination with droperidol 10 mg or haloperidol 20 mg. If the emergency is extreme, use diazepam 10 mg IV or haloperidol 10 mg IV as an alternative.

Medication

Medication remains the mainstay of acute treatment. The choice of medication is largely determined by the side-effect profile and the preferences of the individual clinician. It is important to involve carers and the person in the plans for management at an early stage to ensure that the fears of relatives can be met and they are provided with appropriate support, and that the person understands why particular steps are being taken.

DRUGS USED IN SCHIZOPHRENIA

The first effective drug to be used for the treatment of schizophrenia was chlorpromazine (Largactil).

Since then, a wide range of similar medications with differing potencies and side-effect profiles has been developed (see Table 7.1). It is best to become familiar with a small range of these that will cover differing situations. The initial choice of medication and dose depends on the severity of the problems, the degree of sedation required, the size of the individual and any other medical complications that are known.

MECHANISM OF ACTION

The action most closely correlated with antipsychotic activity is the ability of the medication to antagonize the Dopamine 2 (D_2) receptor which can be found principally in the limbic system.

Most antipsychotic drugs are relatively non-specific in their site of action, and their actions at other sites may contribute to their antipsychotic activity, although the degree to which this occurs is uncertain. Relatively more specific D_2 receptor antagonists are now available, e.g. sulpiride (Dolmotil). The specificity leads to a more favourable side-effect profile.

SIDE-EFFECTS

- acute dystonic reactions
- akathisia
- parkinsonism
- tardive dyskinesia
- neuroleptic malignant syndrome
- postural hypotension
- cardiac dysrhythmias
- hyperprolactinaemia
- galactorrhoea
- infertility
- weight gain
- photosensitivity
- agranulocytosis
- reduction of the fit threshold
- precipitation of glaucoma
- constipation
- urinary retention
- sedation

The side-effect profile can be predicted from the activity of the drug at receptors other than the D_2 receptor.

Anti-dopaminergic (extra-pyramidal) symptoms

Extra-pyramidal side-effects are mediated through the D_1 receptor.

TABLE 7.1 Relative dosage and side-effect profile of some commonly used antipsychotics

	Maximum dose (mg/day)	Anticholinergic activity	Extra-pyramidal activity	Postural hypotension	Sedation
Sulpiride	2400	***	*		
Thioridazine	600	***	*	**	**
Chlorpromazine	1000	**	**	**	**
Haloperidol	100	*	***	*	*
Fluphenazine two weekly as a depot	100	*	***	*	**

*Relatively mild side-effects.
**Moderate side-effects.
***Marked side-effects.

Acute dystonia

This is commonest in young men. They develop problems such as tongue protrusion, torticollis, grimacing and a painful state in which the body is in full extension (opisthotonos). The problems may largely effect the eyes, which roll upwards. The symptoms can be rapidly relieved by intramuscular or, *in extremis*, intravenous anticholinergic medication such as biperiden or procyclidine.

Akathisia

This is an unpleasant internal sense of being unable to keep still, causing the person to rock restlessly to and fro from one foot to the other.

Parkinsonism

The person is stiff and unmoving with an expressionless face and tremor. They have a shuffling gait and lose their arm swing. The symptoms may be relieved by anticholinergic medication such as procyclidine.

The most effective treatment for the above problems is to reduce the dose of the drug.

Tardive dyskinesia

This is a late-onset syndrome which only develops after medication for a protracted period. Between 20 and 40 per cent of people with schizophrenia treated in this way develop the syndrome. It is difficult to manage, and can continue even after the medication has been stopped. Its features are odd facial movements, usually around the mouth, which can become quite grotesque and lead to problems with eating. Choreoathetoid movements of the limbs and trunk occur. The syndrome is most common among women and the elderly. About 50 per cent of cases resolve on stopping the medication.

Amenorrhoea and galactorrhoea are also dopamine-mediated side-effects.

ANTI-ADRENERGIC EFFECTS

Postural hypotension

Postural hypotension is perhaps the most dangerous of these effects, especially in the elderly, in whom it can lead to falls and serious injury. Nasal congestion and failure of ejaculation may cause problems for some people.

Sedation

Sedation may be a desirable consequence of drug administration. It is mediated through both noradrenaline and antihistamine activity.

Anticholinergic effects

The medications vary widely in this respect. Problems include constipation, blurred vision, precipitating glaucoma or urinary retention and dry mouth.

OTHER EFFECTS

Weight gain is particularly distressing for many people. Cardiac dysrhythmias can be fatal, especially if high doses are used. The seizure threshold is reduced. Chlorpromazine is associated with photosensitivity and, rarely, with cholestatic jaundice and neutropenia. Thioridazine in high doses (above 600 mg a day) can cause retinal pigmentation.

NEUROLEPTIC MALIGNANT SYNDROME

This a rare but potentially fatal complication which needs to be recognized early if effective treatment is to be instituted.

The clinical picture of neuroleptic malignant syndrome

- rapid onset within 10 days of treatment
- muscle stiffness and hypertonia
- stupor and impaired consciousness
- autonomic nervous system dysfunction, causing rapid pulse, labile blood pressure and high temperature and sweating
- muscle creatinine phosphokinase (CPK) activity is raised
- neutrophilia
- death in 15 to 20 per cent of cases
- treatment is symptomatic

AETIOLOGY OF SCHIZOPHRENIA

Possible aetiological factors in schizophrenia

- abnormalities of dopamine metabolism
- season of birth
- *in-utero* viral infection
- birth trauma
- neurodevelopmental disorder
- genetics
- social dysfunction

All traditional antipsychotics have activity at dopamine receptors, and there is a strong correlation between the clinical potency of neuroleptics and their ability to block dopamine receptors *in vitro*. This is not the case for the other receptors at which they have actions.

The dopamine hypothesis of schizophrenia

- traditional neuroleptics act upon the dopamine receptors
- amphetamines induce a schizophrenia-like psychosis
- disulfiram (which inhibits the breakdown of dopamine) worsens schizophrenia
- L-dopa produces psychotic symptoms
- changes in dopamine receptors have been found at post-mortem

AMPHETAMINE-INDUCED PSYCHOSIS

The amphetamine drugs cause the release of excess dopamine and noradrenaline, and they can induce psychoses which are indistinguishable from schizophrenia. Other dopamine agonists such as L-dopa may also produce psychotic illnesses. Inhibiting the breakdown of dopamine with disulfiram worsens schizophrenic symptoms.

DOPAMINE TURNOVER

There is no consistant evidence of increased dopamine turnover in patients with schizophrenia *in vivo*. Post-mortem studies have shown no overall increase in dopamine for the whole brain, but increases in brain dopamine have often been demonstrated in isolated brain regions.

DOPAMINE RECEPTORS

These have been shown to be increased in people with schizophrenia at post-mortem and in some studies *in vivo*. The recent isolation of further subtypes which are blocked by atypical neuroleptics such as clozapine may help to refine this theory in the future.

Environmental theories

SEASON OF BIRTH

People with schizophrenia are more likely to have been born in the early months of the year, suggesting that some environmental influence is at work.

INFLUENZA VIRUS

The suggestion that there is an excess of schizophrenia in the sons and daughters of Afro-

Caribbean migrants led to the idea that these fetuses were exposed *in utero* to influenza viruses to which their mothers had not developed immunity, resulting in neurodevelopmental abnormality.

BIRTH TRAUMA

There have been suggestions of excess birth trauma among those who develop schizophrenia, but the evidence is scanty.

GENETICS

Sixty per cent of people with schizophrenia have no family history of the illness. If one parent has schizophrenia there is a 15 per cent chance of their offspring developing the illness. If both parents suffer from the disease, then 46 per cent of their children suffer from the illness. The fertility of people with schizophrenia tends to be low. Monozygotic twins have a concordance rate of 42 per cent for schizophrenia, whilst dizygotic twins have a concordance rate of 10 per cent.

Adoption studies

It has been found that adopted-away offspring of schizophrenics develop the disorder at the same rate as those who stay with their parents, and at a much higher rate than adopted-away controls.

Social theories

FAMILY

Whilst the family dynamic may well play a role in the prognosis of schizophrenia (see below), older ideas of the 'schizophrenigenic mother' or other abnormalities in communication within the family have been discredited.

SOCIAL CLASS

Early studies showed that schizophrenia was more prevalent in lower social classes. By looking at the occupations of their parents, it becomes clear that their social class distribution is normal, but that they tend to drift downwards as a result of their illness and towards inner city areas with high levels of deprivation (social drift hypothesis).

Brain changes

There are abnormalities in the ventricular system of all schizophrenics to a greater or lesser extent. Their brains tend to be smaller than those of controls, suggesting arrested development. These changes are more marked on the left side of the brain. These changes have been explained by an abnormality in a 'cerebral dominance gene'.

Epidemiology

There are few cases of schizophrenia in childhood, but the numbers increase rapidly after puberty. The mean age of onset is 25 years for males and 28 years for females. The earlier the onset the worse the prognosis.

The incidence is 15–20 per 100 000 per year, and the prevalence is 0.5 to 1 per cent. Some parts of the world, e.g. Eire and Sweden, have higher prevalence rates.

Table 7.2 The genetics of schizophrenia

Relation to schizophrenic	Likelihood of developing schizophrenia (%)
One parent	15
Both parents	46
Monozygotic twin	42
Dizygotic twin	10
One sibling	10

PROGNOSIS IN SCHIZOPHRENIA

Good prognostic signs

- acute onset
- a stressful event leading to the onset of symptoms
- no family history of schizophrenia
- a family history of depression
- a normal pre-morbid personality (good social and occupation adjustment)
- marked affective disturbance
- confusion

Poor prognostic indicators

- early onset
- insidious onset
- marked negative symptoms
- enlarged ventricles on CT/MRI scanning
- low IQ
- poor insight
- high expressed emotion family
- long episode

Prior to the introduction of effective treatments, about 20 per cent of people with schizophrenia recovered from their acute illnesses, but the majority became permanent residents in hospital.

With modern treatments, over a period of 5 years about 10 per cent of people will remain so ill as to need intensive nursing and medical intervention. About 20 per cent will recover for good, and about two thirds will follow a path between relatively good health and acute relapses.

Early indicators of relapse in schizophrenia

- insomnia
- feeling anxious, fear of being alone
- lack of interest, and depression
- inability to make decisions
- feeling distant from the world
- increasing preoccupation with a few thoughts

Relapse prevention

MEDICATION

Without medication the rate of relapse over 1 year is about 80 per cent. If the person is compliant with medication the rate is reduced to 33 per cent. Over a longer period, 65 per cent of people taking medication will relapse. Using drugs with fewer side-effects (e.g. sulpiride) may improve compliance. For those who show poor compliance, long-acting depot medication is available (e.g. flupenazine decanoate). This requires the person to receive regular injections (generally at intervals of 2 to 4 weeks). The side-effects of the medication are the same as those when it is given orally.

A number of processes will modify the impact of medication.

CULTURAL BACKGROUND

Schizophrenia in Third World countries and more rural communities shows a better outcome than that in industrial societies.

LIFE EVENTS

Any life event, be it good or bad, puts the person with schizophrenia at risk of relapse. This is in contrast to the depressed person, for whom loss or negative events are more likely to precipitate a relapse.

THE FAMILY

People with schizophrenia who had more than 35 hours of face-to-face contact with their families were found to relapse more rapidly than those who had less contact. If the family was characterized by high levels of Expressed Emotion (EE), a negative, critical and hostile approach to the person, and they were not taking medication, the rate of relapse within a year reached nearly 100 per cent. Medication provided some protection against the high EE, but for those who took their medication and did not see so much of their family the rate fell to 15 per cent. Many studies have shown the value of family work in reducing EE and relapse rate in schizophrenia, but these interventions are not yet available in all local services.

SOCIAL ENVIRONMENT

The asylums of old were associated with degrading and unstimulating environments. These contributed to the poor long-term outcome for many people. Whilst people with schizophrenia need stability in their lives, isolation from social stimulation leads to greater relapse rates and a much poorer quality of life.

Improving the person's supportive network has been shown to be of benefit.

Work training in modern relevant skills (e.g. computer literacy) can also go a long way towards improving self-esteem and gaining a foothold in the employment market.

PSYCHOLOGICAL TREATMENTS

A wide range of treatments have been tried with this group. The development of social skills for those who feel uncomfortable with others has been used over many years. More recently, activities such as cognitive behavioural models, designed both to reduce symptoms and to cope better with day-to-day life, have been used. Whether these techniques can be extended to a wide range of sufferers is not yet clear.

Summary of measures for relapse prevention in schizophrenia

- increase compliance with medication
- family management
- social interventions
- individual psychological treatments
- close monitoring

CHRONIC SCHIZOPHRENIA

CASE 7.6

A 68-year-old man was visited at home at the request of his community psychiatric nurse. He had been diagnosed as suffering from schizophrenia 40 years previously. He was unshaven, and his clothes had not been changed for 4 months. The flat was filthy; he slept on a sofa with a torn blanket. A home help brought him food and he only occasionally went out to buy tobacco. He was indifferent to our presence and gave only monosyllabic answers to questions. Regular injections of fluphenazine (Modecate) kept his hallucinations under reasonable control.

Schizophrenia is a chronic relapsing illness, with episodes of acute disturbance punctuating its course. Large numbers of people with schizophrenia develop so-called 'Negative Symptoms', including apathy or loss of volition, flattening of affect and poverty of speech. This has been called Type II schizophrenia, in contrast to the florid symptoms of delusions and hallucinations of Type I (Table 7.3). Type II is associated with a poor prognosis, increased ventricular brain ratio, 'soft' neurological signs and cognitive impairment, such as disorientation with regard to time. These have been shown to correlate with abnormalities of the dorsolateral prefrontal cortex on positron emission tomography (PET) scans. Negative symptoms respond poorly to traditional neuroleptics, but may respond to novel antipsychotic medication.

TABLE 7.3 Type I and Type II schizophrenia

Type I	Type II
Delusions	Lack of volition
Hallucinations	Poverty of speech
Thought disorder	Poverty of affect
Good response to neuroleptics	Neurological signs
	Cognitive impairment
	Changes on brain CT scan
	Poor response to neuroleptics
	Dorsolateral prefrontal cortex abnormality

TREATMENT-RESISTANT SCHIZOPHRENIA

CASE 7.7

A 32-year-old man had been resident on the ward for 3 years. He had been diagnosed as suffering from schizophrenia 6 years previously. He was continually subjected to voices in the third person of a derogatory nature. He believed he was a psychiatrist and therefore in the right place. He spent much of his time in his room writing equations to prove the existence of God. Without regular prompting he would neglect his personal hygiene and eating. At times, when highly aroused as a result of the voices, he could become aggressive.

About 10 per cent of people with schizophrenia have severe intractable disorders which mean that they need continuing hospital care because their symptoms are so disabling. Many more continue to experience hallucinations and delusions, but these are sufficiently well controlled for them to be able to live in the community.

For those who do not respond to conventional neuroleptics, a number of strategies are available. Initially the diagnosis should be reviewed and any organic cause excluded. A second neuroleptic may be used at a therapeutic dosage for a minimum of 6 weeks. High-dose neuroleptics have been used. The dose is pushed up to the person's maximum tolerated dose, but this does have a number of dangers, including sudden death due to cardiac dysrhythmias or hypotension, severe extra-pyramidal side-effects and a paradoxical worsening of behaviour. This strategy has little basis in terms of receptor theory.

Atypical neuroleptics

The commonly used neuroleptics with activity at the D_2 receptor have been described above. For those who do not respond to these, a number of antipsychotic drugs which act in a differing fashion are available.

Clozapine

Clozapine is not a new drug, but was withdrawn from use following the deaths of a number of people from neutropenia. It has been reintroduced in recent years. Between 30 and 50 per cent of people who have not responded to traditional neuroleptics respond to clozapine. It has a good side-effect profile, with no anti-cholinergic and few extra-pyramidal problems. However, it can cause excess salivation, sedation, hypotension and seizures. Two per cent of people develop agranulocytosis which is potentially fatal, and 80 per cent of these cases occur within 18 weeks of starting treatment. Every recipient must have weekly blood tests for the first 18 weeks, and every 2 weeks thereafter. This practical consideration may limit the use of the drug, since many people refuse to have weekly venepuncture. The drug has a weak affinity for D_2 receptors, with greater activity at noradrenergic and serotonergic sites (5HT). The mechanism of action is unclear, but perhaps lies in the balance of its effects at these various receptors.

Risperidone

This drug is a potent central serotonin antagonist (5HT), and also has some activity at the D_2 receptors. It may relieve negative as well as positive symptoms. It does not have the major haematological side-effects of clozapine, but is probably less effective in treatment-resistant schizophrenia than clozapine.

Electroconvulsive therapy (ECT)

This is rarely used for treatment of schizophrenia. However, it may be useful in refractory cases and for those in a catatonic stupor. Interest in this treatment is being revived in the USA.

Alternative therapeutic manoeuvres

A wide range of options have been described as useful in this category, but few have received thorough investigation. Methyl folate can enhance the effect of neuroleptics, and a wide range of mood stabilizers have been tested. These perhaps only treat a concurrent mood disturbance and do little to treat the core symptoms.

Summary of strategies for treatment-resistant schizophrenia

- review diagnosis and exclude an underlying organic cause
- try treatment with a second neuroleptic of a different family at a therapeutic dose for at least six weeks
- use an atypical neuroleptic, e.g. clozapine or risperidone
- ECT
- psychological strategies, e.g. cognitive behavioural therapy
- lithium, carbamazepine, benzodiazepines (in high doses) and beta blockers (also in high doses) have all been used

---

COMMUNITY CARE AND SCHIZOPHRENIA

Care in the community for the chronically mentally ill

Formerly, many people with schizophrenia spent most of their lives in institutions. Since the late 1950s the number of psychiatric beds has

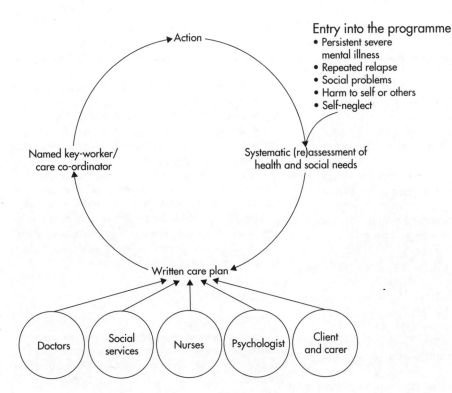

Entry into the programme
- Persistent severe mental illness
- Repeated relapse
- Social problems
- Harm to self or others
- Self-neglect

Action

Named key-worker/ care co-ordinator

Systematic (re)assessment of health and social needs

Written care plan

Doctors   Social services   Nurses   Psychologist   Client and carer

FIG 7.1 The care programme approach.

dropped dramatically, and a number of forces have contributed to this. It was suggested that many of the negative symptoms seen in schizophrenia were a result of the asylum itself; effective biological treatments were meant to eliminate the need for long-term care, and there has been a politically driven move to close large expensive asylums and opt for a community-orientated approach. Unfortunately, policy-makers failed to take into account the fact that care in the community is actually more expensive than residence in a mental hospital. The closure of mental hospitals has been fostered by successive governments, but problems continue to exist as the medical and social needs of the people are looked after by two different agencies (the National Health Service and the Department of Social Security) in the UK. Increasingly, bodies are working together to produce a 'seamless service' for those with chronic mental disorders, but much greater co-operation and provision of resources such as day care, hostels and sheltered housing are required.

The care programme approach (Figure 7.1)

The Care Programme Approach is the cornerstone of the Department of Health's policy for care of the severely mentally ill in the community, and is based on the principle that effective inter-agency work is essential to ensure that vulnerable people do not slip through the net of care. The majority of people involved in the care programme approach suffer from schizophrenia, but other groups, such as those with brittle manic depression, will also be represented.

Section 117 of the Mental Health Act 1983 requires health and social services in conjunction with voluntary agencies to provide after-care for certain categories of detained people, i.e. those detained under Section 3 and those detained under 'forensic sections' (mentally disordered offenders). In practice, the principles of the care programme approach and Section 117 after-care are the same.

The aim of this after-care is to minimize the likelihood of relapse after discharge, and to support mentally ill people in the community by reducing the risk of people losing contact with services and maximizing the effect of any intervention. The essential elements of the programme include:

- systematic assessment of both health and social care needs;
- preparing a written care plan agreed between professional staff, the person themself and carers;
- allocation of a key worker who is required to keep in close contact with the person, to monitor whether the programme of care is being delivered, and to take immediate action if it is not;
- regular review of the person's progress.

The criteria for inclusion in the care programme approach register are: a diagnosis of persistent and severe mental illness and any of the following:

- history of repeated relapse of mental illness due to a breakdown of the provision of medical or social care in the community
- individuals with severe social disability or major housing difficulties as a consequence of their illness
- individuals who require multi-agency involvement and care co-ordination
- a history of severe suicidal risk or self-harm, severe self-neglect or violence and thus danger to others as a consequence of their illness

In 1994, the Department of Health introduced Supervision Registers for mentally ill people. The criteria for inclusion are similar to those for the care programme approach register, but there is an emphasis on the risk of:

- committing serious violence;
- suicide;
- severe self-neglect.

In 1996 the process was taken a stage further with the introduction of Supervised Discharge Orders which enable the person to be returned to hospital in the event of a breakdown of community care.

PSYCHOTIC CONDITIONS RELATED TO SCHIZOPHRENIA

Schizoaffective disorder

As the name suggests, a diagnosis of schizoaffective disorder is made when there is a period of illness

during which there are concurrent symptoms of both schizophrenia and a major mood disorder (either mania or depression). This is to be distinguished from the many people with schizophrenia who become depressed. The mood disturbance must have been present for a significant portion of the person's illness. Poor work record and inadequate social functioning can occur, just as they do in schizophrenia. There is an increased risk of suicide, but the negative symptoms are not usually so severe as in schizophrenia. The long-term prognosis lies between that of schizophrenia and the affective disorders. Schizo-mania is more common in young adults, whilst schizo-depression is more common in the older age group. There is a greater risk of schizophrenia in first-degree relatives and of affective disorder in a larger circle of relatives.

TREATMENT

In addition to psychological and social approaches, drug treatment is used involving both an antipsychotic and an antidepressant or antimanic agent, depending upon the presentation. Many patients respond well to lithium (often supplemented by a neuroleptic).

Diagnosis of schizoaffective disorder DSM-IV

- there is a continuous period of illness during which the person has both schizophrenia and an affective disorder
- during this period delusions and hallucinations have been present without prominent mood disturbance
- the mood disturbance is present for a substantial part of the illness
- there is no organic cause of the illness

Features of schizoaffective disorder

- both schizophrenic and mood disturbance are present
- fewer people go on to have residual symptoms
- the outcome is intermediate between that of schizophrenia and affective disorder
- younger people have schizo-mania, older people have schizo-depression
- there is an excess of schizophrenia and affective disorder in their relatives
- treatment is with both an antidepressant and an antipsychotic

Delusional disorder

In this disorder the person has one or more delusions, but does not have any other symptoms that would lead to a diagnosis of schizophrenia. If hallucinations are present they are very closely related to the delusions and are often not very prominent. Some people cope very well with this disorder and never come into contact with services, whilst others may be severely disabled. This depends very much on the content of the disorder. Care must be taken to ensure that the idea being presented is indeed delusional and not explainable in terms of the culture of the person.

Delusional disorder often has its onset in middle or late life, and the course is difficult to predict, lack of insight of the person being a barrier to effective treatment.

SUBTYPES OF DELUSIONAL DISORDER

Somatic (monosymptomatic hypochondriacal delusions)

The person believes that there is a grave problem with his or her bodily form or function.

CASE 7.8

A 28-year-old man was referred to the clinic by the dermatologists to whom he had presented with concerns about possible infestation of his groin and upper thigh. Examination was normal, although he described burning sensations such that he had to remove his clothing and bathe the area. He believed this was due to a 'bug' he had contracted when on holiday. He responded well to treatment with pimozide.

Frequently the person with this disorder believes that they emit an unpleasant smell from their bodies and they adopt extreme measures to eliminate it. Delusions that their body is misshapen have led people to seek surgery for remedy of the problem, only to become distressed at the results, or to switch their attention to another part of the body.

Erotomania (de Clerambault's syndrome)

The sufferer believes that some person, often someone they have never met, is in love with them. The evidence for this may be very bizarre ('I knew he was on the aeroplane and he signalled to me by moving the wings'). Usually the object of desire occupies a higher status than the pursuer. If the pursuit becomes obsessive it can become a serious disruption to both the person's life and that of their putative lover. The disorder might bring the person into contact with the police.

Grandiose type

The affected person tells you that they have been involved with important work or that they have great talent, often not fully recognized by the public at large ('I was at the Prime Minister's right hand through all that legislation').

Jealous type (Othello syndrome)

The sufferer believes that their partner is being unfaithful to them. They come to this conclusion not on the basis of any firm evidence, but from trivial observations which they believe justify their belief (e.g. 'The rug in the back of the car has been moved', 'the neighbour's curtains were drawn in the afternoon'). This delusion has been associated with alcohol abuse and impotence (see Chapter 20 on addiction). This belief can lead to great stress in a relationship, and often causes it to break down. The partner might eventually seek solace in the arms of another, but the evidence the sufferer uses to develop the belief means that it is still delusional, despite the truth of the conclusion. As in Shakespeare's play, there is a risk of violence by the jealous spouse.

Persecutory type

The sufferer believes that they have had some injustice dealt out to them and are being conspired against in a systematic way by some person or organization. This may lead to legal action or direct and sometimes violent action against those who are believed to be the cause of the person's distress.

Shared delusional disorder (*folie à deux*)

This is a rare syndrome in which one partner begins to share the delusional beliefs of the other, who is usually the dominant partner in the relationship. Frequently one partner has schizophrenia. The situation may become chronic, in which case separation of the couple is the only effective treatment.

Brief psychotic disorder (brief reactive psychosis)

In this disorder the onset is very rapid. Florid delusions, hallucinations and disorders of speech and behaviour emerge quickly, often overnight. These frequently occur following some intense stressor such as bereavement or involvement in a disaster or war. The rapidly changing affect of these people can mean that they indulge in seriously injurious behaviour. Brief psychotic disorder usually occurs in young adults, but is relatively rare. Abnormal personality may contribute to its onset at times of stress. It needs to be differentiated from reactions to stress that might be regarded as acceptable in certain cultures (see Chapter 12 on anthropology and psychiatry).

Further reading

Andreasen, N. and Carpenter, W.T.Jr 1993: Diagnosis and classification in schizophrenia. *Schizophrenia Bulletin* **19**, 199–214.

Department of Health 1996: *Building bridges: a guide to arrangements for inter-agency working for the care and protection of severely mentally ill people*. Wetherby: Department of Health.

Kavanagh, D.J. 1992: *Schizophrenia: an overview and practical handbook*. London: Chapman and Hall.

McKenna, P.J. 1994: *Schizophrenia and related syndromes*. Oxford: Oxford University Press.

MOOD DISORDERS

Mood (affective) disorders are common disorders which have a major impact upon both the individual and society. They have been divided into two major groups:

- Unipolar depressive disorders, in which the person only ever has depressive episodes;
- Bipolar affective disorders, in which the person has periods of elevated mood (mania), and also (although not invariably) experiences episodes of depression.

These two disorders will be considered in turn.

UNIPOLAR DEPRESSIVE DISORDERS

CASE 8.1

A 42-year-old woman was admitted to the ward. During the previous 3 months she had stopped her job at a local school and taken to staying in the house. She did less and less, until she eventually stopped dressing each morning. She would sit all day on the sofa smoking, and she no longer derived pleasure from the visits of her children or the company of her friends. She reported feeling tired, unable to concentrate and she felt that life was just too much bother. She considered suicide, but was too apathetic to take any practical steps towards this end. She slept poorly, managing to get only a few hours of sleep at night. In the early hours of the morning she would lie awake, preoccupied with sad ideas. She ate little, lost weight and became constipated. Only at the insistence of her husband did she agree to come into the ward, believing that nothing could be done to help her and that she was undeserving of our attention.

Clinical presentation

Whilst depression may arise after difficult events that represent a loss (e.g. bereavement, job loss, etc.), it can just as often develop 'out of the blue' with no clear precipitant. 'I've nothing to be depressed about' is frequently heard, and whilst this may represent a failure to grasp the nettle of the difficulties of life, it can be true.

Behaviour

RETARDATION

The people you see with depression are likely to complain of a lack of energy and an inability to undertake all the activities that they used to do. They stop visiting friends, going to the pub or cinema, and tend to spend more and more time in their homes shunning company. Everyday tasks become more of a chore and are neglected. Their personal hygiene suffers, and in severe cases they may take to their beds, not getting up even to urinate or defecate. They turn away from the world and do not communicate.

When you see a depressed person, they will often make poor eye contact and have a furrowed brow. Their movements will be reduced and their actions slow. The very depressed person may no longer even be able to cry, or can only produce 'dry' tears. The person may stop eating and drinking, which represents an emergency, particularly in the elderly who are less able to tolerate such privations.

AGITATION

A second group become agitated and indulge in pointless repetitive activity, frequently seeking reassurance from their carers. These people follow their spouses or the nursing staff around, accost you on visits to the ward and are not easily reassured by brief interactions. They may wring their hands or repeatedly wash in an attempt to get rid of imaginary smells.

UNUSUAL BEHAVIOURS

A third group indulges in very bizarre behaviours which do not at first sight appear to be related to a depressive disorder. This only becomes clearer on more detailed assessment.

CASE 8.2

A 54-year old-man presented to the community team with a history of walking backwards, alternating with episodes of an inability to walk, shortly after his second marriage only a year after the death of his first wife. He later admitted to feelings of hopelessness and worthlessness. Following a course of ECT he recovered completely.

Mood

The person's mood is persistently low, and this is displayed in a number of ways. They may spontaneously report this to you, but it is important to obtain a clear idea of what a person means when they say that they are depressed. Depression has passed into lay usage and can cover almost any negative mood state ranging from feeling 'fed up' to profound misery. People will report a loss of pleasure in all activities (anhedonia). The other major diagnostic clues are the content of the patient's thoughts (see below) and the non-verbal features mentioned above.

Speech

People with depressive disorders tend to speak slowly, often with long pauses between your statements and their response. Typically, the response comes just as you have begun your next sentence. Their speech may be very quiet and monotonous, making interviewing in any but the quietest setting difficult.

Thought

People with depressive disorders think slowly, and this is reflected in both the effort they need to put into thinking about things and the speed with which they respond to conversation.

The content of the thought is pessimistic, e.g. 'I am a bad person', 'I am a failure', 'It's my fault I am like this', 'There's nothing anyone can do to help me', 'I have no future', 'There is nothing to live for'.

If you suspect that the person you are assessing is depressed, then you must search for any ideas they have of committing suicide (see Chapter 14 on suicide and deliberate self-harm). Frequently, people dwell on their physical functioning, reporting headaches, aches in the joints or abnormalities of bowel function, all of which are analysed in minute detail. Any chronic pain (e.g. musculo-skeletal pain) becomes more difficult to tolerate when you are depressed. Some people dwell on a small problem or misdemeanour, blowing it up out of all proportion (rumination).

CASE 8.3

A 58-year-old bricklayer became convinced that, because 30 years ago he did a job for cash which he did not declare to the taxman, he was about to go to prison and his family would be thrown out on the street.

These worries may become delusional in intensity, as in the above case. Delusions in depression arise out of the mood state and are said to be mood congruent. Case 8.3 is a typical example of the type of themes people develop. They may have terrible diseases, e.g. cancer or HIV infection (hypochondriacal delusions), or they may believe that they have infected others with some deadly virus, or that they have no money or no clothes. Beliefs in blockage of the throat or bowels contribute to poor food and fluid intake. At the furthest extreme, patients report themselves to be rotting or even dead (Cotard's syndrome).

CASE 8.4

An 84-year-old woman thanked me for coming to see her on a medical ward where she had been investigated for weight loss. She assured me that there was no point in talking, because she was dead and should be buried. She felt that her bed should be used for someone who really needed it. She had stopped eating and drinking, and was treated with ECT, subsequently making a full recovery.

Hallucinations

Hallucinations may occur in all five sensory modalities. Auditory hallucinations are the most common type. Usually the voices talk to the person (second person), telling them what a dreadful person they are or hurling abuse and expletives at them.

Sensations of foul smells which the person believes emanate from them can lead to delusional ideas (see above).

Insight

People frequently recognize that they are unwell. However, those who have mainly physical symptoms may be unaware of the relationship between their mood and their physical symptoms ('If I didn't have the headache, doctor, I wouldn't be depressed') (see Chapter 13 on somatoform disorders). Others, believing in their own wickedness or the impossibility of getting any better, may refuse treatment. For some, the prospect of facing up to and dealing with the issues that underlie their depression make it difficult to engage in therapy of any kind.

Cognitive symptoms

Many depressed people complain of poor memory. This is related to their inability to concentrate, so no new memories are registered. Other complex thought patterns are slowed.

Biological symptoms

The people you see who suffer from depression of a moderate or severe type will complain about a number of problems, which have been designated as 'biological'. It is important to ask about these, as people with biological symptoms are more

likely to respond to physical treatments than those without these symptoms.

The biological symptoms of depression

- early morning wakening
- diurnal variation (worse in the morning)
- poor appetite, and weight loss
- constipation
- loss of libido and sexual interest
- lack of energy

DIAGNOSIS OF DEPRESSION

The term 'depression' can be used in a wide variety of ways, and it is important to note that in the clinical context a depressive disorder or illness represents something more than the unhappiness of everyday human existence or transient dejection caused by a minor setback, frustration or disappointment.

The DSM-IV criteria for a major depressive episode state that there should be five or more of the following:

- depressed mood for most of the day nearly every day
- diminished interest and pleasure
- weight loss of at least 5 per cent
- insomnia almost every night
- agitation or retardation
- fatigue or loss of energy
- feelings of worthlessness or guilt
- inability to concentrate or think
- recurrent thoughts of suicide

The symptoms are severe enough to cause distress or occupational and social impairment.

Subtypes of depression

MILD DEPRESSIVE DISORDER (NEUROTIC DEPRESSION)

CASE 8.5

A 28-year-old woman presented to her GP. Over a 6-month period she had felt increasingly irritable and unable to concentrate at work. A number of changes in the practices at her office placed her in a position of responsibility that she did not feel ready for. This, she claimed, made her miserable and she would frequently just sit staring into space 'worrying about nothing' at work or when on her own at home. If friends came round or invited her out she was able to forget her problems and join in the fun.

In this disorder the severity of the changes in mood and the depressive cognitions are mild, and they are often accompanied by elements of other disorders such as anxiety or phobias (hence the old term 'neurotic depression'). Physical symptoms often occur, but the full picture of classic 'biological' symptoms is lacking. There is usually an issue (work, relationships, etc.) which the person needs some help in coming to terms with or to remedy in order to relieve the symptoms.

MODERATE DEPRESSION

People who fall into this category usually have a greater number of symptoms than those with mild depressive disorder, and the symptoms interfere with their social and occupational functioning to a much greater degree. Biological symptoms are present but not severe.

SEVERE DEPRESSION (MAJOR DEPRESSION, ENDOGENOUS DEPRESSION, MELANCHOLIA)

Case 8.1 is an example of a person afflicted with severe depression. In addition to having many depressive ideas, the person will also have the classic 'biological' symptoms of the illness. The presence of these symptoms has been used in the past to define a category of depression known as Melancholia. Depression of this severity causes a profound disruption of work and social life. Suicidal thoughts are common. Treatment should almost certainly include some form of physical treatment.

PSYCHOTIC DEPRESSION

Cases 8.3 and 8.4 represent cases of severe depression. These people will have biological symptoms, but these can be obscured as the person fails to sleep at all and finds that their depression does not vary during the day. The delusions are secondary to the change in mood (mood congruent) and reflect the pessimistic view of the world and

themselves which the person experiences ('I've no money', 'I've no clothes', 'I've infected my family with AIDS', etc). The hallucinations experienced are commonly of voices talking to the person. These voices usually berate the sufferer and may encourage them to commit suicide ('You whore!', 'You're no good', 'We know what you did to those children').

They may stop eating and drinking, especially if they believe that they are being poisoned, or that their body is damaged in some way. In depressive stupor the person becomes completely uncommunicative, does not move, and urgent treatment is required to preserve life.

Differential diagnosis

The following major syndromes may mimic depression.

REACTIONS TO PARTICULAR STRESSES (ADJUSTMENT REACTION)

In response to acute stressors (e.g. the breakup of a relationship) a person may feel extremely distressed and be unable to see a way forward to cope with the changed circumstances. They may well report being depressed and miserable. Such people need to be helped to see the possibility of coping with change using both the resources they have within themselves and the social network around them.

BIPOLAR AFFECTIVE DISORDER

A history of manic episodes indicates that the patient has a bipolar affective disorder (see below) rather than a unipolar disorder.

SCHIZOPHRENIA

People who experience schizophrenia often become depressed. This can be a reaction to the realization of the problems of the illness, or may be part of the illness itself. Ten per cent of those with schizophrenia commit suicide, and a careful eye for depression must be kept for these changes. The mental state examination will provide an important clue to the development of this complication.

SCHIZO-AFFECTIVE DISORDERS

See above discussion of schizophrenia.

DRUG-INDUCED DEPRESSION

A number of drugs used to treat medical conditions have been associated with depression. Finding alternative treatments can relieve depressive symptoms, although the depression may still require treatment in its own right.

Drugs associated with depression

- reserpine
- beta blockers
- calcium antagonists
- oral contraceptives
- corticosteroids

MEDICAL CAUSES OF DEPRESSION

Many medical illnesses are associated with depressed mood. A distinction needs to be made between those illnesses that have depression as part of their presentation, and people with a physical illness who become depressed because of the impact of the illness on their life (including chronic pain and disability, or the prospect of a shortened lifespan).

Physical illnesses associated with depression

- stroke
- carcinoma (especially of the pancreas and lung)
- diabetes
- thyroid dysfunction
- Addison's disease
- Cushing's disease
- systemic lupus erythematosus
- Parkinson's disease
- multiple sclerosis

See also Chapter 6 on organic states and Chapter 13 on liaison psychiatry and somatoform disorders.

The diagnosis of depression in people with physical illnesses can be difficult. The biological features are obscured (e.g. waking early because your painkillers only last for 6 hours, loss of weight due to a carcinoma). Depression under these circumstances is all too easy to understand ('I'd feel like that too if I had those problems'). A careful assessment of the persons thinking is needed in order to search for depressive ideas (see section below on diagnosing depression in physical illness).

CASE 8.6

A 63-year-old man was admitted with worsening of his chronic chest problems. He also suffered from disabling arthritis and diabetes. His passion in life had been his two budgerigars, and it took some persuading for him to come into hospital as he feared for their welfare. His progress was slow, and initially when visited by the social worker he would ask after the well-being of his birds. As time went by he became less communicative and said that he felt he had no future and wanted to die. He stopped enquiring after his birds. The physicians felt that his attitude was understandable given his physical condition, but were persuaded by the social worker to seek a psychiatric opinion. Treatment with an antidepressant soon restored his spirits. He took an interest in his birds once more, and agitated to get home to resume his care of them.

Diagnosing depression in physical illness

- beware of empathy!!
- biological symptoms are unreliable
- look for depressive cognitions (statements such as 'I deserve to be ill', 'I don't deserve to be treated'), loss of interest in other people (or pets)
- suicidal ideas
- crying
- indecision
- past history of depression

MANAGEMENT OF THE ACUTE PHASE

CASE 8.7

A 43-year-old man was seen at home by his catchment area consultant. He expressed the feeling that he was a terrible person and deserved to die. He felt responsible for the famine currently in the news, because of his associations with the devil. He described voices which urged him to throw himself under a train. He was eating and drinking poorly. He refused to come into hospital or to accept treatment, and had to be admitted for treatment under the Mental Health Act.

Acute management

The acute management of any person who presents to you as depressed depends upon the assessment of their suicide risk (see Chapter 14 on suicide and deliberate self-harm). This must be a familiar routine task for all doctors. If the person is felt to be at risk of self-harm, then you must ensure that they are admitted to hospital where they can be nursed in a safe environment with appropriate levels of nursing care. For some this may mean having a nurse with them for 24 hours a day. Those whose physical condition is deteriorating because they are not eating or drinking should also be managed in hospital. For people with less acute illnesses a setting for treatment must be sought to deliver the care that they need. This will depend upon the type of depression involved, on local resources (e.g. a day hospital providing psychological treatments and monitoring of medication and mental state), the social network of the person and their own preferences for treatment.

Medication

Medication is important in the treatment of the more severe forms of depression and those with biological symptoms. It may also have a role in the treatment of less severe forms of the illness, especially if the person finds it difficult to work in a psychological way.

Classes of antidepressant medication

- *tricyclic antidepressants*, e.g. amitriptyline, imipramine, dothiepin, lofepramine
- *selective serotonin reuptake inhibitors*, e.g. fluoxetine (Prozac), paroxetine (Seroxat), fluvoxamine (Faverin)
- *monoamine oxidase inhibitors*, e.g. moclobemide (Manerix), phenelzine
- *miscellaneous*, e.g. mianserin, trazodone

The choice of medication is largely determined by the side-effect profile and the preferences of the individual clinician. It is important to involve carers and the person with depression in the plans for management at an early stage to ensure that the concerns of relatives are met and the depressed person understands why particular steps are being taken.

DRUGS USED IN DEPRESSION

Tricyclic antidepressants

These drugs, named after their three-ring structure (hence the name), were the first antidepressants to be introduced, 40 years ago, and they remain the most effective.

Mechanism of action

The tricyclic antidepressants inhibit the reuptake of noradrenaline and serotonin (5HT) back into the cell from which they have been released. This increases the amount of neurotransmitter in the synaptic cleft and the length of time for which it is effective. These effects lead to changes in the postsynaptic receptors which closely correlate with the time taken for the antidepressant effect of the drugs to be manifested clinically, i.e. over a period of 7 to 10 days or so. In some cases the response may be delayed by up to 6 weeks. People should be warned that the drugs take some time to work and encouraged to persist with the medication for a reasonable length of time (i.e. about 6 weeks). The drugs must be given at therapeutic doses (e.g. 150 mg dothiepin or amitriptyline) if they are to be effective.

Problems encountered with tricyclic antidepressants

- anticholinergic side-effects, e.g. dry mouth, blurred vision, constipation, ileus, precipitation of glaucoma, retention of urine, delirium
- noradrenergic side-effects, e.g. postural hypotension, sedation
- cardiac dysrhythmias
- lowering of the fit threshold
- inappropriate antidiuretic hormone (ADH)
- anorgasmia
- toxicity (especially cardiac) in overdosage
- abnormalities of liver function
- weight gain

The drugs are metabolized by the liver and largely excreted in the urine. In the case of some tricyclics, e.g. imipramine, the metabolite may have antidepressant activity in its own right.

The choice of antidepressant depends largely on its side-effect profile. Those which have more effect on the serotonergic system (e.g. imipramine) are less sedative than those which have more effect on the noradrenergic system (e.g. dothiepin). The latter may be better for people with agitated depression.

The most commonly experienced side-effects are those due to the anticholinergic actions of the drug. The problems include constipation and even ileus, blurred vision (due to problems with accommodation), precipitating glaucoma or urinary retention and dry mouth. Postural hypotension is perhaps the most dangerous of the adrenergically mediated side-effects, especially in the elderly, in whom it can lead to falls and serious injury. Nasal congestion and failure of ejaculation may cause problems for some people. Sedation, which may be a desirable consequence of drug administration, is mediated through both noradrenaline and antihistamine activity.

The risk of cardiac dysrhythmias means that great caution needs to be exercised when treating those with cardiac problems. Newer tricyclics (e.g. lofepramine) are safer in this respect but not completely without risk.

The toxicity of this medication in overdose needs to be born in mind, as suicide attempts with tricyclics (especially when combined with alcohol) can easily be fatal. Careful monitoring is needed if any suspicion of suicidal intent is held. Tricyclic antidepressants cannot be started at their therapeutic dose, so the dose has to be built up over time (7–10 days). This minimizes unpleasant or dangerous side-effects.

Monoamine oxidase inhibitors (MAOIs)

This class of drug is known to be effective in the treatment of depression, but has a reputation for being of especial value in cases of depression where there are unusual or 'atypical' features, e.g. where there is weight gain or hypersomnia, or where anxious or phobic symptoms are predominant. These drugs also act by increasing the levels of noradrenaline and serotonin in the synaptic cleft, this time by blocking the metabolism of the monoamines by the enzyme monoamine oxidase.

The older drugs in this class (e.g. phenelzine, tranylcypromine) are bound irreversibly to the enzyme, and this has led to particular problems (see below). However, the newer drugs in this class are reversible and selective for the monoamine oxidase A form of the enzyme. This class is known as Reversible Inhibitors of Monoamine Oxidase A (RIMA). Only moclobemide (Manerix) is currently on the market in the UK.

> **Problems of the classical monoamine oxidase inhibitors**
>
> - sudden increase in blood pressure because of the 'cheese' reaction
> - drowsiness
> - gastro-intestinal disturbances
> - headache
> - postural hypotension
> - interactions with morphine, pethidine, etc
> - interactions with anaesthetic agents
> - liver damage
> - interactions with sympathomimetics (e.g. ephidrine in cold cures)

By far the most important side-effect is a catastrophic rise in blood pressure caused by the ingestion of food and drink containing Tyramine. This amino acid is usually dealt with by the monoamine oxidase system in the gut wall. Without metabolism the tyramine is converted into noradrenaline, which raises the blood pressure to dangerous levels. All people taking the non-reversible forms of these drugs must be given detailed dietary instructions (see below) and carry warning cards indicating that they are taking such medication in case they require analgesia or surgery. It is recommended that the drug is stopped at least 2 weeks prior to any elective surgery.

Dietary advice and the MAOIs

> Avoid the following foods:
>
> - cheese (cooked or raw)
> - meat extracts (e.g. Oxo, Marmite, Bovril)
> - well-hung game
> - pickled herrings
> - broad bean pods
> - alcohol (especially Chianti)

The person should continue to avoid these foods for at least 2 weeks after stopping the medicine.

RIMAs do not cause the same problems with diet as the classical MAOIs and generally have a more favourable side-effect profile.

Selective serotonin reuptake inhibitors (SSRIs)

As their name suggests, these drugs selectively block the uptake of serotonin (5HT) alone and have little direct effect upon other neurotransmitter systems.

Their introduction has not been without controversy, but they represent an important addition to the range of drugs available to treat depression. They are probably of equal efficacy to the tricyclic antidepressants.

The major advantage of the drugs lies in their side-effect profile and their relative safety in overdose.

Tricyclics compared with SSRIs

- SSRIs are less sedative
- they have fewer cardiovascular side-effects, making them safe for use by physically unwell patients
- they have no anticholinergic side-effects, so can be used in the presence of glaucoma, prostatic disease, etc

Problems with SSRIs

- gastro-intestinal side-effects, nausea, vomiting and diarrhoea can limit compliance
- appetite loss may be undesirable in depressed people
- agitation and insomnia
- headaches
- fluoxetine (Prozac) requires a 5-week washout before treatment with an MAOI can be started
- cost (they remain more expensive than traditional tricyclics but increased compliance may cancel out this difference)
- inappropriate ADH secretion

The major advantages of the SSRIs lie in their side-effect profile. The lack of cardiovascular toxicity makes them particularly attractive for use in the elderly. Both paroxetine and fluoxetine can be started at the therapeutic dose and in once-daily doses, which is likely to improve compliance. They do have a number of disadvantages. Gastro-intestinal side-effects often limit their use, and for many doctors, especially in primary care, cost is an issue. So far these drugs have been more expensive than the traditional tricyclics.

Miscellaneous

In UK practice perhaps the most commonly used antidepressants after those described above are mianserin and trazodone. Both are relatively sedative in nature, and they have the advantage of a good cardiovascular side-effect profile. Problems with blood dyscrasias and the need to monitor the person's platelet count regularly have meant that mianserin has not really found a place in the routine management of depression. Trazodone, whilst having the standard side-effects of almost all centrally acting drugs, is perhaps most memorable for the side-effect of priapism common to all drugs with alpha-adrenoceptor activity.

CHOOSING AN ANTIDEPRESSANT

Choosing an antidepressant

- clinical picture (mild, moderate or severe)
- with neurotic symptoms (i.e. high levels of anxiety) or agoraphobia (consider MAOI)
- sedative vs. non-sedative
- cardiovascular disease
- tolerance of side-effects
- cost

The choice of antidepressant for a person can be difficult. The most important influence on selection is the clinical picture (see above), followed by the side-effect profile. A person with a retarded depression will not do well with a sedative antidepressant, whereas an agitated person can find it calming. The presence of cardiovascular disease, e.g. dysrhythmias, or the susceptibility of people to effects such as postural hypotension may make you turn to the SSRIs as the first line of treatment (as may other illnesses in which anticholinergic side-effects are undesirable). Cost remains an important issue.

Other drugs used in the treatment of depression

Neuroleptics

(See Chapter 7 on schizophrenia for details.) For people with depression of psychotic intensity it is best to treat with both an antidepressant and a neuroleptic as an antipsychotic medication.

Neuroleptics can also aid sleep and calm the agitation of distressed people who are not psychotic.

Benzodiazepines

These have been used extensively to treat depression in the past. They serve to reduce the associated anxiety and help sleep, but when used alone do little to assuage the underlying disturbance of mood.

Electroconvulsive therapy

Although this treatment has received a bad press in some quarters it is a highly effective method of treating severe depression (with an 80 per cent response rate), and its use can be life-saving. Following general anaesthesia (including a muscle relaxant), a current is passed between two electrodes placed on the person's head (usually bi-temporally, but they can be placed on one side, on the non-dominant hemisphere). The current should be sufficient to induce a grand mal fit with a duration of at least 20 seconds. The modification of the fit makes the treatment safe (even in the very elderly) and complications are rare, the major risk factors being those of anaesthesia.

INDICATIONS FOR ECT

- the person is not eating or drinking
- the person is intensely suicidal
- the intensity of depression is very severe
- other treatment methods have failed
- the person cannot tolerate medication

The indications for ECT are now much more clearly defined than in the past, and it is usually used in cases where a more rapid response to treatment is required than would be achieved with medication alone.

SIDE-EFFECTS OF ECT

- headache
- amnesia for the time around the treatment
- unwanted seizures between treatments
- delirium, especially in the elderly (this can be reduced by using unilateral treatments)
- cardiovascular complications

One of the major concerns about ECT has been the reported induction of memory deficits. These are present for the time around the treatment, but objective evidence for any long-term effects is lacking. Serial MRI scans and animal studies have shown no lasting structural change to the brain following ECT.

MECHANISM OF ACTION

This has not yet been fully elucidated, but the massive outpouring of neurotransmitters during the fit induces similar receptor changes in the noradrenergic system to chronic administration of tricyclic antidepressants.

Psychological treatments

Any biological treatment of a depressive illness needs to be accompanied by psychological interventions. These may be limited to low-key support whilst the physical treatments take effect. For others they need to be very much more extensive and are the mainstay of the treatment. For those without clear indications for medication or who decline the treatment a number of therapies can be used to alleviate the symptoms of depression (see Chapter 16 on psychotherapy).

AETIOLOGY OF DEPRESSION

Genetic influences

In most of the early family, twin and adoptee studies there was an excess of depressed individuals in the biological families of those suffering from a depressive illness. The association holds best for those with more 'biological' depressions. More sophisticated linkage studies have yet to demonstrate any consistent findings to shed light on this relationship.

Developmental factors

Death of or separation from the parents at an early age predisposes the child to mental illness later in life. The effect is not specific for depression, and some studies have failed to demonstrate this connection. The jury is still out on the importance of these early experiences (see below).

Vulnerability factors

Some people are able to bear the stresses and strains of life without developing depression, whereas others cannot. In addition to possible biological vulnerability, a number of social factors have been identified that make exposure to stress and major adverse life events more likely to lead to depression. Identified first in women (by Brown and Harris), they are as follows:

- having the care of three or more young children;
- having no confiding relationship;
- not working outside the home;
- separation from the mother before the age of 11 years.

These vulnerability factors sensitize the person to the effects of so-called 'life events' (LEs). The events of importance in developing depression are those which imply loss or threat to the person, e.g. loss of job, illness, etc. There is an excess of such events in the months prior to the onset of depressive illnesses. It used to be thought that the response to social change tended to be a milder depression without 'biological' features (reactive depression), but this is now known not to be the case, and severe depressions with biological features are just as common after life events.

CASE 8.8

A 40-year-old woman refugee from Bosnia developed a 'neurotic' depression in response to a series of harrowing and life-threatening ordeals, and subsequently responded to a course of antidepressants. Her mood improved, she was better able to care for her family, and began to take up voluntary work with her fellow exiles.

Cognitive theories

Rather than depressive thoughts being secondary to the mood, cognitive theorists argue that these ideas are primary and the mood change secondary. Aaron T. Beck identified three components to the thoughts:

- negative thoughts ('I am a bad student');
- negative expectations ('I can't be a good doctor unless I know everything');
- cognitive distortions, e.g. drawing conclusions from a single detail ('I couldn't do one question so I've failed the whole examination').

Given these habitual ways of thinking, the person is more likely to become depressed if they receive some kind of a setback. Treatment aims to explore the thinking patterns of the person and to get them to identify the patterns that they are using. Having done this, they can then challenge their automatic assumptions and begin to think with a less depressive cognitive set.

Biological theories

THE AMINE THEORY OF DEPRESSION

This has remained the dominant biological theory for many years, arising from observations that people taking reserpine (a monoamine-depleting drug used in the treatment of hypertension) became depressed, whereas people receiving MAOI medications for the treatment of tuberculosis had a markedly improved mood.

The initially simple hypothesis (not enough serotonin and noradrenaline activity in the brain) has become increasingly complex as the number of receptor subtypes has burgeoned and it has been shown that their responses to different treatments, each of which is effective for depression, varies. Simple urine or cerebrospinal fluid (CSF) estimations of neurotransmitter activity have often proved inconclusive, as have the results of neurochemical probing (e.g. with d,fenfluramine). It is likely that the chemical pathogenesis ultimately lies in complex interactions between the serotonin and noradrenergic systems.

Evidence for the amine theory of depression

- tricyclic and MAOI antidepressants increase the availability of amine in the synaptic cleft
- amphetamines causing the release of monoamines can induce euphoria
- monoamine-depleting drugs (e.g. reserpine) induce depression
- serotonin levels are reduced in the brains of suicide victims

ENDOCRINE THEORIES

For some the answer to the genesis of depression lies in abnormalities of the endocrine response to stress at the level of the hypothalamic pituitary axis. Many depressed people fail to suppress their cortisol production following the standard dexamethasone suppression test (DST). The abnormalities of the cortisol response to stress may have an effect on the monoamine system. It was hoped that the DST would become a useful clinical tool in the diagnosis and treatment of depression, but its early promise has not been realized.

BRAIN CHANGES

Unlike people with bipolar illnesses (see below), no consistent findings have been demonstrated on either CT or MRI scanning that either aid understanding of the pathogenesis of the disorder or help in the management of standard cases.

Functional imaging (e.g. PET) has been of more interest, but as yet it is not a clinical tool of any value.

EPIDEMIOLOGY OF DEPRESSION

Depression is a common disorder. Between 13 and 20 per cent of people have isolated depressive symptoms rather than the full syndrome. It is more prevalent in the lower social classes and in women. It is more difficult to estimate the prevalence of minor depressive disorders, as the definitions vary and the methods of case identification are very variable. For moderate to severe depressive disorders about 5 per cent of people will experience an episode in their lifetime. At any given time, 2 to 3 per cent of men and two to three times as many women will suffer from a depressive illness. The rates of depression encountered in general practice are considerably higher than those found in the community at large; 25 to 30 per cent of attenders at general practice surgeries meet the criteria for psychiatric illness, and many of these cases have depressive features. The recognition of these people varies widely between practitioners, but only a very small percentage find their way through to mental health services.

Prognosis in depression

Most episodes of clinical depression remit within 5 to 6 months; however, about 15 per cent of cases go on to experience chronic symptoms. Of those who recover completely a large percentage will relapse at some later time in life.

The outlook for the elderly who become depressed is probably less good than that for members of the younger population. Although many recover from their first episode, the relapse rate is high during the first 2 years after recovery. These patients tend to succumb to physical illness at a greater rate than their non-depressed peers.

Long-term management of depression

TREATMENT-RESISTANT DEPRESSION

Most depressed people will respond to a combination of psychological intervention and first-line biological treatments (e.g. tricyclic antidepressants) given in adequate doses for a reasonable trial period (e.g. 6 weeks). About 10 to 15 per cent fail to do so, and a number of strategies can be employed to increase the rate of recovery:

- ensure compliance by means of blood sampling if necessary;
- increase the dose of the current antidepressant to the limit of the persons tolerance of side-effects. Only nortriptyline has been shown to have a therapeutic window beyond which an increase in the dose is of no value;
- change of antidepressant – if a tricyclic has been used, an SSRI could be substituted, or perhaps a RIMA;
- treatment with ECT – failure to respond to a tricyclic antidepressant reduces the response rate to ECT, but the latter remains an important option under these circumstances;
- augmentation – certain drugs have little effect upon mood on their own, but in combination with an antidepressant appear to have a synergistic effect.

Examples of drugs which have a synergistic effect with antidepressants include the following:

- *lithium* – lithium carbonate is the most commonly used of the augmentation strategies. As outlined below it has a number of drawbacks in clinical practice which may preclude its use;
- *anticonvulsants* – both carbamazepine and sodium valproate can be used in this manner;
- *neuroleptics* – in addition to any central action, the neuroleptics increase the plasma levels of the antidepressants by competing for metabolism in the liver;
- *tryptophan* – this simple amino acid is the precursor of serotonin. It is present in natural foodstuffs, particularly pumpkin seeds, but recent concerns about side-effects (eosinophilic myalgia) have restricted its use. It can be used

with a tricyclic antidepressant and lithium in the classic 'Bridge's cocktail'.

PSYCHOSURGERY

If despite all of the above strategies the person continues to suffer intractable depressive symptoms, psychosurgery should be considered. Subcaudate tractotomy, performed by the insertion of small radioactive rods stereotactically just below the caudate, is perhaps the most widely used and successful operation.

Prevention of recurrence and relapse

Relapse This is defined as the worsening of symptoms following their initial improvement during a single episode of illness. Treatment to prevent relapse is called Continuation Therapy.

Recurrence This is defined as a new episode of the disorder after complete recovery. Treatment to prevent recurrence is called Prophylaxis.

In essence, however, the strategies adopted to achieve and maintain remission are the same, and can be summarized as follows:

- continuation of the medication which resulted in the person getting better for a minimum of 6 months from full recovery (2 years for the elderly);
- continuation indefinitely for those people who have demonstrated that they relapse at regular intervals;
- lithium is effective in preventing relapses in people who relapse despite taking the medication which made them well. It is perhaps even more effective in bipolar illness;
- carbamazepine is also effective in the same people as those who would be considered for lithium;
- cognitive therapy – people who are treated with both medication and cognitive therapy do better than those who are treated with either therapy alone;
- social interventions – long-term support for the more isolated and vulnerable through community workers or day facilities can be of enormous value. This helps sufferers to improve their sense of self-worth and confidence in their place in the world. Assistance in developing skills of use in the world of work can be of major importance.

SOME VARIETIES OF DEPRESSION

Atypical depression

Depressive disorders in which the presenting and most prominent symptom is not a disturbance in mood have been called atypical depressions. The depression is often fluctuating, and they may find that under some circumstances they are able to enjoy themselves. They often feel worse in the evening and have difficulty in getting to sleep. Once asleep, they sleep for very long periods and at times will sleep during the day (hypersomnia). They overeat (particularly sweet foods) and gain weight. Lassitude and fatigue are common and there are often phobic or anxiety symptoms.

The place of this concept in current classifications is debatable. People belonging to this group are said to respond preferentially to MAOIs.

Seasonal affective disorder

Some people respond to the turning of the seasons with alterations in mood. The autumn, with its shortening days, can induce depressive disorders which continue over the winter months until the days become lighter. These disorders often do not come to the attention of the medical profession, the person affected 'soldiering on' until the spring days. People with this disorder are frequently women (female:male ratio of 6:1), with onset in the mid-twenties. The depression is often accompanied by hypersomnia and hyperphagia (oversleeping and overeating).

The mechanism underlying the mood disorder remains unclear, but it is probably related to changes in the circadian rhythms induced by the changes in the length of daylight hours. Melatonin is probably the mediator of these changes.

Treatment has been by traditional methods (antidepressants, etc.), but also by the use of special lights which mimic the qualities of natural daylight. These are used to lengthen the day artificially and so maintain the biological rhythms. This treatment is best if given in the mornings.

Recurrent brief depressions

There is a group of people who experience brief bouts of intense depression which last for 2 to 5 days and occur every 2 to 5 weeks. These episodes would meet the criteria for major depressive episodes except that they are very short. They are very disruptive to the working and social life of the person who is suffering from them. It has been suggested that these people are at high risk of suicide.

Treatment of recurrent brief depressions is probably best achieved with SSRIs.

ECONOMICS OF DEPRESSION

For the person who becomes depressed there are a number of costs both to themselves and to society.

The direct costs of treating moderate to severe depression in the UK have been estimated at £222 million (and in the USA $2.1 billion). This consists of clearly identifiable costs such as drugs, doctor's time, in-patient time, and so forth. The indirect costs (lost wages and productivity, caring by the person's family and early mortality) are difficult to calculate, but are clearly enormous.

Treatment strategies must bear these figures in mind. If the doctor is faced with the possibility of using equally effective treatments (e.g. SSRIs and tricyclics), the natural response is to take the cheaper option. If the cheaper option has increased numbers of side-effects and therefore poorer compliance, it is likely that this may cost the doctor and society more in the long term than a more expensive option that ensures good compliance. If suicide by overdose is much more common with one form of treatment than with another, the relative costs of these treatments must be weighed against this issue. Considerations such as these are only now beginning to be taken into account when choosing the options for treatment in a given case.

BIPOLAR AFFECTIVE DISORDER

CASE 8.9

A 24-year-old man said that he had begun to feel full of energy for about 4 weeks before he 'borrowed' and crashed a four-wheel-drive car into the bollards of a pedestrian precinct. He was arrested after a brief fracas with the police. He said that he had felt more energetic and lively than for a long time. He slept very little, turning up at his friends' houses at all hours of the day and night 'to party'. He was unable to understand why they did not wish to join him. He spent a lot of money on drink and became involved in fights in bars, especially at closing time when he wanted to carry on drinking. He believed that he had 'a right' to the car and that it was perfectly all right to take it and drive at high speeds. He said he knew that he was a very good driver and would not crash.

When a person experiences an elevation of mood, they are described as experiencing hypomania. This usually alternates with periods of low mood (depression), hence the name Bipolar Affective Disorder.

The episode of elevated mood is known as hypomania. If the episode is severe and has psychotic features (delusions and hallucinations), it is known as Mania.

The depressive swings of mood are identical to those of unipolar depression, and are managed in the same way (see above).

Presentation of hypomania and mania

BEHAVIOUR

The behaviour of the person will reflect the elevation in mood. They will usually have a great deal of energy which is difficult to contain. They will walk about during the interview and not settle. They may flout the usual conventions of the interview and begin to question you ('Why do you wear a bow tie?'). They are disinhibited and tactless, sometimes making perceptive and hurtful comments. Their dress may echo their mood, being bright and garish, or it may reflect their careless use of money and be way beyond their apparent means. This tendency to spend money can be very damaging, especially when facilitated by credit cards.

People with hypomania and mania display voracious appetites for food, drink and sex. Sometimes they can be so distracted that they forget to eat. Promiscuity during an attack with a careless attitude to safe sex and contraception can be disastrous. The sense of being right and knowing best can lead to difficulties when the person's wishes are thwarted. Their tolerance is limited and frustration of their aims quickly leads to arguments and violence. For some people this irritable behaviour is much more noticeable than the elevation in mood.

SPEECH

People speak rapidly ('pressure of speech'). It is hard to interrupt them and get a word in edgeways.

MOOD

The person's mood is grandiose, elevated and expansive. They will never have felt better in their lives, they feel full of energy and vitality and they are loathe to relinquish the feeling.

THOUGHTS

The person's thoughts go fast, crashing over each other in a torrent. It may be difficult to follow their thoughts as new ideas, concepts and subjects follow faster and faster ('flight of ideas'). In extreme cases it is impossible to follow the patient's train of thought.

The person develops any number of ideas and delusions secondary to the mood state. They may believe that they have special powers to influence the course of political events or nature (e.g. a 28-year-old woman found herself able to control the earthquakes in Japan). They may have made great discoveries (e.g. a 67-year-old man found the cure for HIV in a packet of processed cheese), or be chosen for special purposes by God (e.g. a 34-year-old man had been put upon the earth to rid it of witches). Some believe that they have become God or are his offspring and must act to save the world. Under such influences it is easy to see how thwarting of the person's aims by family, the police or psychiatric services can cause problems.

PERCEPTIONS

Some people describe heightened perception. Colours are more vivid and tastes more piquant.

Auditory hallucinations in which voices are heard talking to the person (second person) are the commonest type of hallucination. Usually they say what a fine and splendid person they are (mood congruent) and may be interpreted as the voice of God.

COGNITION

Failure to concentrate is the most obvious cognitive abnormality as the persons mind 'flies off' in all directions and is distracted by the events going on around him or her. This can also lead to poor memory, as events are not registered.

INSIGHT

For mild episodes of mania (hypomania), insight can be retained. Some people like the feeling that highs give them and are able to keep them carefully regulated with medication. Others find that they are more creative when their mood is elevated. They find ways to release this energy when ideas are needed and then damp down the mood when the development of the concept requires concentration and sustained attention.

Features of mania

- abnormally elevated mood or irritability
- grandiosity
- boundless energy and reduced sleep
- over-talkative (pressure of speech)
- racing thoughts
- poor concentration and application to the task in hand
- overactivity, especially in pleasurable but potentially harmful areas (e.g. sex, drinking, spending money)

Differential diagnosis

Drug-induced state Especially in association with the use of amphetamines, Ecstasy and cocaine.

Organic state Rarely, dementia or a delirium can present with elevated mood. Thyroid dysfunction, multiple sclerosis, HIV and syphilis may present in this way.

Schizophrenia Among manic people 15 per cent have first-rank symptoms, but a careful review of the symptomatology and the history should make the diagnosis clear.

Schizoaffective disorder If the person meets the criteria for the diagnosis for both disorders then they qualify for this category (see Chapter 7 on schizophrenia for details).

Mixed mood state See below.

AETIOLOGY OF MANIA

Genetics

Twin studies support an important genetic component to the development of bipolar illnesses. A concordance rate of about 75 per cent in monozygotic twins and about 54 per cent in dizygotic twins has been shown.

Amine theory

Crudely stated, the amine theory of affective disorders (see above) suggests underactivity in depression and excess activity in mania.

There is some evidence to support this view. The metabolites of noradrenaline are found to be increased in the active phase of the illness and return to normal levels once this has been treated.

Abnormalities of serotonin suggest that it might act as some kind of trigger for the manic episode, but are not sufficient in themselves to cause the problem.

Dopamine is involved in the process, but the mechanism is unclear. Amphetamine-releasing dopamine (but also noradrenaline) can improve mood, and neuroleptics (e.g. haloperidol) are effective in managing mania.

The relationship between amines and mania

- the levels of noradrenaline metabolites are raised in the acute phase
- a serotonin-related mechanism may trigger the episode
- dopamine is involved in ways that are unclear

Psychological theories

CASE 8.10

A 68-year-old man was admitted to the ward a month after the death of his partner. He was speaking rapidly, telling me that he was related to royalty, he had won several million pounds on the National Lottery, and that his dog had powers to communicate intelligibly not only with himself but also with his dead friend in ways that the author could not understand.

Unlike the situation for depression, there is a paucity of psychological theories of the development of mania, apart from the view that the flight into mania ('manic defence') protects the person from the realities of a situation. Only when the mania has settled can the difficult work of coming to terms with the loss or situation be done.

EPIDEMIOLOGY OF MANIA

- The mean age of onset is about 30 years
- The lifetime risk of developing mania is 0.6 to 1 per cent
- The excess of women is not so marked as in unipolar depression

---

COURSE AND PROGNOSIS OF MANIA

The first episode of bipolar affective disorder usually occurs much earlier than is the case for unipolar depression. The bouts tend to be more frequent.

If left untreated, most episodes will resolve within 3 months and rarely last longer than 6 months. However, they can carry a significant mortality from exhaustion if not treated.

The risk of recurrence is particularly high (over 50 per cent) if the disorder begins before the age of 30 years. Ten to twenty per cent of sufferers have three episodes of depression before they develop manic illnesses.

It is not clear whether all of these represent the manic phase of a true bipolar illness, or whether they are the result of treatment by antidepressant medication or ECT for depression (so-called Bipolar II illness). Over time, manic episodes become less frequent whilst the depressive swings increase in frequency. The prognosis is much better than for schizophrenia, but there is wide variation, some people having their lives repeatedly disrupted, whilst others experience only a single episode.

TREATMENT OF MANIA

Usually the person who is manic will have to be admitted to hospital, since their behaviour is too disruptive to be contained in a community setting. This may have to be done under Mental Health legislation as such people feel so well that they are not likely to agree to be in a constraining environment.

Nursing this group can be difficult. The grandiose ideas and rapid changes in directions of thought and action can be dangerous for the person, and restraint can provoke violence. Hypomania might be managed at home if the person has someone else there and they are prepared to take regular medication.

ACUTE DRUG TREATMENT

For the uncomplicated case two drugs are the mainstay of treatment. Emergency treatment may require parenteral medication (see Chapter 7 on schizophrenia).

Haloperidol

Haloperidol (see Chapter 7 on schizophrenia for details) has the effect of sedating the person rapidly, which can be a useful adjunct to the longer term antimanic properties of the drug. It is the treatment of choice for severe mania.

Some clinicians use chlorpromazine, despite its greater range of side-effects.

Lithium

Lithium (as a carbonate or bicarbonate) is also an effective antimanic agent in its own right. It can take 5 to 6 days before it begins to have an effect on the person's mental state. This is a major drawback, particularly if the person is aggressive or violent. It is suggested that lithium might not induce a depressive swing following the manic episode, as haloperidol is prone to do.

Lithium is better tolerated than haloperidol, leaving the person more alert, but it needs careful blood monitoring and physical work-up for which the person may not give consent.

Mechanism of action

Lithium is rapidly absorbed and replaces sodium (Na^+) and potassium (K^+) in the cells. This alters the flux of both magnesium and calcium across the cell membrane. Lithium is filtered by the kidney and only partially reabsorbed.

Mechanism of action of Lithium

- changing the concentrations of Na^+ and K^+ within the cell
- changing the dynamics of Mg^{2+} and Ca^{2+}
- changing the responsiveness of Na/K^+-ATPase
- changing the permeability of the blood–brain barrier
- changing the sensitivity of the dopamine receptors
- decreasing the uptake of noradrenaline into cells
- altering the sensitivity of beta-adrenoceptors

Interactions

The major drug interaction is with haloperidol when either drug is used at a high dose. Confusion, tremor, extra-pyramidal and cerebellar signs have been reported and have led to permanent cerebral damage.

Co-administration with thiazide diuretics can cause a dangerous rise in the serum and intracellular levels of lithium.

The physical work-up for lithium

- urea and electrolytes
- creatinine clearance
- full blood count (FBC)
- thyroid function (including TSH)
- electrocardiograph (ECG)
- pregnancy test

Acute side-effects of lithium

- gastrointestinal side-effects
- tremor
- weight gain
- muscle weakness
- leucocytosis

The long-term side-effects

- weight gain
- hypothyroidism
- nephrogenic diabetes insipidus (5 per cent of cases)
- ECG changes

The toxic effects of lithium (e.g. diuretics, diarrhoea, surgery)

- ataxia
- nystagmus
- delirium
- coma
- death

Fetal abnormalities
- Awareness of this problem is vital.
- Women of reproductive age must be counselled and adequate contraceptive advice provided.

Monitoring lithium levels
- Aim for a serum level of 0.6–0.8 mmol/L.
- Measure levels each week until stable.
- Thereafter measure levels every 6 weeks.
- Measure urea and electrolytes, and thyroid function and full blood count (FBC) every 6 months.

Lithium as a prophylactic agent
Lithium is used as a prophylactic agent in bipolar affective disorder, but is also effective in unipolar depressive disorders.

It acts to reduce both the frequency of the episodes and the severity of the swings. Serum levels of 0.6–0.8 mmol/L are adequate for most people.

Indications for lithium prophylaxis

- three or more episodes of mania within 2 years
- severity of the manic disorder
- augmentation of tricyclic antidepressants in resistant depression
- prophylaxis in unipolar depression

In addition to lithium, carbamazepine and sodium valproate have both been shown to be effective in prophylaxis against bipolar illness in those individuals who cannot tolerate lithium for some reason. For those who have rapid cycling disorder (see below) sodium valproate is perhaps even more effective than lithium.

Carbamazepine

This is a tricyclic compound which, as an anticonvulsant, inhibits fast sodium channels, but it also influences the release of noradrenaline and noradrenaline-induced adenylcyclase activity, which are more closely related to its mood-stabilizing effects.

It has little effect on the serotonin system.

Treatment-resistant mania

In some cases the first-line treatments with haloperidol or lithium are not effective. Many other drugs have been used under these circumstances, including combinations of lithium and carbamazepine. The most effective alternatives are benzodiazepines (particularly clonazepam) and sodium valproate, both of which have activity at the γ-aminobutyric acid (GABA) receptor, but many others have been used.

Drugs used in resistant mania

- combinations of lithium and carbamazepine
- clonazepam
- verapamil
- beta blockers
- ECT is sometimes used *in extremis*, and appears to be an effective treatment

Rapid-cycling bipolar affective disorder

This is defined as more than four episodes of severe affective disorder in a year.

- it is more common in women
- it is more common in those taking antidepressants
- it is associated with thyroid disorder
- it responds to treatment with sodium valproate

People who have rapid changes of mood are difficult to stabilize, as you always feel you are reacting to the changes rather than thinking ahead of them to provide an effective strategy to combat the changes. Rapid cycling is more common in women than in men, and it is more common when antidepressants and neuroleptics are used to control the ups and downs. It is related to thyroid abnormalities, which may be subtle and revealed only by subnormal responses to thyrotrophin-releasing hormone (TRH) tests. Thyroxine or triiodothyronine (T_3) can be effective in such cases.

Sodium valproate is probably more effective than lithium in stopping these rapid cycles.

Secondary mania

One important cause of mania has already been mentioned. It can be induced as a result of treatment with antidepressants for a depressive disorder. In late life more brain changes are found in patients than in younger individuals (especially subcortical abnormalities), suggesting that organic factors are more important in late-onset cases. Mania may also be induced by head injury, stroke or drugs (e.g. amphetamines).

Mixed mood states

When you see a person with mania you will get the impression that depression is never far below the surface. This is often shown in fleeting glimpses of despair or brief episodes of crying, and is even more obvious in some people who have rapidly alternating moods and will move from elation to profound depression in a matter of hours. Diagnosis is very difficult, as the clinical picture can change so fast. It is thought that elderly people are more likely to have depressive features as part of a manic presentation.

Further reading

Beck, A.T. 1976: *Cognitive therapy and the emotional disorders*. New York: International Universities Press.

Feighner, J.P. and Boyer, W.F. (eds) 1991: *Diagnosis of depression*. London: John Wiley & Sons.

Goldberg, D. and Huxley, P. 1992: *Common mental disorders*. London: Routledge.

Goodwin, F.K. and Jamison, K.R. 1990: *Manic-depressive illness*. Oxford: Oxford University Press.

9 ANXIETY DISORDERS

CASE 9.1

A 43-year-old man came to out-patients. He had recently been promoted to a foreman's post and was now involved with meetings with the managers of the small factory where he worked. He became very tense, sweaty and light-headed prior to any meeting. He felt unable to speak, his heart would pound loudly and he felt sure that everyone could hear it beating. He believed something terrible was about to happen. On occasions he would feign a coughing fit as a pretext to leave the room. If he managed to stay in the room the symptoms would subside, but he often had to leave, and the symptoms would then slowly die away.

The anxiety disorders share several common features. At their core is a sense of fear and dread which is not appropriate to the situation and impairs the person's everyday functioning. Case 9.1 represents a fairly typical set of symptoms, but these can be many and varied. These feelings can occur in a generalized, persistent way, or in discrete episodes which build rapidly to a peak and subside again over the following 10 to 15 minutes (a panic attack).

Anxiety is a common feeling in response to stress of any kind, such as conflicts of loyalty or duty within the family or at work, especially if there is no escape from the situation (are you reading this to revise for an exam?). Increases in circulating adrenaline and noradrenaline levels under conditions of stress have an important survival function. The stimulus to run or fight in the face of threat remains important in today's world. When feelings of apprehension, fear and tension become overwhelming or occur in inappropriate circumstances then they become maladaptive. It is estimated that 2 to 4 per cent of the population suffer from disabling anxiety symptoms.

Symptoms of anxiety

Somatic symptoms:

- cardiac – palpitations, pounding in the chest, rapid heart beat
- pulmonary – shortness of breath, choking and hyperventilation
- abdominal – butterflies in the stomach, nausea, frequent and precipitant bowel motion
- urinary – urinary frequency
- neurological – headaches, dizziness, light-headedness, tingling in the fingers and around the mouth (paraesthesia)
- autonomic – feeling cold, hot flushes, sweating, shakiness

Cognitive symptoms:

- apprehensiveness
- terror
- fear of death
- fear of losing control (fainting, vomiting, fitting)
- fear of going mad
- a desire to run away
- fear of a serious medical problem (heart attack, stroke or AIDS)
- derealization

Classification of anxiety disorders

- generalized anxiety disorder
- panic disorder
- agoraphobia
- specific phobia
- social phobia
- obsessive-compulsive disorder
- post-traumatic stress disorders
- substance-induced anxiety
- anxiety due to a medical condition

Biology of anxiety

The following neurotransmitter systems are involved in anxiety:

- noradrenaline;
- serotonin (5HT);
- gamma-aminobutyric acid (GABA).

NORADRENALINE

This neurotransmitter is closely related to the central and peripheral effects of anxiety. Drugs that enhance its release (e.g. yohimbine) lead to an increase in anxiety, whereas drugs which reduce its release (e.g. clonidine) decrease anxiety levels.

SEROTONIN (5HT)

A reduction in the levels of 5HT reduces anxiety.

GAMMA-AMINO BUTYRIC ACID (GABA)

GABA is extremely widely dispersed throughout the brain, and it acts as an inhibitory neurotransmitter. When the GABA receptors are blocked, symptoms of anxiety appear, whereas stimulation of the action of GABA leads to a reduction in anxiety.

It is unlikely that any one neurotransmitter is responsible for all the changes seen in the anxiety disorders, but a number of pathways interact to develop the symptoms.

PHARMACOLOGICAL TREATMENT OF ANXIETY

Benzodiazepines

Benzodiazepines have been shown to be extremely effective in the treatment of anxiety, to the extent that 500 million people in the world have taken them at some time in their lives. It is estimated that 1.5 per cent of the UK population have taken them for at least a year, and often for a great deal longer.

The drugs act by enhancing the action of GABA. The GABA receptor is complex, but appears to have a very specific binding point for benzodiazepines. Alcohol and barbiturates also affect the GABA receptor, but act at different sites on the receptor.

The drugs are used as both anxiolytics and hypnotics, and there is little difference between the drugs that are used in these different ways. It is best to become familiar with a few of the many varieties on the market (e.g. diazepam, temazepam, lorazepam).

SHORT-TERM ADMINISTRATION

In the short term these drugs are very effective anxiolytics. They may cause some drowsiness, especially when active metabolites accumulate (e.g. diazepam, chlordiazepoxide). It is best to limit treatment to several weeks or less in order to deal with specific problems or events (e.g. the holiday flight to Marbella). These drugs should only be used when the anxiety is severe. Using them intermittently helps to reduce the problem of dependence.

Side-effects of benzodiazepines

- addiction
- sedation
- slowing of reaction times (especially when taken with alcohol)
- depression of respiration
- confusional states
- ataxia
- memory problems

Good practice with benzodiazepines

- short-term use
- use to deal with specific problems or events
- use only in cases of severe anxiety
- intermittent dosing
- lowest effective dose

LONG-TERM ADMINISTRATION

The problems of long-term administration

- tolerance
- dependence (physical and psychological)
- rebound effects

Tolerance

People usually develop tolerance to the side-effects but also to the therapeutic anxiolytic qualities of the drug. This can lead to ever escalating demands for the drug, and to its abuse.

Dependence

Physical
Sudden withdrawal of the drug can lead to delirium, paranoia, sensitivity to light or sound and odd sensations of bodily movement (kinaesthesia). The person may become anxious and irritable, and sleep poorly. Epileptic fits can be intractable unless they are treated quickly.

Psychological
People will often not tolerate reductions in the medication, and will either 'doctor shop' to get further supplies or resort to the black market. This may be due to the fear of withdrawal or rebound symptoms when the dose is reduced.

Rebound effects

Stopping a benzodiazepine can lead the person back to their original state, often with a worsening of the symptoms for which the drug was prescribed in the first place. Rebound insomnia is perhaps the most commonly met. This often happens when people are admitted to hospital and their medication is stopped.

Avoiding rebound and withdrawal effects

The best way to avoid these problems is to engage the person in a therapeutic alliance to stop the drug. The reasons for stopping should be explored in some detail, and alternative strategies for managing the anxiety (see below) learned before any attempt is made to reduce the medication.

When reducing the medication it is best to use a benzodiazepine with a long half-life (e.g. diazepam) rather than one with a short half-life (e.g. lorazepam). The rate of reduction should be slow and, within reason, at the person's own pace. Try to avoid being carried away by their initial enthusiasm. Too quick a reduction, with rebound symptoms, has ruined many withdrawal programmes. Close monitoring and support of the person throughout his or her withdrawal is very important. Small frequent meals to avoid hypoglycaemia and adrenaline release should be encouraged, as should regular exercise.

Continuing help once the person is off the drug, to avoid its restitution, is an important part of therapy.

BUSPIRONE

Buspirone has been introduced into practice relatively recently. Its primary site of action is the 5HT1a receptor. It is an effective anxiolytic, but takes time to work (as do antidepressants), which tends to limit its use in clinical practice.

BARBITURATES

The use of barbiturates as anxiolytics has been superseded by the use of newer drugs.

TRICYCLIC ANTIDEPRESSANTS

The more sedative antidepressants can be used at lower doses to treat anxiety symptoms. If there is evidence that the patient is depressed either secondary to the anxiety or as a primary problem, full therapeutic doses need to be used.

NEUROLEPTICS

In relatively low doses, neuroleptics can be used to help to alleviate anxiety symptoms. Given that they do not induce dependence, they are often preferable to benzodiazepines (e.g. promazine or thioridazine), but prolonged use may lead to tardive dyskinesia (see Chapter 7 on schizophrenia).

BETA-BLOCKERS

These can be useful in some milder cases, where they are able to damp down some of the cardiac symptoms and tremor associated with anxiety. Atenolol is the most suitable drug, as its low fat solubility reduces central side-effects.

RELATIONSHIP BETWEEN ANXIETY AND DEPRESSION

There are two schools of thought:

- that anxiety and depression are different expressions of the same neurochemical disorder (unitary position); or

- that they are distinct entities (binary position).

UNITARY POSITION

- There is considerable overlap in symptoms between the two disorders.
- People with anxiety disorders frequently have a history of depression.
- People with a history of depression and anxiety disorders have increased numbers of relatives with both disorders.
- Both anxiety and depression respond to tricyclic antidepressants.

BINARY POSITION

- Sleep and appetite disturbances are more often associated with depression.
- Depressed people have a better prognosis than anxious ones.
- Sleep studies show different rapid eye movement (REM) sleep changes in anxiety and depression.
- Neuroendocrine differences exist between the two disorders.

MEDICAL DISORDERS, DRUGS AND ANXIETY

Anxiety may be a response to being told about any diagnosis, but some medical disorders include anxiety as part of their symptomatology:

Medical causes of anxiety

- hyperthyroidism
- phaeochromocytoma (noradrenaline-producing tumour)
- cardiac dysrhythmias and failure
- insulinomas (hypoglycaemia)
- respiratory dysfunction (chronic obstructive airways disease (COAD), asthma, etc.)

In addition to medical disorders causing anxiety symptoms, drugs may also produce similar types of symptoms.

Intoxication

- amphetamine
- cocaine
- alcohol
- phencyclidine (PCP)

Therapeutic concentrations

- thyroid replacement therapy
- selective serotonin reuptake inhibitors
- insulin
- sympatheticomimetics (in cold remedies)
- bronchodilators
- analgesics (especially opioid-based types)
- caffeine

Withdrawal symptoms

- alcohol
- opiates
- benzodiazepines

When investigating the underlying causes of anxiety it is important to exclude a number of medical problems and the use and abuse of both legal and illegal medications. It can be that two problems coexist, e.g. the anxious person who drinks to calm his nerves, but the anxiety gets worse as withdrawal phenomena start, or the person with respiratory difficulties who becomes anxious as his breathing becomes more laboured, and so begins to hyperventilate.

SPECIFIC ANXIETY DISORDERS

Panic disorder

CASE 9.2

A woman aged 23 years presented to out-patients with a 6-month history. She had led a normal life up to that time, with no evidence of major psychological dysfunction. Working at her word processor she became increasingly tense and felt that her heart racing and she was unable to breathe. She tried to cry out but was unable to do so. Eventually she got to the toilet where the feelings slowly subsided. She went to her GP, who could find no reason for the attack, and she returned to work. Over the following weeks she had four further attacks which occurred in different places and at different times of day. She was unable to concentrate at work and took time off. She worried that the attacks might recur and was concerned about what might happen to her when they did. She went out less and consequently lost much of her social network.

For those suffering from Panic Disorder the symptoms of anxiety occur in discrete attacks (panic attacks) that are erratic in timing and without situational cues. This leads the affected person to worry about the next attack and to make substantial changes to their usual activity (e.g. stopping work and leisure activities). Each person varies in the frequency of the attacks that they suffer. They may well present to emergency services or to physicians with concerns about their physical health (see Chapter 13 on liaison psychiatry and somatoform disorders) (A woman aged 20 years was convinced that she was developing a brain tumour due to the blurred vision and paraesthesiae she developed during each attack, and she repeatedly presented to emergency services demanding head scans). It is estimated that 50 to 60 per cent of people develop depression secondary to the panic attacks and the effects they have on their life. They may also display elements of other anxiety disorders, particularly agoraphobia (20 per cent of cases) (see case described above).

About 2 to 3 per cent of people will develop panic disorder during their lifetime, with onset in late adolescence or early adulthood.

AETIOLOGICAL THEORIES

Genetic

First-degree relatives of those with panic disorder have a five times greater likelihood than members of the general population of developing the disorder.

Biochemical

Panic attacks can be easily induced in this group by yohimbine, and this suggests an abnormality of noradrenergic receptors, as does the effectiveness of treatment with imipramine.

Hyperventilation

Some people can induce panic attacks by hyperventilation. Spontaneous attacks are believed to arise from involuntary hyperventilation.

Cognitive

Concerns about physical illness are more common in anxious patients who experience panic attacks than in those who do not. This suggests a spiralling effect in which anxiety leads to physical symptoms, which lead to anxiety, which leads to physical symptoms, which lead to anxiety....

TREATMENT

Drug treatment

Treatment with benzodiazepines is the most rapid form of short-term relief for panic disorder, but over a longer period tricyclic antidepressants, especially imipramine, are more effective and do not cause the problem of dependence. Many people experience a transient worsening of their symptoms as treatment starts, which can be discouraging, but if helped through this phase they frequently do well.

Cognitive behavioural treatment

Breaking the spiralling thought patterns of the person is the aim here, by learning to control the symptoms and reattribute them so that the panic does not develop.

Obsessive-compulsive disorder

CASE 9.3

A soldier spent half an hour each morning ensuring that his hair was parted exactly in the centre. Parting it first on one side and then on the other, he continued until he felt that it was more or less correct, but it was never to his satisfaction. He had a compulsion to do things four times. On getting up he would dress and undress four times, and vice versa on retiring. He always had to begin doing things with his right hand or foot. The customary procedure in the army is 'by the left, quick march'.

Most people find that spontaneous thoughts can intrude into their minds without causing distress, but for those suffering from obsessive-compulsive disorder these thoughts disrupt the normal flow to an intolerable degree. The affected person attempts to exclude the intrusive thoughts from their mind. For some people this can take the form of internal debates (obsessional ruminations) about the pros and cons of some simple action, which are endlessly and inconclusively reviewed.

OBSESSIONS

These are repeated ideas that come unbidden into the mind of a person, despite attempts to force them out (e.g. the names of all the railway stations on the line between Sidcup and Charing Cross).

COMPULSIONS

These are actions a person feels compelled to undertake, often increasing their anxiety levels. Such actions are often repeated a magical (ritual) number of times.

Obsessive rituals or compulsions are activities that the person affected feels that they have to undertake. These activities are thought to be senseless, but if they are not completed then the person becomes very anxious. Some have an obvious relationship ' to the obsessional thought (e.g. handwashing to combat contamination, or checking the gas), while others appear to have little to do with the thoughts (a girl failed her examinations because she was unable to resist the need to fill in all the letters on the question sheets, and so did not have time to complete the answers). Some rituals are carried out in order to magically prevent an imagined disaster.

The anxiety caused by the thoughts can be assuaged by the ritual actions for some, but for others who know how foolish and shameful the ritual is, their anxiety levels can rise (e.g. the man who felt compelled to retrace his steps when halfway down the tower of Pisa).

Depression is often found in this group of people.

The onset of the illness usually occurs in the early twenties.

AETIOLOGY

It is difficult to identify the aetiological factors in this disorder. There appears to be some genetic component to the illness, but others have rather suggested that the rituals are avoidance responses and ultimately serve to reduce anxiety. This reduction in anxiety is the reward that perpetuates the behaviour. Some people develop these symptoms following head injury or encephalitis.

TREATMENT

Behavioural methods are the mainstay of treatment for this group. Graded exposure to a feared situation (e.g. a dirty lavatory), and teaching anxiety control whilst preventing the anxiety-reducing ritual (e.g. handwashing), known as response prevention, is successful in 50 per cent of cases.

Antidepressants

Tricyclic antidepressants (especially clomipramine) and SSRI antidepressants (e.g. high-dose fluoxetine) have been used to treat this disorder. They provide some success, but relapse is frequent after the drugs have been stopped. If there is a significant depressive component to the illness this must be treated in its own right.

PROGNOSIS

Most cases improve within a year. When the disorder lasts for longer than a year the course is fluctuating and often has a poor outcome, especially if the symptoms are severe and the onset is early. If the obsessive symptoms develop as part of a depressive illness the prognosis is much more favourable.

Phobias

Features common to all phobias
■ anxiety only occurs in certain circumstances
■ it is out of proportion to the perceived threat
■ it is recognized as being excessive by the patient
■ the patient avoids the situation that gives rise to anxiety
■ anticipation of that situation leads to anxiety

SIMPLE PHOBIAS

Simple phobias are common. These are fears that are above and beyond the perceived threat, and are believed to be irrational by the person experiencing them. Common phobias such as spider phobia (arachnophobia) cause little disruption to life in the UK, but are more disabling in Australia. Other phobias (e.g. fear of flying in the businessman) may severely restrict the affected person's ability to carry out their normal life.

CASE 9.4

A 28-year-old woman with a small baby presented to out-patients having developed the fear that her kitchen cupboards would fall off the walls and damage her child. She kept out of the room as much as possible, and as meal times approached she became increasingly tense. This phobia had developed at a time of stress within her marriage. She recognized that it was silly, as the cupboards had been up for nine years and there was no reason why they should fall now. She was taught some relaxation techniques and, with a small amount of cognitive psychotherapy, the problem resolved.

Treatment

Learning relaxation techniques to control the anxiety is the core of treatment. Once these have been mastered, exposure to the feared situation can begin. This exposure is graded until the person can tolerate the feared situation. The plan should be negotiated with the person so that each stage is felt to be achievable but still represents a significant step forward. For example, the following steps might be used to overcome spider phobia:

step 1 – imagining a spider;
step 2 – looking at a picture of a spider;
step 3 – seeing a spider from a distance in a jar;
step 4 – coming closer to the jar;
step 5 – handling the jar;
step 6 – seeing the spider out of the jar;
step 7 – handling the spider.

For very specific problems (e.g. a once-a-year holiday flight or a trip to the dentist), benzodiazepines can be given.

SOCIAL PHOBIA

CASE 9.5

A man aged 24 years became anxious when out with friends in the street. He was worried that he might do something embarrassing or that his friends would look on him in a poor light. He was afraid of shaking, blushing and sweating. He began to go out less with his friends, frequently walking behind the group to avoid conversation. He would always buy the first round in the pub so that he did not have to find a seat in the group but could sit a little apart from them on his return.

> Social phobia is characterized by fear of social situations in which:
>
> - the affected person is exposed to the gaze of others; and
> - they fear that they may do something embarrassing

Social situations are avoided or a companion is sought to help them in these situations.

The major problem in diagnosis of this disorder is distinguishing it from the personality difficulties of the chronically shy. There must be a discrete onset, usually following a bout of anxiety. People with social phobia usually have social skills but need to undergo relaxation training and a combination of cognitive therapy with exposure to the feared situation.

AGORAPHOBIA

CASE 9.6

A 74-year-old man was seen at home following a referral from his GP. He had a number of medical problems and had become depressed and irritable since the death of his dog. His wife had sat through the interview contributing little. When asked whether she visited family or friends she replied 'Oh no, I've not been out for 15 years. I'm agoraphobic'.

> ### The symptoms of agoraphobia
>
> - a fear of being in situations from which escape might be difficult or embarrassing
> - a fear of being in situations where help might not be available in the event of calamity or embarrassment
> - avoidance of these places

When away from home or in crowds the person develops anxiety symptoms, often with a fear that something awful will happen to them (e.g. that they might faint or lose control of their bowels or bladder). This fear can develop following an episode of anxiety in a public place. Afterwards, the possibility that the attacks might occur is sufficient to develop the anxiety (anticipatory anxiety).

The symptoms usually develop in the person's twenties or thirties and frequently do not come to the attention of professionals (see above), especially if a spouse supports the affected person and the need to go out is very limited. About one in 1000 people suffer from disabling agoraphobia. The disorder is more common in women than men.

Aetiology

- Psychoanalytical – a form of protection against unacceptable sexual or violent urges.
- Biological – as for all the other anxiety-related syndromes.
- Personality – dependent people are more prone to this disorder.

Treatment

- Exposure to the situation with anxiety management.
- Anxiolytics: used in the short term for specific events.
- Tricyclics: useful if there are high levels of depressive symptoms.
- Monoamine oxidase inhibitors.
  Note that there is a high rate of relapse if the medication is stopped.

Prognosis

If agoraphobia persists beyond 1 year the prognosis is poor. The course is likely to be punctuated with depressive episodes.

Generalized anxiety

CASE 9.7

I worry about everything. I haven't got anything to worry about, no money difficulties, a good husband; I've got my health. I shouldn't do it but I do. I know where the children are and I know they are safe, but what if something happened, you read about things, don't you?

People with generalized anxiety disorders worry in an unrealistic or excessive manner about things which others, and often they themselves, realize they have no real need to worry about. The basis of this disorder is outlined above.

Post-traumatic stress disorder

CASE 9.8

A woman aged 68 years was referred by her GP. A man had entered her flat 4 months previously, pushed her to the floor and stood on her back. He had demanded money, and while he was getting this she pressed her alarm button, at which point he ran, aiming a kick at her dog, which swallowed its teeth and later died. She had become nervous and depressed, and she lay awake at night listening for noises on the landing outside her flat. She found it difficult to go out, and avoided any groups of youths she saw in the street. She had a sensation that there was someone in the flat and she was about to be grabbed, as in the assault. She would jump at the least noise.

For people who are exposed to or witness a traumatic event there is usually a period of numbness and shock followed by short periods of anxiety and depression before they return to normal and begin to go about their everyday life once more.

COMMON REACTIONS TO STRESS

Psychological symptoms

- fear and worry
- feeling scared and miserable
- irritability
- feeling numb and detached
- loss of interest
- being jumpy and easily startled
- avoiding reminders of the incident
- 'action replays' in the mind
- feelings of guilt

Physical symptoms

- sleep problems
- bad dreams
- poor appetite
- shakiness and sweating
- tiredness
- poor concentration
- nausea and diarrhoea
- loss of sex drive

When these symptoms occur it is important to remember that they are normal, and to talk about the stressor rather than sweep it under the carpet. Using alcohol tends to delay the resolution of these feelings, whilst keeping the person's usual leisure activities is helpful.

A small group of people become 'stuck' in a recurring set of symptoms which continue over a long period of time. This syndrome is known as Post-Traumatic Stress Disorder (PTSD).

Features of post-traumatic stress disorder

- exposure to an event perceived as an extreme threat to oneself or others
- intrusive thoughts, feeling and perceptions related to the event (reliving the events in flashbacks and dreams)
- recurrent dreams related to the event
- avoidance of situations likely to trigger memories
- decreased interest in other matters
- increased vigilance
- hyperarousal with enhanced startle response
- sleep disturbance
- poor concentration

TRAUMATIC EVENTS

The events which produce this profound effect are ones that involve either threat to oneself or witnessing threat to others. Classic examples are large-scale disasters such as the Hillsborough Stadium Disaster in which many football fans were crushed to death. PTSD was found not only in those who were directly involved in the crush, but also in other spectators in the stadium and viewers of the television pictures if they had relatives in the stadium. Health care workers caught up in the aftermath of these situations can also develop the characteristic symptoms (see above list of features of PTSD).

This syndrome has been known in various guises for a long time. It was first recognized in relation to war (combat neurosis), and much work in the USA has focused on the veterans of the South East Asia conflict.

In addition to these large-scale public disasters, personal disasters, mugging, rape and assault can be equally likely to produce the symptoms.

The above cases demonstrate many of the cardinal symptoms of PTSD. The disorder is more common in the elderly, young children and those with a past history of psychiatric problems, but much of the research on the disorder has been conducted on the military, where one study found that 58 per cent of veterans of the South East Asia conflict had symptoms of PTSD, if not the full syndrome.

TREATMENT

Treatment takes a number of forms. Medication may be useful to treat severe anxiety and depressive symptoms, but unless the core problems are addressed patients are likely to relapse. A programme of psychotherapy, including anxiety management and exposure to the cues producing anxiety, and working through the feelings that the trauma has evoked, is needed.

Further reading

Marks, I.M. 1980: *Living with fear*. New York: McGraw Hill.

Marks, I.M. 1987: *Fears, phobias and rituals. Panic, anxiety and their disorders*. Oxford: Oxford University Press.

Nutt, D. and Lawson, C. 1992: Panic attacks. A neurochemical overview of models and mechanisms. *British Journal of Psychiatry* **160**, 165–78.

Snaith, P. 1993: *Clinical neurosis*. Oxford: Oxford University Press.

10 EATING DISORDERS

ANOREXIA NERVOSA

CASE 10.1

A woman aged 21 years was brought to the ward by her father. She had been unwell for the last 4 years, and she weighed only 4 stones (25.2 kg). She was angry and distressed, saying that there was no reason for her to be in the hospital and she would be all right if left alone. She ate little, often inducing vomiting, saying that she felt full and bloated. Despite her emaciated appearance she believed herself to look overweight, but was unable to say just how thin she would like to have been. She had gone through a period of using laxatives, and for some time had been taking her mother's diuretics in order to lose weight.

Diagnostic criteria for anorexia nervosa

- refusal to maintain a weight that is at least 85% of the minimum normal weight for the person's age, height and build
- intense fear of gaining weight or becoming fat
- a disturbance of the way in which the body is perceived
- amenorrhoea

People who suffer from anorexia nervosa frequently suppress their appetite in order to achieve a body weight that is significantly below the standard for their height, age and build. They are intensely fearful of being 'fat', even when they are grossly emaciated. They perceive themselves as fat despite the fact that their ribs are clearly visible and they have little muscle bulk. The other cardinal feature is amenorrhoea.

The disorder occurs mainly in young women (only 5 to 10 per cent of cases are men). It begins in adolescence, often after a schoolgirl has become over-concerned about 'puppy fat' and has begun to diet zealously. This rigorous dieting frequently masquerades as 'vegetarianism'. The woman may supplement self-imposed food restriction with other methods of losing weight, including energetic exercising and the abuse of appetite suppressants, purgatives and diuretics. Depression is common.

Associated physical findings

- emaciation
- bradycardia and hypotension
- hypothermia
- lanugo (fine downy hair on the body)
- peripheral oedema
- dental enamel erosion from persistent vomiting

Laboratory abnormalities

- anaemia and leucopenia
- dehydration
- hypothyroidism
- vomiting can induce a metabolic alkalosis
- liver function tests are abnormal
- low oestrogen or testosterone levels, depending on the sex of the individual

The prevalence of anorexia nervosa appears to be increasing, and it is now estimated to affect 1 to 2 per cent of schoolgirls and students. Social factors associated with anorexia nervosa include a cultural preference for a slim build, with intense advertising pressure from the fashion and 'slimming' industries. Certain occupations, such as ballet dancers, seem to be at greater risk. Psychologically at least some people with anorexia nervosa appear to be responding to the insecurities and loss of personal control associated with adolescence, and they assert their sense of personal autonomy by means of rigid control of food intake and consequently of weight.

About 20 per cent of people with anorexia nervosa make a full recovery. A further 20 per cent tend to suffer a severe unremitting course. The mortality is high (at least 15 per cent). Suicide is a common cause of death. Those who present later (after the age of 18 years) have a worse prognosis. The remaining 60 per cent have a chronic fluctuating course with periods of remission and intermittent restoration of menstruation. Many women with anorexia nervosa go on to develop bulimia nervosa (see below).

The prognosis in anorexia nervosa can be summarized as follows:

- later presentation has a poorer prognosis;
- 20 per cent of cases make complete recoveries;
- 20 per cent of cases have a chronic unremitting course;
- 60 per cent of cases have a chronic fluctuating course with remissions.

Treatment of anorexia nervosa

Admission to hospital is indicated if the person is severely depressed and at risk of suicide, or if their weight has fallen below 65 per cent of their standard body weight. Restoration of weight can only be achieved by the establishment of a sympathetic rapport between the anorexic person and the nursing and medical staff. The aim is to achieve an agreed target weight which will be between the persons own 'ideal' and the standardized norm. Three gently supervised meals a day, aiming for a total daily calorie intake of 2000 kcal, is the usual regime. In the early stages the person may be nursed in bed, and careful surveillance for self-induced vomiting or for hiding food is required. Individual and family psychotherapy are essential elements of the regimen. Above all,

it is important to reassure the sufferer that there is no intention of making them exceed the agreed weight.

Some units use an operant behavioural programme in which the person is rewarded with privileges such as being allowed to watch television or exercise if they are making satisfactory progress. If behavioural programmes of this type are introduced, it is important to avoid presenting them in a way that could be interpreted as punitive, since this simply reinforces the anorexic person's sense of oppression.

Management of anorexia nervosa

- admit to hospital the very depressed or suicidal, and all those below 65 per cent of their standard body weight
- agree a target weight between the person's 'ideal' and the standard weight
- reassure the person that this target weight will not be exceeded
- provide individual and family psychotherapy
- beware of behavioural regimens

BULIMIA NERVOSA

CASE 10.2

A woman aged 26 years presented to out-patients. She was anxious and depressed, and she felt unable to perform her day-to-day activities. Her days were dominated by food. She was unable to balance how much she ate, and she would feel compelled to eat large amounts, only to feel so disgusted with herself afterwards that she had to vomit to rid herself of the food. Unless she had got this balance right she was unable to go out.

Bulimia nervosa is characterized by recurrent binge eating, with feelings of loss of control, together with self-induced vomiting and/or the use of purgatives to control weight. Despite the 'dietary chaos', body weight remains fairly constant. As with anorexia nervosa, there is a morbid preoccupation with bodily dimensions and shape. The person's sense of self-worth depends to a large degree on their perception of their weight and body shape. The sufferer is consumed with guilt and self-disgust after each episode of binging, and depression is a common feature of the disorder. Repeated vomiting can cause potassium depletion with weakness, renal damage and even cardiac arrhythmias. The enamel of the teeth becomes eroded by the gastric acid.

Diagnostic features of bulimia nervosa

- recurrent binging, with lack of control of eating during the binge
- repeated vomiting, purging, etc., in order to reduce weight
- self-evaluation is influenced by body shape and weight

The prevalence of the disorder is 1 to 3 per cent in adolescent and young women. It usually begins in adolescence or young adulthood after an episode of dieting. Frequently the disorder is long-standing before treatment is sought. For many sufferers the course is a chronic relapsing one with episodes emerging at times of stress.

Management of bulimia nervosa

Cognitive behavioural therapy is the treatment of choice. The person is asked to identify those moods, feelings, situations and activities which tend to trigger bouts of overeating. Common precipitants are boredom, loneliness or feelings of rejection. People are helped either to avoid these triggers or to find more constructive strategies for dealing with them. If depression is severe, then antidepressant medication might be beneficial. In some cases selective serotonin reuptake inhibitors (SSRIs, e.g. paroxetine) help to reduce the frequency of binging even in the absence of a depressive illness, but relapse is rapid once the drugs have been withdrawn.

Further reading

Brownel, K.D. and Fairburn, C.G. 1995: *Eating disorders and obesity: a comprehensive handbook*. New York: Guilford Press.

Hsu, L.K.G. 1990: *Eating disorders*. New York: Guilford Press.

11 POST-PARTUM PSYCHIATRIC DISORDERS

CASE 11.1

A woman aged 38 years with no previous psychiatric history gave birth to a baby boy after a long and difficult labour. The couple had been waiting for a child for the previous 6 years. A junior doctor who was known to have an interest in psychiatry was asked to see the woman 3 days after delivery. She was tearful with a rapidly fluctuating mood, concerned whether she was fit to be a mother, and quite overwhelmed by the experience of childbirth. There were no overt signs of major depression, psychosis or delirium. She settled down over the next couple of days with support from the midwives, and became ready to face the challenge of her new baby.

Having a child produces some of the most profound physiological changes that a woman can experience. It can also cause emotional reactions of astonishing force for both of the parents, who have to adapt and realign their lives and relationship to the presence of the child. It is small wonder, then, that childbirth is associated with a number of psychiatric disorders.

Psychiatric disorders associated with childbirth

- maternity blues
- puerperal psychosis
- chronic depressive disorder

MATERNITY BLUES

These occur in 50 to 70 per cent of women, especially on the third or fourth day after delivery (see Case 11.1). There is lability of mood, tearfulness, tension and irritability. The cause of these changes is unknown. Maternity blues resolve spontaneously and do not require any specific treatment beyond support and reassurance. They are more common in the first pregnancy, in those depressed during the last trimester and in those with a history of premenstrual tension (PMT). They are not related to complications at delivery.

Features of maternity blues

- onset occurs 2 to 3 days after delivery
- resolves rapidly
- characterized by lability of mood, tearfulness and irritability
- more common following first delivery, in those depressed during the last trimester, and in those with a history of PMT

PUERPERAL PSYCHOSIS

CASE 11.2

A woman aged 18 years gave birth to her first child uneventfully. She returned to her parents' flat where 14 days later she began to take less good care of the baby, and stayed out late in a bar when she had told her parents she was going to the shop. She was elated and grandiose, believing she and her child had been chosen for special purposes. However, she claimed that some people were out to stop her mission and damage her and the baby. She knew this was so because she heard God telling her this and had seen it on television. She was admitted to a mother and baby unit where small doses of haloperidol soon resolved her symptoms and she was able to care for her child normally.

Psychotic illnesses occur following one in every 500 births. They are commonly affective in nature (see Case 11.2), but in 20 per cent schizophrenia-like illnesses occur. Some have an 'organic flavour' with disorientation, but these have become rare since the decrease in puerperal sepsis. The onset is usually in the first couple of weeks following delivery. Such disorders are more common in primipara and in those with a previous or family history of psychotic illness.

These illnesses carry a risk of suicide, and it is important to detect the development of delusional ideas about the baby (e.g. that it is a dangerous monster, or the Devil) as these can lead to the mother harming the child.

The mother and child should be managed in a specialist mother and baby unit wherever possible. Here the nursing staff are trained to care for the babies, in addition to their mental nursing skills. This helps to preserve the developing bond between mother and child at a time when separation may be critical. Conventional treatments for depression, mania or schizophrenia are used (including ECT) and the prognosis for immediate recovery is good, but there is a high risk of recurrence (15 to 20 per cent), especially in subsequent pregnancies, which should be monitored closely.

Features of puerperal psychosis

- frequency of 1 in every 500 births
- more common with first child, or in those with previous or family psychiatric history
- affective, schizophrenic and 'organic' forms
- short-term response to treatment is good
- 15 to 20 per cent of cases experience a relapse at next delivery
- 50 per cent subsequently develop non-puerperal depressions

About 50 per cent will develop depressive illnesses later in life that are not puerperal.

MILD TO MODERATE DEPRESSION

A depressive illness starting about 2 weeks after childbirth is experienced by 10 to 15 per cent of women. There is often a history of previous depression, recent adverse life events and marital conflict. These problems occur in vulnerable mothers who find the adjustment to their new routine difficult and who lack social support. Psychological and social interventions are most important, with medication indicated for those whose symptoms are severe and persistent. A small number (5 per cent) develop persistent dysphoria.

Features of mild to moderate depression

- 10 to 15 per cent of cases develop depression
- commences 2 weeks after the birth
- usually occurs in vulnerable mothers who lack social support
- social and psychological interventions are important
- medication is needed if symptoms are persistent or severe
- 5 per cent of cases develop chronic illnesses

PSYCHOTROPIC DRUGS IN PREGNANCY AND POST-PARTUM

Great caution must be exercised in the prescribing of psychotropic drugs in pregnancy and during breast-feeding.

Lithium

Lithium should not be prescribed in pregnancy or during breast-feeding for the following reasons:

- lithium taken during the first trimester can cause cardiac malformations in the fetus (atrialization of the right ventricle);
- during pregnancy the clearance of lithium by the kidneys steadily increases, but it falls

abruptly just after delivery, causing a dangerous rise in serum lithium levels;

- lithium is secreted in breast milk, and if the infant develops diarrhoea, serum lithium levels rise sharply and can rapidly reach toxic levels.

All patients of childbearing age must be counselled about these risks and appropriate contraception discussed.

Tricyclics and neuroleptics

There is no conclusive evidence that neuroleptics have a teratogenic effect, but they should only be prescribed if there are strong indications. Occasionally neonates show side-effects of the drugs taken by their mothers, including extrapyramidal signs, and cardiovascular dysfunction and withdrawal phenomena from tricyclic antidepressants.

Neuroleptics and tricyclic antidepressants are secreted in the breast milk in small quantities. If possible, breast-feeding should be avoided, but if the mother insists on it, the drug should be given in divided doses and the baby's condition should be carefully monitored.

Benzodiazepines

Benzodiazepines taken late in pregnancy can cause floppy infant syndrome or withdrawal symptoms in the neonate.

Psychotropic drugs that cross the placenta

- tricyclic antidepressants
- SSRIs (there is no evidence of harm caused by these drugs, but caution is recommended by the manufacturers)
- Lithium
- Carbamazepine
- Barbiturates
- Benzodiazepines
- Neuroleptics
- Clozapine
- Opioids

Psychotropic drugs secreted in the breast milk

- Amphetamines
- Tricyclic antidepressants
- Barbiturates
- Neuroleptics
- Lithium
- Benzodiazepines.

The pregnant drug addict

Opiates cross the placenta (see above), and the fetus becomes dependent upon them and suffers withdrawal symptoms if the mother stops taking them. Withdrawal may precipitate fetal distress, induce premature labour or cause the death of the fetus. The fetus is also susceptible to overdoses. There is a high incidence of prematurity and low birth weight.

Ideally the pregnant addict should be weaned off opiates, using methadone cover, at least 2 months before the expected date of delivery. Gradual reduction of the methadone dose prevents fetal distress or premature labour. If the mother refuses to withdraw from opiates or if the expected date of delivery is too close, then she is offered the lowest possible dose of oral methadone necessary to prevent withdrawal symptoms (i.e. 25 mg daily or less). If the mother is receiving a prescription for opioids, these can be continued in labour in order to provide analgesia. There is no specific contraindication to epidural analgesia.

If the mother is HIV-positive she should be counselled about the increased risk to herself of the development of AIDS if the pregnancy continues, and the very high risk of the baby being born HIV-positive as well.

The abstinence syndrome in the neonate includes hyperactivity, irritability, restlessness, tremulousness and sometimes convulsions and vomiting. If the mother is taking methadone the withdrawal syndrome may not develop in the neonate for 48 to 72 hours. The withdrawal symptoms in the neonate are treated with low doses of chlorpromazine.

Features and management of the pregnant drug addict

- opiates cross the placenta
- the infant may suffer withdrawal problems, premature birth or death
- it is best to detoxify the mother at least 2 months before the expected date of delivery, or to maintain her on low-dose methadone

Further reading

Brockington, I.F. and Kumar, R. 1982: *Motherhood and mental illness.* London: Academic Press.

Kumar, R. and Brockington, I.F. 1988: *Motherhood and mental illness II: Causes and consequences.* London: Wright.

PART

3

SPECIAL TOPICS

12 ANTHROPOLOGY AND PSYCHIATRY

A 32-year-old woman of West African origin was admitted to hospital under Section 2 of the Mental Health Act. She had presented as a result of increasingly bizarre behaviour in her flat. She had daubed religious symbols in red paint on all the doors, kept the curtains closed and could be heard wailing late into the night. She was hostile and largely mute on admission. She was treated with antipsychotics and settled on the ward, but continued to say little about her experiences. The psychiatrists treating her were unsure if this represented a first schizophrenic illness or a way of expressing distress which was culturally sanctioned. Her brother later said that she was sent by the family to train in this country, but her college course had not gone well and her current employment as a secretary was also causing problems. She felt increasing pressure from her family, who perceived her performance abroad as one of failure, but did not regard her behaviour as in any sense understandable despite these social pressures.

The social sciences can help clinicians to understand the effect on mental health of (1) environmental factors and (2) social change.

Social factors influencing mental health

ENVIRONMENTAL FACTORS

- Poverty
- Racial discrimination
- Poor housing
- Poor health care

SOCIAL CHANGE

- Unemployment
- Migration
- Urbanization

The contribution of anthropology has been to define the influence of culture on views of causation and appropriate treatment of mental disorders. When the cultural backgrounds of the patient and the clinician are divergent, they might not share basic assumptions about the probable origin, nature and treatment of mental disorders (see Case 12.1).

CULTURAL INFLUENCES

Culture has been defined by Cecil Helman (a GP and anthropologist) as a set of guidelines by which the individuals of a particular society view the world, experience it emotionally and behave in relation to other people, to the supernatural and to nature.

Culture is transmitted down the generations by language, symbols and rituals. Cultures are neither static nor homogeneous, and the differences between members of one cultural group can be as great as the differences between members of different cultural groups. It is important not to blame culture for economic and social hardship and racial discrimination. Thus overcrowding might be due to poverty and/or discrimination in housing, rather than to the 'extended family'.

The influences of culture include:

- patients' illness behaviour;
- the content of delusions and hallucinations;
- attitudes of the family and community;
- assumptions regarding the recognition and aetiology of illness;
- the appropriateness of treatment.

Arthur Kleinman (an anthropologist and psychiatrist) has developed the concept of Explanatory Models in order to understand the cultural influences each person brings to his or her illness. In non-industrialized small-scale societies, social causes of both mental and physical illness (e.g. envy, the evil eye, witchcraft) and supernatural causes (e.g. malign spirit possession) are common explanations for sickness. In Western societies, aetiologies tend to be physiological (e.g. imbalance, deficiency, heredity) or environmental (e.g. viruses, allergens). These aetiological explanations are not mutually exclusive, and for many patients the explanation is multi-factorial.

Explanatory Models incorporate:

- culture-specific ideas of aetiology, pathophysiology, treatment and prognosis;
- the contributory role of the individual in relation to the illness;
- the contributory role of the individual's social milieu in relation to the illness.

CASE 12.2

The mother of a teenage Turkish Cypriot with paraparesis due to a paravertebral neurofibroma refused to allow surgical intervention. The clinical team attempted to explain that the operation had to be carried out immediately if the boy was to be spared irreversible paraplegia. When the distressed mother persisted in her refusal, a psychiatrist was called in to deal with her 'hysteria'. Through an interpreter, the psychiatrist managed to elicit her 'explanatory model'. According to a Muslim folk tradition the patient has to wear a talisman for a prescribed period before resorting to the Western biomedical approach. The psychiatrist explained the urgency of the situation to the local imam, who intervened to persuade the boy's mother that recourse to

supernatural healing had to give way to surgery in this particular case if the boy were ever to walk again.

Idioms of distress

These are culturally standardized ways of expressing grief, unhappiness, frustration, guilt and helplessness. Each culture has its own language of distress which mediates between the subjective experience of impaired well-being and social acknowledgement of this internal state. Culture also determines which symptoms are regarded as abnormal, and how they are shaped into an illness which entitles the individual to enter into the 'sick role'.

The language of distress, if unfamiliar, might make you think that your patient is suffering from a psychotic illness:

- bewitchment: paranoid delusions;
- possession: passivity phenomena;
- vivid fantasy: hallucinations.

Each of these 'symptoms' can only be correctly interpreted within its cultural milieu.

Talk of witchcraft might simply be an attribution, i.e. a culturally shaped explanation for misfortune, including affliction with physical or mental illness. Western biomedicine deals with the 'how' of disease but, unlike many traditional systems, it ignores the question of 'why' that particular person has become ill at that particular time. All cultures recognize insanity. Universal stereotypes of madness are based on behavioural criteria.

Universal aspects of madness include:

- unprovoked violence;
- incomprehensible speech;
- gross self-neglect;
- purposeless self-injury.

Universality vs. cultural specificity

Those psychiatric disorders with largely biological bases, such as schizophrenia and bipolar affective disorder, occur with relatively uniform frequency in all cultures. The form and pattern of these disorders is universally recognizable. The content of hallucinations and delusions obviously varies, and often reflects and articulates local preoccupations, symbols, images and icons. Electronic bugging devices might form the content of hallucinations and delusions in industrial societies, while concern about neglected ancestors might preoccupy a psychotic patient in developing areas of the Third World. Both the patient's and the local community's understanding of the cause and the appropriate treatment will also be culture-specific. We talk of 'stress' and 'breakdown' (engineering metaphors), in contrast to a villager in Mali or an ultra-orthodox Jew who might attribute a psychotic episode to violation of a religious taboo or failure to carry out a cleansing ritual ('personalistic' explanations).

Somatization

This is the cultural patterning of psychological discomfort ('dysphoria') into the language of bodily distress which employs the idiom of physical ill health, especially pain, weakness and fatigue. It cannot be regarded as a purely non-Western phenomenon, since it is commonly found in those who have little ability to 'psychologize', i.e. to express worry, depression and anxiety verbally (see Chapter 13). The expression of psychological distress in Western cultures depends much upon the language of the mind/body split. Where the relationship between mind and body is conceived differently (as in the Indian subcontinent), a different, usually somatic, language is employed to express psychological distress.

Culture and psychiatric diagnosis

Understanding the cultural background of your patient is important not only in order to avoid over-diagnosis, but also to avoid under-diagnosis and failure to treat a very ill person (see Case 12.1 above).

Common pitfalls

- A particular religious belief or ritual which is acceptable in your own culture becomes labelled as delusional in another culture.
- Bizarre behaviour of your patient from an unfamiliar culture may be wrongly attributed to 'culture' rather than individual psychopathology.
- Distress due to interpersonal conflict (marital tension or parent/child conflict) might be inappropriately dismissed as being due to 'culture' (arranged marriages or puritanical child-rearing).

Witchcraft as attribution, content or precipitant

A distressed person from a cultural background where beliefs in witchcraft are not uncommon, such as West Africa, may claim to be the victim of witchcraft. In these circumstances you should consider the following four possibilities.

- The person may have suffered a misfortune – e.g. an untimely bereavement, serious accident, or severe physical or mental illness – which they *attribute* to malevolent envy.
- The person may have become acutely anxious or terrified because they have reason to believe that a rival has used witchcraft against them. They may then present with severe reactive depression or even a brief reactive psychosis (witchcraft fear as *precipitant*).
- The person may experience a psychotic illness in which hallucinations or thought removal, thought insertion, or thought broadcasting are *attributed* to witchcraft.
- Witchcraft may provide the *content* or themes of delusions and/or hallucinations.

Migration and mental illness

Immigrants have higher rates of mental illness than either the population of their country of origin or that of the host country. Examples include alcoholism in Irish immigrants to England, paranoid psychosis in East European refugees, and schizophrenia in migrants from the new Commonwealth to the UK. Various issues have acted as confounding factors and inflated these figures:

- misinterpretation of cultural beliefs;
- the immigrants are mostly young men, i.e. those most at risk of psychotic illness.

Explanatory hypotheses include:

- selection – restless marginal people migrate in the hope of solving their personal problems;
- stress – migration itself causes problems of language, accommodation, employment, isolation and conflict.

These two major hypotheses have been proposed for the increased rate of illness in immigrants. Selection and stress may work together in some individuals. Refugees undergo a 'cultural bereavement' with permanent and traumatic loss of their roots. They will also have been subjected to a great deal of physical and emotional trauma and deprivation.

CASE 12.3

A woman aged 54 years from South America presented to the emergency clinic. Weeping and wailing loudly, she threw herself around the room. An artist in her own country, she had been held and tortured by the regime in power. She later escaped and had been living in the UK for 4 years. She kept in contact only with compatriots, and had undergone extensive therapy for the effects of her torture, but with little effect. She continued to display disturbed behaviour, making it hard for her friends to care for her.

Further reading

Dein, S. and Lipsedge, M. 1995: Negotiating across class, culture and religion: psychiatry in the English inner city. In Opaku, S. (ed.), *Clinical methods in transcultural psychiatry*. Washington: American Psychiatric Press.

Littlewood, R. and Lipsedge, M. 1987: The butterfly and the serpent: culture, psychopathology and biomedicine. *Culture, Medicine and Society* **11**, 289–335.

Littlewood, R. and Lipsedge, M. 1989: *Aliens and alienists: ethnic minorities and psychiatry*. London: Routledge.

13 LIAISON PSYCHIATRY AND SOMATOFORM DISORDERS

The relationship between physical and mental disorders is a complex one. There is no doubt that in all populations there is a strong association between physical illness and psychiatric illness (especially in the elderly), which can take a number of forms.

CASE 13.1

A 72-year-old man was admitted urgently to a health care of the elderly ward with a serious respiratory infection. He was unable to give much history on admission, but he recovered well with an antibiotic given intravenously. He was seen each day by the junior doctors, but just before the consultant's round in his second week of admission he attempted to cut his wrists with a fruit knife. This was because of pain in his calf due to vascular disease. The doctors kept telling him how good his chest was and gave him no time to talk about his other problems. He did well following a lumbar sympathectomy and antidepressant treatment.

RELATIONSHIP OF PHYSICAL TO PSYCHIATRIC ILLNESS

This can take a number of forms:

■ coincidental (a person with schizophrenia contracts influenza);

■ the physical illness causes the psychiatric symptoms (e.g. delirium or depression secondary to hypothyroidism);

■ the psychiatric illness is presented as a physical one (somatization);

■ the psychiatric illness causes the physical problems (e.g. dehydration in depression, alcohol abuse, deliberate self-harm);

■ the psychiatric symptoms stop treatment for a physical illness (e.g. a demented man with retention of urine cannot give informed consent for a prostatectomy);

■ the relationship between the two is unclear (e.g. a person who, after a stroke, fails to mobilize and is miserable);

■ the treatment of the physical illness causes psychiatric disorder, or vice versa (e.g. digoxin causing delirium or fluoxetine induced syndrome of inappropriate antidiuretic hormone secretion (SIADH)).

On medical wards the level of recognition of psychiatric disorder by the surgeons and physicians is frequently low. It is estimated that 20 per cent of people in medical wards have significant psychiatric morbidity, including alcoholism, but only a small proportion of these are referred for specialist advice.

Reasons people are not referred to psychiatrists

- the recognition of psychiatric problems is limited because:
  a. recognition and treatment of organic disease is considered to be sufficient
  b. education is limited
  c. doctors are not used to dealing with emotional issues
- The usefulness of recognizing psychiatric problems is not appreciated because:
  a. psychiatric problems are not regarded as treatable
  b. recognition of psychiatric issues causes more problems
  c. psychiatric problems are not believed to influence organic disease
- The usefulness of psychiatrists is not appreciated because:
  a. working relationships are poor
  b. they talk a different language
  c. they might appear to offer no solutions
- There is not time to explore issues of a psychological nature on busy medical wards

The role of the liaison psychiatrist

The role of the liaison psychiatrist

- to make links with other disciplines
- to identify psychiatric disorder
- to assess its relevance to any existing organic disorder
- to provide a management plan for the individual in consultation with the physicians and surgeons
- to communicate with all staff so that this plan can be executed
- teaching

The psychiatrist working on medical wards has a number of roles, none perhaps more important than establishing the links between the disciplines involved with the care of the patients. However, these extend much further, as outlined above.

Common reasons for referring to a liaison psychiatrist

- no organic cause for the physical ailment is found
- the ailment continues despite 'appropriate' treatment
- behavioural disturbance on the ward
- overt psychiatric disorder
- patient appears to be unable to manage at home

SOMATIZATION DISORDER

CASE 13.2

A woman aged 34 years presented to her family doctor with vague complaints of pain in the legs. Her file was thicker than all those of the rest of the clinic put together. Over the previous 15 years she had been investigated by urologists, gynaecologists, endocrinologists and several gastroenterologists. She had been cystoscoped twice, endoscoped twice, had been given a barium enema, four abdominal ultrasound examinations, two laparoscopies and examinations under anaesthesia, in addition to numerous plain X-rays and blood tests.

Problems caused by somatization

- excessive use of health resources
- moving from doctor to doctor, or from hospital to hospital
- complaints are not assuaged by negative findings
- hostility develops between patients and doctors
- patients and doctors fail to appreciate the importance of psychological factors in developing symptomatology

Somatization is an important concept for all clinicians. In 20 per cent of attenders in primary care there does not appear to be an organic basis for the symptoms reported, and for psychiatrists in liaison services in general hospitals one third of their referrals will be for cases involving somatization.

The essential nature of somatization is the expression of psychological stress through bodily symptoms. This may occur in the presence of physical illness, but the symptoms expressed are out of proportion to the perceived illness.

Presentation

People who somatize present to medical services with physical complaints which the doctor is unable to explain in organic terms. Either no abnormality is found, or only minor abnormalities which do not account for the intensity of the symptoms. This finding and its explanation frequently lead to animosity between the sufferer and the doctor.

The presentation may be acute, e.g. with chest pain to an Accident and Emergency department, but is more likely to be insidious, with repeated consultations and referrals until it is realized that a somatization disorder is present.

Epidemiology

Whilst somatization of a mild nature is frequently seen in primary care, the more severe forms of hypochondriasis and somatoform disorders are rare. It is suggested that in some cultures emotional distress is much more commonly shown as physical distress, perhaps because the western dichotomy of mind and body is not universally recognized.

Sensations occurring as a result of stress and of previous experience of illness lead to the belief that the person has a physical illness. This abnormal interpretation is then maintained through a series of reinforcements (Figure 13.1). Why any particular individual should do this is unclear, but a number of factors may contribute.

SOCIAL FACTORS

In some cultures it is unacceptable to express psychological distress, so physical manifestations of emotional turmoil or conflict are more likely. In order to see a doctor you need a physical complaint to legitimize your visit.

ENVIRONMENTAL FACTORS

Early experiences of your own and family illness contribute to 'illness behaviour' in later life. At times of illness, parents take more notice of a child

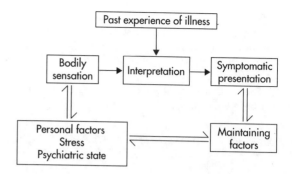

FIG 13.1 Maintaining factors in Somatization Disorder.

or a husband takes more notice of their spouse. An unacknowledged desire to get attention or recapture the warm feeling of parental concern contributes to future behaviour.

PERSONAL FACTORS

The personality of the individual, their coping strategies or the presence of a psychiatric illness all contribute to the development of the syndrome.

MAINTAINING FACTORS (Figure 13.1)

Doctors do a great deal to maintain people in this role with repeated investigations and consultations. There is often a failure to provide clear explanations and appropriate treatment early in the career of the somatizer. Other doctors may respond positively to the person when he or she is ill and not when they are 'well'. Some illnesses serve to reduce family discord. The presence of a personality or psychiatric disorder will help maintain the behaviour.

Diagnosis

Somatization is a common presentation of other psychiatric disorders. Depression is the most common of these, but anxiety disorders also present in this way (see Chapter 8 on mood disorders). The rapid heartbeat of a panic attack or paraesthesia following hyperventilation can suggest physical illness. Rarely, schizophrenia may present in this way.

CASE 13.3

A 21-year-old man was referred to an open-access endoscopy clinic. He had reported abdominal pains to his family doctor. When his history was taken in greater detail he revealed that he believed these to be due to a radio receiver planted in his abdomen which could control his mind and actions.

These other psychiatric disorders must be ruled out before the diagnosis is made.

Management of Somatoform Disorder

When engaging the person in treatment, it is necessary to explore:

- the person's attitude to the referral;
- the person's reactions to previous treatment;
- the person's attitudes to his or her symptoms;
- what people actually do (diaries may be of use here).

This group of people is difficult to engage in treatment. 'You think I'm mad', 'It's not all in my mind' and 'You think it is not real' are all common responses to the suggestion that the person should see a psychiatrist.

In order to engage the person, you must be prepared to listen in a sympathetic manner to their complaints and gauge their reaction to the referral. It is useful to bring up the issue of stress, how it can make physical problems worse, and how you might be able to help the person to learn to cope with such problems more effectively in the future. People are often caught in a vicious circle in which (1) increased physiological arousal (e.g. increased heart rate) leads to (2) focusing the person's attention upon the effects of that arousal, leading to (3) increased checking (e.g. taking the pulse again and again). Explorations of their disappointments with the medical profession and correction of their mistaken beliefs about these can be of help.

A period of self-monitoring (diary-keeping) in order to look at the events, feelings and thoughts that occur around with the physical symptoms can help to identify the factors that are maintaining or exacerbating the problem.

Treatment depends upon these maintaining factors. The thrust of all treatments is to look at coping strategies and cognitive approaches to the reassignment (relabelling) of the physical experiences.

This can be achieved by simple demonstrations (e.g. to show how tense muscles cause pain, try holding this book on your outstretched arm for 3 minutes), as well as by more complex explorations

of trigger situations (e.g. family rows). Any psychiatric illness present should receive treatment independently.

Principles of treatment

- acknowledge that the symptoms are not 'imaginary'
- give the person information about basic physiology
- elicit from the person the observations that have led them to conclude that they have a serious illness
- monitor health-related thoughts in the light of their new knowledge
- keep a written record of the activities and situations which are associated with the physical problems
- give instruction in relaxation techniques, assertiveness and graded exposure to difficult situations

Maintaining factors

- family discord
- psychiatric illness, e.g. depressive illness, anxiety state
- personality disorder
- social and occupational problems

Poor prognostic features

- absence of anxiety or depression
- strong belief in a physical cause
- chronic symptoms
- symptoms not made worse by stress
- no life events prior to the onset of the symptoms

SUBTYPES OF SOMATOFORM DISORDER

General subtypes include:

- somatization disorder;

- conversion disorder;
- hypochondriasis.

Specific subtypes include:

- somatoform pain disorder;
- body dysmorphic disorder;
- chronic fatigue syndrome.

SOMATIZATION DISORDER (BRIQUET'S SYNDROME)

See Case 13.1.

Features of somatization disorder

- multiple complaints in several physical systems
- no physical basis demonstrated
- several years in duration
- onset generally below the age of 30 years
- the person frequently consults the doctor about these problems
- the person has changed their lifestyle as a result of this

People who suffer from a wide range of persistent physical complaints without an underlying organic cause represent a considerable drain on resources and are difficult to deal with at all levels of medical expertise. They suffer greatly and may develop iatrogenic complications.

Aetiology

Aetiological factors

- heightened awareness of bodily sensations
- misinterpretations of bodily sensations
- family illness during childhood
- separation and loss during childhood
- genetic factors

The aetiology of the disorder is complex and multifactorial. The evidence for genetic influences is limited, and it is perhaps better explained as learned behaviour towards illness.

Treatment

Treatment is limited. It is recommended that a single physician looks after the person over a long period of time, so that they are able to listen sympathetically to the person and not respond to each new symptom with a medical investigation or referral. A cognitive therapy approach helps to change the attribution from a morbid cause to a normal, physiological response.

CONVERSION DISORDER (HYSTERIA)

CASE 13.4

A 55-year-old woman claimed to have suddenly become blind. She was born in India, but now lived in the UK with her husband and four children. The husband drank heavily and was frequently violent within the family home. Her physical examination was unremarkable. On the ward she sat quietly and would talk calmly about the severity of her visual problems. She was able to find her way about the ward without accidents. She said that there were no problems in her home life.

CASE 13.5

A middle-aged man was brought into the Accident and Emergency department by the British Transport police. He had been found in a dazed state at a London train station, and was unable to recall his name, age, address, family or profession. Using a combination of suggestion and intravenous diazepam he regained his memory. It transpired that he was from Manchester and had learnt that morning that he had contracted a venereal disease. He took the next train to London while experiencing a fugue state which gave him temporary respite from his predicament.

In conversion disorder there is an alteration or loss of physical functioning. Episodes of loss of function are usually acute, but can become chronic. Such episodes frequently follow a stressful event which the person is unable to resolve. Taking on the sick role provides a way of reducing the psychological tension (primary gain). In addition, this creates a short-term resolution of the problem, and the person also receives the attention of others (secondary gain). The patient may show little concern for himself or herself, despite the severity of the loss of function (*la belle indifférence*).

This form of illness appears to be increasingly rare in western/urban medicine, but remains common in more rural communities.

Treatment has been by hypnosis, psychoanalytical techniques, behavioural treatments to reduce positive reinforcement, and diversion away from the physical problems to the psychological ones. Physiotherapy may be needed if the problem involves a limb, to ensure that full function is maintained.

Features of conversion disorder

- loss of function
- reduction in psychological distress (primary gain)
- resolution of stressful situation
- attention from others (secondary gain)
- indifference to the loss (*la belle indifférence*)

HYPOCHONDRIASIS

CASE 13.6

A 59-year-old man came to the clinic asking for help because he had been 'rapidly going downhill for 10 years'. He had multiple physical complaints ranging from problems with his bowels to the loss of fat from the back of his head, which he believed was indicative of a serious health problem. He repeatedly visited his family doctor to seek reassurance or further investigation.

The central feature of hypochondriasis is that the person experiences his or her bodily sensations as being due to illness when in fact they are quite normal. Having made this attribution they then seek reassurance about the sensations. The severity of this condition varies enormously. At one end of the spectrum it involves one-off consultations, while at the other it involves repeated trips from one physician to another, with invasive investigations and the potential for serious iatrogenic damage.

Hypochondriasis may be secondary to another psychiatric problem (e.g. depression) which needs to be treated in its own right.

Treatment with serotonergic antidepressants only leads to limited success unless there is a large depressive component. More recently, cognitive behavioural psychotherapy has been used to treat the condition. Chronic hypochondriasis can cause exasperated doctors to overlook the development of grave physical illness.

CASE 13.7

A man aged 45 years had a long history of hypochondriasis. His wife, GP and psychiatrist were dismissive of a new complaint of abdominal pain. His weight then decreased alarmingly and he was found to have an inoperable carcinoma of the pancreas.

SOMATOFORM PAIN DISORDER

Pain is a common complaint, and it is frequently difficult to find the source of the problem or to relate the severity of the subjective complaint to any discernible lesion.

CASE 13.8

A 28-year-old woman attended the back clinic. She had experienced pain in her lumbar region over the last 4 years. She had married a rather unsatisfactory partner, believing that with her level of incapacity no one else would have her. They had a child whom she could not pick up, and whom she could only play with for short periods. She was spending more and more time on the sofa and doing less about the house. She rarely went out and as a result she saw few people. Her mood became depressed.

Assessment of pain

- sensory component
- affective component
- behavioural effects
- effects on lifestyle
- psychological coping strategies

The assessment of pain explores a number of elements. It requires a view not only of its sensory component (mild, severe, etc.) but also of the affective component (punishing, cruel, etc.). It is important to see how people respond to their pain (e.g. how much time they spend in bed, how much medication they take) and what effect the pain is having on their overall lifestyle (have they lost a job, friends, etc.?). The psychological strategies the patient has used to date provide a baseline from which more effective ones can be built.

Treatment of chronic pain

This can be achieved by behavioural, cognitive, and relaxation methods.

Behavioural methods

These aim to promote healthy behaviours and to reduce pain behaviours, but make no direct assault on the pain itself. This treatment is received as an in-patient, under which circumstances pain behaviours are ignored and healthy behaviours rewarded with social reinforcement in combination with an ever progressing exercise programme.

Cognitive approaches

A number of methods that aim to alter the experience of pain have been used, often accompanied by relaxation training.

Relaxation methods

Relaxation techniques can help the patient both to understand and to control their bodily feelings.

BODY DYSMORPHIC DISORDER

CASE 13.9

A woman aged 26 years presented to the plastic surgeons after multiple requests to her family doctor for referral. She believed her nose was too large and this resulted in her failure to advance at work and to maintain a long-term relationship. She had experienced a difficult upbringing in a turbulent family, making her distrustful of close relationships and lacking in confidence. Although it was repeatedly pointed out that her nose was quite normal, and she admitted there was a possibility that these other factors may have had an influence on her problems, she continued to sue for corrective surgery.

Body dysmorphic disorder includes a whole spectrum of beliefs. There are few of us who would not change some part of our anatomy given the chance, but this is rarely (although increasingly in some cultures) pursued surgically. At the other end of the spectrum it fades into monosymptomatic hypochondriacal delusions (see Chapter 7 on schizophrenia).

This preoccupation with a subjectively perceived abnormality can lead to unnecessary surgery with all its attendant risks. This group is rarely seen by psychiatrists.

FATIGUE

CASE 13.10

A 24-year-old man worked out or played sport each day. He had previously been fit and well and had experienced no serious illness or injuries. After a 2-week period when he had influenza and did nothing active he went straight back to training at his old level. He rapidly became fatigued, his muscles ached and he was unable to complete his programme. This happened several times. He became distressed and did less and less. Each time he attempted his old schedule he failed once more. He believed that he was still infected and needed an antibiotic to cure him. An explanation of the effects of inactivity and a graded activity programme slowly returned him to his previous level of functioning.

Fatigue is a common complaint in all populations. Ten per cent of primary care attenders report fatigue as one of their symptoms. The person who complains of being tired all the time ('TATT') is difficult to deal with in the limited time available to most family practitioners.

CASE 13.11

A married woman aged 45 years with three children in their teens came to the surgery complaining of being 'tired all the time'. She was overweight and believed that her problem was 'glandular'. It emerged that she was working as a cleaner to support the family whilst her husband and older child were out of work. Her mother-in-law, who had dementia, was sleeping poorly, and the youngest child was having problems at school. Exploration of these problems and referral of the mother-in-law for assessment by the old age psychiatrists helped both to relieve the fatigue and allowed her to see it as understandable in the situation, and not the result of a medical illness.

Causes of fatigue

- chronic or acute illness (e.g. anaemia, multiple sclerosis, HIV infection, thyroid dysfunction)
- iatrogenic causes, e.g. diuretics, beta blockers
- psychiatric disorder, especially depression
- chronic fatigue syndrome (CFS)

CHRONIC FATIGUE SYNDROME (CFS)

A high proportion of those with chronic fatigue lasting for more than 6 months will have a psychiatric diagnosis, principally depression and somatization disorder. The majority of the cases will be women with an onset in their early thirties.

CASE 13.12

A woman aged 27 years found herself taking increasing amounts of time off work because of vague physical symptoms. She felt tired, unwell and weak, and had headaches. She felt dull in her mind and was unable to concentrate, and eventually lost her job and found herself spending more and more time in bed doing nothing. She relied on friends to do her shopping and household chores. She repeatedly called out her family doctor, demanding investigations and medications for this state. Any attempt to relate her state to the stresses she was under at work or to engage her in a gradual plan of exercise were unsuccessful.

Symptoms of CFS

- fatigue
- headache
- exercise-induced malaise
- aching muscles
- sensorimotor disturbance
- high levels of depression and somatization disorder
- impaired cognition
- unexplained fevers
- no identifiable organic cause

Aetiology

Abnormalities identified in CFS

- minor abnormalities on magnetic resonance imaging (MRI)
- minor abnormalities on single-photon emission computerized tomography (SPECT)
- abnormalities of immune function
- evidence of retrovirus infection

The aetiology of CFS remains unclear. The organic factors outlined above may be of importance, but psychosocial variables are paramount. Sufferers often come from an environment in which activity and business are the dominant way of life ('yuppie flu'), and where illness is viewed as a legitimate reason to slow down. Those coming to hospital frequently have higher levels of psychiatric morbidity and a strongly held belief that the symptoms are related to some as yet undiscovered pathogen. The average person suffers from a viral infection about four times a year, but the symptoms (feeling tired and weak) usually resolve spontaneously within a couple of weeks.

Treatment

Treatment with antidepressants, even for those without overt depression, has been suggested. A cognitive behavioural approach to developing a programme for gradually increasing activity and to exploring the attribution of symptoms has also been shown to be effective.

Prognosis in chronic fatigue syndrome

- Psychiatric syndromes at onset
- Belief in the organic nature of the illness.

The concept of chronic fatigue

The prognosis is better if there are clear psychiatric syndromes (e.g. depression or anxiety) and the person accepts that there may not be an organic basis to their illness.

Several lines of development have come together in the concept of CFS.

Neurasthenia

Neurasthenia was common among certain classes in the nineteenth century. Women with the disorder took to their beds or sofas and lived out their lives in a recumbent pose, as it was believed that they should rest and refrain from the overstimulation of the modern world (see Charlotte Perkins Gilman's in *The Yellow Wallpaper* or Signora Neroni in Trollope's *Barchester Towers*). Although retained in some diagnostic systems (most notably the Chinese version), it is now rare in western society.

Benign myalgic encephalomyopathy (Royal Free disease)

Similar symptoms occurred in epidemics and were thought to be due to hysteria.

Post-viral fatigue syndromes

This is particularly prevalent following Epstein Barr (glandular fever) infections.

Benign myalgic encephalomyopathy and post-viral fatigue syndrome came together in the 1980s as CFS.

FACTITIOUS DISORDERS (MUNCHAUSEN'S SYNDROME)

CASE 13.13

A woman aged 27 years presented to the Accident and Emergency department with an acquaintance who claimed that she had restrained the woman from jumping from a balcony. The friend then promptly left the department. The woman claimed to have just returned from America and found her gay lover dead on the floor of their flat. She was extremely agitated, claiming that she wished to die, and she was histrionic in her behaviour. She was admitted to the ward where she settled quickly. Over the next few days she told inconsistent stories of being in the army and the national netball team. She gave no contact numbers or next of kin, but she later talked about her probation officer, who was traced. The woman had been in numerous hospitals with a similar history and was on probation following a knee operation in a private hospital, for which she had claimed the army would pay. Following the operation the army denied all knowledge of the woman, and she was tried for fraud.

Features of factitious disorder

- intentional production of medical symptoms (physical or psychological)
- produced in order to enter a sick role
- not produced for financial gain, to obtain drugs, etc. (see discussion of malingering)
- can be by proxy

This is a relatively rare condition named after the fantastical weaver of tales, Baron Munchausen. The person produces symptoms, often of a vague and changing nature, in order to enter the sick role. Physical symptoms are most common, and may be seen as exacerbations of an earlier physical illness. During the interview patients agree with almost any symptom proposed to them, and develop fantastic tales about their background (pseudologica fantastica). Such people end up having numerous investigations and operations as a result of their presentations to hospital. These repeated hospitalizations lead to breakdown of family ties, social networks and employment. Problems usually start in early adulthood and run a chronic course. Parents may present their children as having physical symptoms (Munchausen's by proxy). These people are not producing symptoms in order to avoid legal responsibility, or to obtain drugs or money (malingering). The aetiology is not clear, but the patients usually have a severe personality disorder.

MALINGERING

Malingering is defined as the conscious production of physical symptoms for gain.

CASE 13.14

A man aged 32 years presented to the Accident and Emergency department giving a classic history of appendicitis and mimicking the signs of that disorder. He was give an intramuscular injection of pethidine and was last seen running out of the hospital gate in the direction of the nearest shopping centre.

Careful histories are needed in order to distinguish this group of people from those with 'genuine' medical conditions, somatoform disorders or factitious disorders. The dividing line between them is often difficult to detect.

PREPARING A COURT REPORT

Any medical practitioner may be required to write a report on a patient for medico-legal purposes. The general practitioner may be required to prepare a report at the request of a person's solicitor in connection with a compensation claim for personal injury suffered in a road traffic accident or an accident at work. The injury might be mainly of a psychiatric nature, such as post-traumatic stress disorder or a phobic anxiety state. The report covering psychiatric aspects of the sequelae of an accident should include the following:

■ details of the solicitor requesting the report;
■ the purpose of the report;
■ the length of time for which the person has been under the care of the general practitioner;
■ details of documentation made available to the report-writer, including their own or others' handwritten reports;
■ a summary of the person's complaints and the clinical observations made at each interview;
■ details of the treatment prescribed;
■ details of the person's medical and psychiatric history;
■ details of substance or alcohol abuse;
■ details of the person's own account of the trauma or incident;
■ description of the immediate physical and mental consequences, as well as the longer term consequences.

The summary should include a description of the person's psychiatric state and general level of functioning during the period shortly before the accident, if this is known. This should be contrasted with injuries and symptoms which have developed as a result of the accident or incident. A medical practitioner might be requested to provide a report about one of his or her patients who has been charged with a criminal offence. A report which is to be used in criminal proceedings has a similar format to a report that is to be used in a compensation case.

Further reading

Bass, C. and Potts, S. 1993: Somatoform disorders. In Granville Grossman, K. (ed.), *Recent advances in psychiatry 8*. Edinburgh: Churchill Livingstone, 143–64.

Creed, F., Mayo, R. and Hopkins, A. (eds) 1992: *Medical symptoms not explained by organic disease*. London: Gaskell.

Straus, S. (ed.) 1994: *Chronic fatigue syndrome*. New York: Marcel Dekker.

14. SUICIDE AND DELIBERATE SELF-HARM

SUICIDE

CASE 14.1

A man aged 23 years was admitted to the ward following a visit to his home by his doctor. He had a 3-month history of increasing social withdrawal, and he sat on his bed with his knees drawn up saying little and making little eye contact. He refused food and slept poorly, and told the staff life was not worth living and that he had no future. There were no precipitating factors that had led to his state. He left the ward after 3 days without the knowledge of the staff and threw himself under a train at the nearby railway station.

Epidemiology of suicide

The suicide rate in the UK is about 10 per 100 000 members of the population. In all age groups the rate is higher in men than in women (12 vs. 6 per 100 000). The incidence increases with age, but the magnitude of the difference has been decreasing in recent years. There has been a marked increase in the number of young men committing suicide, which might be associated with higher levels of unemployment and homelessness. Divorce and widowhood also correlate with suicide. Suicide is commoner at the extremes of the social scale, involving unskilled workers and professional people more often than members of the intermediate classes.

In summary, suicide is more common in men, the elderly, the divorced and widowed, and social classes I and V. It also occurs more often in spring.

Suicide and psychiatric disorder

As one might imagine, suicide is most common in depressive illnesses: 15 per cent of people who have major depressive illnesses will go on to kill themselves. Suicide is also remarkably common in schizophrenia, which has a suicide rate of 10 per cent. Because schizophrenia is so much rarer than depression, only about 3 per cent of those committing suicide have a diagnosis of schizophrenia, whilst the majority have a diagnosis of depression. Alcoholism is the second commonest disorder associated with suicide, being present in 20 per cent of cases. Personality disorder is present in 30 to 50 per cent of those who commit suicide, particularly those with alcohol- and drug-related problems.

Relationship between suicide and psychiatric disorder

- depression is the commonest diagnosis
- 15 per cent of depressives go on to kill themselves
- alcoholism is the second commonest diagnosis
- 10 per cent of schizophrenics commit suicide
- personality disorder is detected in about 40 per cent of those committing suicide
- substance abuse is common in the younger suicides

The methods used to commit suicide varies with gender. Sixty-six per cent of female suicides result from self-poisoning, usually with analgesics (especially paracetamol) and antidepressants. By contrast, only 30 per cent of male suicides are by self-poisoning, whilst another 30 per cent are by inhalation of carbon monoxide from car exhausts. The remainder are carried out by a variety of physical methods, e.g. hanging, drowning, shooting, or throwing oneself in front of a car or train.

Assessment of suicide risk

Successful suicide is unlikely to be based on a sudden impulse, and tends to be planned in advance. The majority of those who commit suicide have recently given some warning to their family and friends, and about 50 per cent have consulted their general practitioner or a psychiatrist in the week before their death. The assessment of suicide risk is a basic skill that all doctors should learn. Any patient who is considered to be depressed or to have a psychotic illness should have their risk of suicide assessed. Do not be afraid to ask about suicidal ideas or plans. The person may be very relieved to know that these fearful thoughts are not taboo, and to be able to talk about them. The person who has no suicidal thoughts will soon tell you this, and is unlikely to take up the idea and attempt suicide.

If the distressed person gives a direct statement of intent, then this is the clearest indication of risk. From asking about the person's general view of life, it is no great leap to ask about more definite plans to commit suicide.

General aspects to be considered

- Does the person have a depressive illness or schizophrenia?
- Does the person have alcohol problems or other substance abuse history?
- Is there a history of previous suicide attempts (especially in the last 6 months)?
- Have they recently been discharged from hospital?
- Is the person socially isolated and lacking supportive relationships?
- Are they unemployed?
- Do they have a chronic painful medical condition?
- Have there been recent adverse events in the patient's life?

Any one of the above is associated with an increase in suicide risk, and provides a frame into which the patient's statements can be placed to give an overall indication of risk.

Management of the suicidal patient

Having obtained an idea of the person's likely risk of suicide, the management plan depends upon a number of issues:

Issues to be explored with the depressed patient

- Do you get any pleasure in life?
- Would you be better off dead?
- Have you ever thought of killing yourself?
- Have you made any preparations to do so?
- Can anything be done to help you?
- Do you have any future?

Issues to be explored with the suicidal patient

- Have you made plans about how you would kill yourself?
- Have you prepared for this in any way (for example, by saving tablets, obtaining piping for the car exhaust, writing letters or notes of explanation)?

Issues affecting the management plan

- the seriousness of suicidal intent
- the severity of the accompanying psychiatric disorder
- past history
- available community resources

If a significant suicidal risk is present, the patient should almost always be managed in hospital, unless social and community mental health resources are very good indeed. In such circumstances the patient and carers must be able to contact mental health professionals easily and quickly, as the situation may change rapidly. Drugs should only be given in small amounts, daily if necessary, and frequent review of the patient is necessary.

If the person requires admission to hospital this may have to take place under the Mental Health legislation, as such people often refuse to be admitted.

The prevention of harm to a patient in a hospital ward can be difficult. Staffing may be limited, other people may need greater input, and the quiet depressed person may be neglected. For each patient the degree of surveillance necessary must be determined and appropriate levels of nursing provided, even if this means someone being at the person's side for 24 hours a day.

In addition to this fundamental level of care, the person should receive appropriate physical treatment for his or her mental disorder (given the length of time antidepressants take to exert their effect, ECT should be considered in the depressed patient who is actively suicidal).

In addition, appropriate supportive psychological treatments must be provided to examine the problems that the person is facing and how these might be addressed in the future.

Management of the suicidal person in hospital

- prevention of self-injury
- suitable levels of supervision
- physical treatment for their mental disorder
- appropriate psychological intervention

DELIBERATE SELF-HARM

CASE 14.2

A woman aged 18 years was brought into the emergency room. She had taken 15 paracetamol tablets and drunk a bottle of vodka at a party. She had had an argument with her boyfriend earlier that evening and he had left her. She was crying noisily and resisted any medical interventions for some time, saying that she wanted to die. When seen the next morning she felt very unwell, but in the interim had been reconciled with her boyfriend and regretted what she had done. She returned to her parents' home later that day.

The above case is something of a caricature (although the case of a real person) of the typical person presenting with deliberate self-harm. The term 'self-harm' separates this group from cases in which the suicide attempt has failed. The act is impulsive and takes place in response to some acute stress. It serves to readjust the dynamics of the situation back towards the status quo which had been upset (in this case, the return of the boyfriend).

These events must not be dismissed as trivial, because the risk of completed suicide in the year following an episode of deliberate self-harm is 1 to 2 per cent, i.e. the risk is 100-fold greater than in the general population.

Self-poisoning accounts for 90 per cent of cases of deliberate self-harm (frequently accompanied by alcohol consumption), the remainder being accounted for by lacerations to the wrist or forearm.

In cases of self-harm, the drugs most frequently ingested, in order of frequency, are as follows:

- anxiolytics;
- hypnotics;
- analgesics (aspirin and paracetamol);
- antidepressants.

General features of acts of deliberate self-harm

- more common in women than in men (by a ratio of approximately 2:1)
- more common in young people
- peak for women at 15–30 years of age; later for men
- more common in the lower social classes
- more common in cities
- unemployment is common, especially in men
- 20 per cent of people repeat the act within 1 year
- 1 to 2 per cent of people die of suicide within 1 year

Factors associated with repetition of deliberate self-harm

- previous act of deliberate self-harm
- previous psychiatric treatment
- alcohol and drug abuse
- personality disorder
- unemployment
- a forensic record
- lower social class

Deliberate self-harm is more common in women, and particularly young women. People who present with deliberate self-harm are often unemployed and live in cities.

Assessment

The important issue to explore with the person is the degree of suicidal intent that they feel, and whether they are suffering from a psychiatric disorder.

Assessing suicidal intent of an act of deliberate self-harm

- Was the act carefully planned and prepared?
- Could the person reasonably expect to be found after the act?
- Did they leave a note?
- Have they put their affairs in order?
- Did the patient want to die at the time?
- Did they think that what they did would kill them (even if it is patently clear to the knowing physician that it would not)?
- Have they sought help for the problem afflicting him or her?

Management

The most important initial consideration is the person's physical well-being. People need appro-

priate medical attention before any psychiatric assessment is made. This may mean supporting staff on a medical ward whilst medical investigations and treatments take place.

The presence of serious suicidal intent usually means that the patient should be managed in hospital (see above). In many cases, little or no action needs to be taken because the acute situation will have resolved itself. Those in whom factors predicting repetition are recognized or who have longer term problems may benefit from psychotherapy. Repeated self-mutilators often find it difficult to express their emotions in words (hence the physical act of cutting), and may find it difficult to use more than low-key supportive approaches.

Steps to be taken

- ensure the person's physical well-being by means of medical treatments
- admit people with serious mental illness
- admit people who still have suicidal intent
- examine the risk of the act being repeated
- give psychological interventions appropriate to the stresses that the person is experiencing

Further reading

Hawton, K. and Catalan, J. 1987: *Attempted suicide; a practical guide*. Oxford: Oxford University Press.
Royal College of Psychiatrists 1994: *The general hospital management of adult deliberate self-harm*. London: Royal College of Psychiatrists.

15 PSYCHOSEXUAL PROBLEMS

INTRODUCTION: CONCEPTS AND DEFINITIONS

Sexual function can be understood using a biopsychosocial approach. Genital performance is a biological activity; the relevant structures respond to patterns of nervous stimulation of central origin that are themselves determined by cerebral and mental processes responsive to social and environmental cues.

Adequate genital functioning requires:

- intact local structures
- adequate vascular supply
- adequate peripheral nervous control
- appropriate hormonal modulation
- functioning connections with the central nervous system

Four interrelated systems can be discerned in the cerebral, psychological and behavioural processes involved in sexual and intimate relationship activity (Figure 15.1).

Gender identity is the experience of the self as male, female or ambivalent; it is the private expression of *gender role*, the ways in which an individual expresses himself or herself in public as male, female or ambivalent.

Sexual preferences are the kinds of people or representations of or substitutes for people to

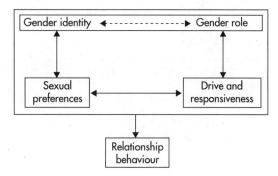

FIG 15.1 Sexual and relationship behaviours.

whom or to which an individual may be erotically responsive. In discussing sexual preferences it is helpful to distinguish between acts and status. Sexual acts may be possible without emotional attachment, whereas sexual status refers to the morphology of the sex organs of the person with whom one might fall in love. According to this view, many people are capable of falling in love with males and females, and are hence correctly designated bisexual. In most societies a small number of people appear to be exclusively homosexual in their sexual preferential status.

Sexual drive and responsiveness is a cumbersome phrase; it may refer to different processes which it is important to specify in the individual case.

'Sexual drive' may point to:

- the urge to begin sexual activity;
- the frequency of various forms of sexual expression;
- the ease or difficulty with which an individual may respond in a sexual situation;

- the satisfaction or otherwise associated with sexual activity.

The term 'libido' is best avoided, since its exact meaning in any context is usually unclear.

Specifically sexual (i.e. genital) activity can only be fully understood in relation to the interactions and affiliative relationships of which it forms a part. Very common indeed are problems which can be understood at least in part as involving a disjunction between sex and affection. For instance, a person may be able to have sex with someone they do not love, and unable to have sex with a loved partner.

SYSTEM DISTURBANCES

Interactions and relationships

As stated already, it is not appropriate to regard a sexual (i.e. genital) problem as if it were a disturbance of body parts unconnected to behaviour with a partner.

Relationship problems may be defined in four ways.

1. By phase of relationship

Problems may arise at the following stages:

- during development of relationships;
- during maintenance of relationships;
- during the dissolution of relationships.

A continuing relationship, once developed, passes with time through phases, each of which has particular duties, opportunities and susceptibility to particular problems. Thus a marriage may progress from an initial childless phase through the phases of child-rearing and of 'grown children leaving home' to retirement and involution. At any point, relationship dissolution requires only one of two partners to decide that the relationship should end.

2. In terms of the number of people involved

Often, more than two people who may be sexual or affiliated partners are involved in a problem, e.g. when a person is separated from his or her spouse but not divorced, and has another liaison; other problems involve people who have never had close emotional and/or sexual relationships.

3. By type

Most relationship problems involve:

- conflict;

- communication difficulties;
- uncertain or differing degrees of commitment.

Conflicts involve areas of shared concern, e.g. parenting, wider family relationships, sexual activity, housing and household issues, money, use of time, or wider moral, political or religious issues. Failure or lack of communication skills usually accompanies clinical presentation of couple problems; a couple with good communication skills is more likely to resolve conflicts without consultation.

4. In terms of stability or instability of the relationship and individuals' satisfaction or dissatisfaction with it

Relationships may be thought of as stable or unstable, and satisfying or not satisfying. Therefore a relationship may be:

- stable and satisfactory;
- stable and unsatisfactory;
- unstable and unsatisfactory;
- unstable and satisfactory.

Relationship problems

- the phase of the relationship
- the number of people involved
- the type of problem experienced
- the stability of the relationship

Most clinical work is concerned with 'stable and unsatisfactory' relationships. For obvious reasons, 'satisfactory and stable' relationships are rarely the source of difficulty, and 'unstable and unsatisfactory' relationships are the most likely to dissolve. Some interesting problems involve relationships which are 'unstable, yet satisfactory'.

Sexual preferences

Discussion of sexual preferences, and what should be defined as problematic in this area, is often guided by emotion, ideology or prejudice, rather than science, always in relation to current local laws. Sometimes society or its agents define a behaviour as a problem (e.g. some instances of attraction experienced by an adult male for prepubertal children), while the individual concerned sees no problem in following his or her sexual urges, and may consider that society is inappropriately constraining their sexual expression. In most societies, the majority disagree with paedophiles, and paedophilia is rated as socially unacceptable, whatever those drawn to this behaviour may think. A balanced view of this matter is that sexual preferences reasonably attract disapproval if they involve actual physical harm to or abuse of others, with coercion or without consent. A person might disapprove of rape, but not of sadomasochism between consenting adults, or fetishistic behaviour.

In the case of heterosexual and homosexual preferences, disapproval of the latter has often been noted, with attempts to identify homosexuality as an illness or perversion. In recent years it has become clear that there are no scientific grounds for rating homosexual status *per se* as anything other than a normal variant, like left-handedness. As such it no longer appears in any generally accepted classification of diseases. Clinical experience suggests that the same range and types of relationship and sexual function problems may arise in homosexual and heterosexual individuals. The clinician has the duty to try to sustain a clear science-based view amidst the various punitive and homophobic myths which permeate some thinking in this area.

In nosological terms, anomalies of sexual preference are classified as '*paraphilias*'. They are often associated with a compulsive attraction coupled with chronic conflict about the tendency, which may be experienced as profoundly shameful.

Features of paraphilias

- abnormality of sexual preference
- compulsive attraction
- chronic conflict and shame

Gender identity problems

A person's 'core gender identity' is formed and fixed by the age of 3 or 4 years. Normally, chromosomal, gonadal, and internal and external genital sex are congruent with the psychological sense of self as male or female. However, this congruence may be disturbed. For instance, in the disorder of Testicular Feminization, the male fetus (XY chromosomal structure) is androgen insensitive

and therefore develops a female phenotype ; this individual develops a female gender identity and grows into a (sterile) female. This condition indicates that chromosomal sex can be overridden during development by other influences, with the production of a gender identity that is discordant with chromosomal sex.

In the clinical syndrome of *transsexualism* (primary gender dysphoria), the individual experiences himself or herself from early in life as a person whose body has the wrong anatomy. It is important to realize that it is this way round; the problem is experienced as being with the body, not the mind. Thus the male-to-female transsexual may experience a heterosexual attraction to men, and may rightly complain to a listener who refers to their erotic attraction to men as homosexual that they have not understood anything at all about their story. Indeed, the case of transsexualism demonstrates that gender identity and sexual preferences are separate (although interconnected) systems, since both male-to-female and female-to-male transsexuals may be heterosexual or homosexual. In properly selected cases, the surgical components of a gender reassignment programme are some of the most successful surgical interventions in the whole of medicine.

Drive problems

The main point to note here is that people's sexual behaviour varies enormously. While many adults in established relationships engage in sexual behaviour one to three times weekly on average, the range is from never or once every few months to several times daily. For the clinician, the message is that no assumptions should be made about the sexual activities of any person without detailed enquiry. Sexual frequency *per se* is not a problem unless someone rates it as such. Common problems in this area are:

- a mismatch between the desired frequencies of sexual behaviour of established partners;
- an unwanted loss (or, less commonly, excess) of sexual interest, or 'drive'.

Problems in this area may affect:

- the preliminary behaviours leading to coitus (proceptive phase);
- the achievement of orgasmic responses (the acceptive phase);
- the achievement (or prevention) of pregnancy (conceptive phase).

SEXUAL DYSFUNCTIONS

Sexual dysfunctions constitute by far the commonest problems in the sexual domain. Professional people probably only deal with a small proportion of the sexual dysfunctions which occur, and it seems likely that some degree of sexual dysfunction affects most people at some stage in their lives. As with all sexual problems, dysfunctions are usually accompanied by relationship concerns or difficulties.

Sexual dysfunctions make sexual intercourse difficult, impossible, inefficient or unrewarding. They may be primary (when the function in question has never been satisfactory) or secondary (when difficulty follows a period of effective behaviour), and more than one dysfunction may coexist in a couple. They may be defined in terms of the arousal and response phases of sexual responsiveness (Figure 15.2). In addition, there is the syndrome of vaginismus, which occurs in women and consists of a spasm of pelvic muscles preventing penile entry. Vaginismus is not directly related to the sexual response cycle, as women with this disorder may have no problems with sexual arousal and response and are often orgasmic.

Also often considered in the same context as sexual dysfunctions are drive problems, the most common of which is loss of desire, as already noted, although increased sexual desire may also be a problem.

Erectile impotence is the commonest sexual dysfunction seen in clinical practice, although premature ejaculation and failure of lubrication and/or orgasm in the female are also common. Primary erectile failure and primary ejaculatory failure are rare and usually attributable to physiological causes. Impotence has attracted increased attention in recent years on account of the availability of useful physical treatments. Hence, assessment of the cause of an impotence problem is nowadays of considerable practical importance. Three principles are helpful:

- it is not a question of psychological *or* physical causation, but rather an estimate of how much of which sort of factor is causing the problem;
- if the history is of gradually increasing loss of erection, particularly with a history of previously adequate erectile function, then some degree of physiogenesis should be assumed;
- a multifactorial aetiology should be assumed until proved otherwise.

	AROUSAL	RESPONSE
MALE	Erectile impotence	Premature ejaculation Retarded ejaculation
FEMALE	Lubrication failure	Anorgasmia

FIG 15.2 Varieties of sexual dysfunction.

The following case indicates one common way in which several factors may combine to produce a clinical problem.

CASE 15.1

A 50-year-old business man consulted because of gradually increasing erectile failure over the past 3 years. His business had failed 4 years previously and his wife had divorced him 6 months later. Three years ago a routine medical examination had disclosed significant hypertension for which a beta blocker had been given, and the patient had been advised at the same time to reduce his alcohol intake from the 30 units weekly which he had been consuming for the previous 5 years.

This history suggests five factors that could be plausibly related to erectile difficulty: work and marital stress (psychological factors), and hypertension, its drug treatment, and alcohol (physical factors). Other common organic contributors to impotence are diabetes and antidepressant drugs.

Some common drugs causing sexual dysfunction

- alcohol
- alpha and beta blockers
- thiazide diuretics
- calcium-channel blockers
- ACE inhibitors
- tricyclic antidepressants
- anxiolytics

In the assessment of impotence, valuable information may be obtained by an investigatory intra-cavernosal injection of papaverine. This may produce erections in neuropathic and psychogenic cases, but rarely does so in cases of vasculogenic impotence. Continuing self-administered papaverine (or the more recently introduced, and more expensive, prostaglandin E_1) has become a popular treatment, but it is ill advised without a comprehensive psychosocial assessment and opportunities for the user, and preferably also his partner, to discuss the implications of the method.

Other physical treatments that are already established or currently being explored include the following: a vacuum device which, when placed over the penis, encourages erection by removing air from the space surrounding the penis; trinitrin patches placed on the penis; and the surgical insertion of semi-rigid penile rods.

The physical components of treatment fit easily into a general counselling framework in which the individual's or couple's concerns are shared. It seems likely that the outcome of any intervention for impotence, including physical treatments, is better if the partner is involved and if the relationship between the person and their partner is satisfactory. The same is true for all sexual dysfunctions, for which the same general counselling approach offers a satisfactory framework for specific measures. Apart from impotence, specific measures may be particularly helpful in cases of premature ejaculation and vaginismus.

The general counselling approach used in UK psychosexual clinics owes something to the work of Masters and Johnson, adapted to different cultural and social conditions. The basic principles are that:

- sexual behaviours which are desired but which do not occur, or which occur too often, should be defined in detail;
- treatment goals should be clearly defined;
- treatment goals may be approached gradually so that patients are guided to practise desired behaviours in a programme designed to replace failure experiences with successes, and anxiety with enjoyment.

'Homework' or 'practice' between sessions is usually essential, and may entail improved couple communication and negotiation about altered use of time, using couple therapy techniques.

GENERAL COMMENTS

One of the most striking changes in psychiatric and medical practice in the last 25 years has been the increased ease with which people consult in growing numbers about sexual and relationship difficulties. The onus is on clinicians to provide effective interventions; at present it appears that there is considerable room for improvement. It seems likely that increased effectiveness will depend on better ways of assessing and helping with relationship problems rather than the purely sexual aspects of behaviour.

It has also become obvious to practitioners in this field that the attention paid to cultural aspects of sexual and relationship problems has often been inadequate, and that intervention methods derived from those of the Americans Masters and Johnson are culture-bound and inapplicable to many couple and family arrangements now familiar in multiethnic Britain. For example, a person may have had children by different partners rather than living in stable monogamy, or have had a marriage arranged for them by their parents rather than on the basis of an individual decision, perhaps after a period of unmarried cohabitation, or they may view sexual contact with others as requiring no commitment to them as other people or any expectation of affectionate involvement. Such circumstances are bound to affect the approach which clinicians should take in addressing sexual complaints, and the effectiveness of interventions. Any view of sexual difficulties which ignores the relationship context in which sexual behaviour takes place or is attempted is bound to be inadequate.

Further reading

Bancroft, J. 1988: *Human sexuality and its problems*, 2nd edn. Edinburgh: Churchill Livingstone.

Crowe, M.J. and Ridley, J. 1990: *Therapy with couples*. Oxford: Blackwell.

Davenport-Hines, R. 1990: *Sex, death and punishment*. London: Collins.

Dominian, J. 1979: *Marital pathology*. London: British Medical Association.

Duck, S. 1988: *Relating to others*. Milton Keynes: Open University Press.

Ford, C.S. and Beach, F.A. 1952: *Patterns of sexual behaviour*. London: Eyre and Spottiswoode.

Gregoire, A. and Pryor, J.P. 1993: *Impotence. An integrated approach to clinical practice*. Edinburgh: Churchill Livingstone.

Spence, S.H. 1993: *Psychosexual therapy*. London: Chapman and Hall.

INTRODUCTION

'Psychotherapy' should be understood as meaning 'psychological treatments', i.e. activities designed to help people (treatments), whose effects are mediated through conversation and interaction between people.

In ordinary life, people influence each other by a range of interactive behaviours, such as listening, understanding, communication, friendship, falling in love, and persuasion. Psychological treatments are built on the foundation of such human processes by the addition of professional, scientific and technical knowledge and practice to create systematic 'packages' of rationally based procedures that are open to scientific scrutiny.

RANGE OF PSYCHOLOGICAL TREATMENTS

Psychological treatments should be thought of as belonging to two major groups.

Adjuvant therapies

Psychological influence is inevitable when help-seeker and help-provider meet. Sometimes, these influences can for practical purposes be ignored, usually because they simply work in the smooth service of the investigation or intervention of current concern. Sometimes, however, they are of crucial importance, for example when an initially reluctant patient needs, in the doctor's judgement, to be persuaded to undergo something unpleasant or life-threatening. These secondary psychological influences may be intentionally promoted by the clinician, or they may occur without the clinician's awareness, in which case their (beneficial or harmful) effects are therefore less well understood and apparently more unpredictable.

Specific interventions

These are procedures whose form, content and use are designed to bring about particular changes which can in principle be specified at the start. Regrettably this is not always done in practice.

Psychological treatment interventions should be distinguished conceptually from social interventions which may lead to behavioural change (e.g. moving house or changing jobs), which are often made at the same time. Treatments should also be distinguished from other ways of producing behavioural change through interaction and conversation, such as interrogation, torture and even 'brainwashing', which of course have no place in a professional help-providing system.

CONCEPTUAL AND SCIENTIFIC BASES OF PSYCHOLOGICAL TREATMENTS

Conversation

Psychological treatments require an acknowledgement of the conversational basis of clinical activity. Hence the sciences that are applicable to conversation are relevant, such as social psychology, sociology, anthropology and linguistics. Scientific approaches might, for instance, focus upon information processing in the therapeutic interaction, or upon the fact that conversations take place according to rules, with the interactants occupying social roles which are reciprocal to one another. In most forms of psychotherapy, it is essential that the therapist and the patient understand each other's vocabulary, and an important initial phase may be devoted to the development of what has been called 'a shared language of meaning' (Hobson, 1985).

Social roles

A role is a position in a social organization. Individuals learn to occupy many roles in various social systems. The family is a social system, and people may be involved in educational or work systems, and so on. When they seek help for health problems, they enter the medical social system. Roles are always reciprocal to other roles, and each role has its expected behaviours, rights and obligations.

Being a patient is reciprocal to being a doctor (or nurse or other health professional), and seeking psychological help involves occupying some version of the patient role. With many psychological treatments, it is inappropriate for the patient to be relatively passive as in 'the acute sick role', because in the case of acute illness the patient is in the hands of professionals whose instructions are to be obeyed. Patients may have to be taught the role behaviours expected of them in psychotherapy. Often something close to being a 'student' in relation to a 'teacher' defines what is required.

Frames of reference

When therapist and patient meet, the interaction derives its form and content from three kinds of influence.

1. The interaction has ordinary human qualities, each person tending to act as they do habitually in ordinary life. Two processes, relating to conversational rules and to person perception, are particularly important.

Conversation tends to take place according to rules governing behaviour such as taking turns to talk, and patterns of eye gaze (which communicate messages of interactive import, such as 'I am going to stop speaking soon'). Psychiatric illnesses may interfere with the ability to keep to conversational rules, which may then require specific attention.

'Person perception' means that when two people see each other, each immediately develops an impression of the other, which adds to the perception of obvious characteristics such as gender, age (roughly), and style of dress, evaluative ideas such as attractiveness. These ideas may be modified by increasingly close acquaintance, but an evaluative component will remain because it is inevitable in all interactions and relationships that people regard each other with some degree of favourableness, likeability and so on. These ideas must be acknowledged in therapy and may be an immensely important focus within treatment. One reason for this is that ordinary people tend to arrive at adulthood with broadly favourable views of themselves and their parents, from which they have derived a tendency to think well of others. Psychiatric patients and individuals seeking psychotherapy often have negative views of self and/or others, changing which is often an important therapeutic theme.

2. In addition to 'ordinary human' qualities, the therapist–patient interaction has characteristics derived from the professional nature of the meeting. Thus, while the conversation takes place according to rules, these rules differ from those of interactions between friends or neighbours. Because it is a professional system, the conversation is asymmetrical, with self-disclosure expected from only one party (the patient), the other reciprocating by attentive listening and informed questioning and other behaviours to guide patient self-disclosure. This arrangement tends of itself to introduce distortions into the perception each person has of the other, those distortions of the therapist by the patient often being very important in the substance of therapy.

3. Patient and therapist bring into their conversation about the patient's problems their own ideas about what these problems are – their nature, origin and significance. These frames of reference exist in both patient and therapist. The patient's

ideas will depend on what he or she happens to know, and may vary from superstition, 'lay psychology' or culturally derived or religious notions to sophisticated psychological theories. The therapist will, as a professional, bring some 'expert' view to bear on the matter. There are many systems of thought applicable to behaviour, which vary in popular appeal, philosophical cogency, and degree of empirical support. Each practitioner has the duty to be informed about plausible and perhaps useful approaches, justifying the use of those which inform personal work with patients. A vital contribution to the validation of therapeutic approaches is to be made by the measurement of therapeutic outcomes.

Formulation

This is the crucial part of the assessment process. In general psychiatric work, the history taking and examination provide a *description* of the abnormalities and phenomena which allows a *diagnosis* to be made. In the assessment for psychotherapies these approaches need to be supplemented by *problem statements* which lead to an *explanation* in terms of whichever frame of reference the assessor judges may lead to a useful intervention plan that is acceptable to the patient. What is required is a view of present difficulties which can be shared with the patient and which offers hypotheses about origins and causes which can lead to hope of future change and a strategy for achieving this.

Therapist–patient relationship

As noted above, the therapist–patient interaction involves conversational rules which differ from those that govern the formation of ordinary friendship. The therapist is required to *attend* to what the patient says and generally to express an accepting attitude, to attempt to see things from the patient's point of view and to understand their wishes, ideas and feelings.

These requirements *alone* tend to distort the patient's perceptions of the therapist as an ordinary human being, and to allow the therapist to be ascribed qualities according to the patient's wishes, needs and personal biography. As patient and therapist spend more time together, the interaction develops into a relationship in the sense that the interacting parties increasingly feel that they know each other, but once again the patient's

perceptions of the therapist tend to be distorted as the self-disclosure continues to be one-sided. This process was called *transference* by Freud, who pointed to the childhood origins of tendencies to ascribe inaccurate characteristics to others in interactions. Of course, therapists as human beings also have the capacity to ascribe characteristics inappropriately to patients, a process which is called *counter-transference*. Distortions of both sorts have also been called *parataxic distortions* by the American Harry Stack Sullivan.

Therefore, clinicians need to learn to identify and monitor the qualities of the therapist–patient interaction and relationships. This is important throughout clinical practice, but is essential in all psychological treatments because the patient's difficulties are often manifested by changes in aspects of the patient–therapist relationship. The monitoring is by introspection during the actual clinical sessions.

TREATMENT DIMENSIONS AND SPECIFICATION

An adequate description of a psychological treatment requires consideration of 10 dimensions, in relation to the formulation of what is to be treated with what end in view. That is, what happens in treatment, and its outcome, may vary with all 10 factors. Keeping track of these complexities requires adequate techniques for measuring therapeutic outcomes, and for relating this information to treatment processes (i.e. what happens within interventions).

Location

The setting in which the treatment takes place may have major effects on both process and outcome. Most therapy in the UK occurs in hospital clinics or community mental health facilities on an outpatient basis, or in consulting rooms which may be in the therapist's home. An increasing amount of treatment occurs in general practitioner surgeries or health centres. Rarely, therapy occurs in the patient's own home.

Economic background

Psychological treatment implies an agreement between therapist and patient about what is proposed should happen (this is sometimes called a contract, but it is professional and moral rather than legal, even though it may be specified in writing and may have considerable influence on both parties). This agreement tends to differ markedly if therapy is paid for by the patient rather than free at the point of receipt.

Some arrangements for public health funding may impose delay before treatment can begin, e.g. if a health authority has to give permission for a patient to be seen, which may delay assessment. Such delay may materially affect the treatment process and outcome. Funding rules in private or public sectors may impose limits on the amount of therapy which may be given. This has resulted in increasing interest in time-limited therapies whose costs can be calculated more easily than in cases where therapy is open-ended.

Space and time

Basically, therapy consists of conversation which may focus upon matters of great personal intimacy and sensitivity. For this to proceed as smoothly as possible, therapy needs to occur in suitably appointed and private premises with appropriate furnishings, especially reasonably comfortable chairs. The way in which the chairs are arranged affects the experience of the interaction and requires careful thought. People feel very uncomfortable if they are either too close to the people they are talking to, or too far from them. The interaction is also affected if people cannot see each other's facial expressions and movements, and it is usually good practice to have the chairs set at an angle of about 120 degrees to each other. It is rarely helpful for the therapist to sit behind a desk.

Treatment can be very difficult if there is not adequate privacy and comfort. This is very commonly the case in general hospital wards, and special arrangements are usually required when therapy is requested for a general hospital in-patient (e.g. with a psychosomatic problem).

The timing of treatment sessions is important. Often therapy may need to take place outside working hours, which may entail a changed therapist timetable. When patients are seen very early in the morning or late in the day, problems may arise because clinic structures (e.g. receptionist or record staff) may not be available.

Quantity of treatment

The issue of how many sessions of what length are needed to produce what effects with which types of patient is a crucial question for service planners and managers. This is because hours of professional time represent the building blocks out of which services are constructed, and for which money is paid.

Time-limited therapies specify the number of sessions at the outset. A *brief* therapy may include up to about 16 sessions, and there is considerable current interest in therapies which may be effective in about 4, 8 or 10 sessions, and some work suggests that in some categories of patient one or two sessions of an appropriate length may be helpful. In many therapies, sessions usually last for between 45 and 60 minutes. Sessions are often longer than this (around 90 minutes) with group, couple and family methods, and shorter (15 to 30 minutes) in cognitive behavioural therapy, except when particular techniques are used which require very long sessions. There are reports of good results being obtained with a small number of very long sessions in several therapeutic modes.

It is common for treatment sessions to take place weekly, but there is no generally cogent theoretical reason for this, and sessions may be more frequent (e.g. in psychoanalysis) or less frequent (e.g. in family therapy). More research is needed on this point.

Treatment mode

Psychotherapies are available in four modes: individual, couple, group and family. Couple therapy means that two people involved in a relationship are treated together, and family therapy similarly involves the whole family, although it may be difficult to define exactly who should count as a family member. Group therapy may involve people who do not know each other beforehand, but share a common problem, or some group members may know each other (e.g. a group treatment of four or five married couples), or a group may include people with different problems and without previous acquaintance. Groups with variable membership may also occur on in-patient wards, where the aims are often related more to the functioning of the organization than to the problems of individuals.

How to decide whether an individual would be best treated on an individual basis or as part of an interpersonal system (in a couple or family) is an important question on which research is needed.

As already stated, the interaction between therapist and patient has characteristics derived from ordinary interaction processes. This is true for couples, groups and families as well as for individuals, and in these modes *the interaction processes peculiar to them occur and may materially affect outcome*. For example, when a couple is seen together, some of the interaction involves the couple as a *whole*, functioning as more than the sum of its parts (which defines a *system*). Families also function as whole systems. In groups, processes occur which are also explicable in terms of the group functioning as a whole.

Content

This heading includes the rationale of treatment, and procedures peculiar to it. These are described below.

General effects

The effects of psychological therapies can be thought of as both general and specific. There is good evidence that many treatments with very varied theoretical bases, some logically incompatible with others, may benefit many patients, provided that the therapist believes in it. The communication of hope appears to have curative properties. The ability of the therapist to communicate interest, enthusiasm, expectations of improvement and value-free concern also contributes to therapist effectiveness. In any particular therapy, an attempt can be made to estimate how much of what occurs is explicable in terms of non-specific influences (i.e. influences which occur across therapies).

Specificity

This is the other side of the 'general effects' coin. Specific factors are those peculiar to that therapy. They are likely to follow from the treatment's rationale, and to be aimed at specifiable changes. In practice, it may be important to check that they actually happen and also that, if they do, then the effects that occur are attributable to them. This requires continuing records of process, because a relationship between therapists' reports of what they do and what they *actually* do cannot be assumed.

Outcomes

Psychological therapies stand or fall by their effects. Outcomes can be considered in four categories, and all should be measured in a comprehensive assessment. The results may be good in one sense and bad in another. The outcome may be (a) *clinical* (e.g. symptom reduction), (b) *social* (e.g. improved work adjustment, or housing, or starting a new close relationship), (c) *administrative* (e.g. reduced service usage, or cost of care) and (d) *consumer* (e.g. patient self-report of benefit from meeting the therapist).

Outcome can be assessed by repeating measures before and after therapy, and perhaps also at a later follow-up. It is important for measures to reflect the problems for which the patient sought help, even though the methodology may be difficult if treatment aims are for problems, mental structures or behaviours presumed to 'underlie' 'manifest' symptoms. Frequently, patients present for help with distress which signals that they have been unable to cope with life problems. Distress often tends to subside with time, so that psychological therapy might often be largely expectant if distress reduction is a main therapeutic aim. Treatment directed at 'underlying' factors is often best begun when the patient feels better from their most acute state.

Process

Processes in therapy should be checked for general effects and also for specific content. Session records should be written as soon as possible after sessions have finished, to summarize the therapist's view of what has happened. Patient accounts may complement these records and may highlight quite different session events! Audio or video recordings of therapeutic sessions are an invaluable guide to process assessment.

TREATMENTS: ADJUVANT MEASURES

Four kinds of psychological process accompanying clinical practice are of widespread significance and should be understood by every doctor.

Alleviating distress

The emotional distress which accompanies illness, disability and death tends to be reduced when the distressed person is *attentively listened* to, which contributes to a healing sense of being able to *share* the experience with another person. The process cannot be hurried, and its duration should be measured in hours or days rather than in minutes.

Giving information

Throughout clinical practice, patients need to know what is the matter with them, what may or should be done to them, and what may happen in the future. Knowing what to do, or different possible things that one might do, is the start of rational decision making. Knowing all the possibilities makes sensible decision making more likely. Time to talk to the doctor is essential.

To be sensibly acted upon, the information must be successfully communicated. This is often better done in written or recorded form than in words. It is very difficult for patients to remember accurately more than a small part of what is said to them during clinical interviews.

Information should be presented in an unhurried manner, and repeated as often as necessary to ensure understanding. Explaining anatomical or pathological terms so as to convey their meanings accurately is a difficult art and requires practice.

Support and coping

Within clinical practice, *support* is often talked about but rarely defined; it amounts to interactive behaviours which have the effect of making it easier to do difficult things. A sense of support can be transmitted by friendly non-verbal communications such as smiles, nods and gurgles, and by encouraging or sympathetic statements such as 'come on, you can do it', 'it will be over soon', etc. The experience of support tends to increase a person's ability to mobilize their personal, emotional, intellectual and volitional resources to deal (i.e. to cope) with life's vicissitudes.

Irrational aspects of interaction

Emotions and ideas emerge in clinical situations as understandable responses to aspects of the situation, and also because unreasonable or inappropriate responses may also be triggered in response to them. The emergence of 'parataxic distortions', mentioned previously, arising from the social role arrangements in consultations is one example. Irrational elements of experience are usual when serious aspects of life's major themes of death,

aggression and sex are manifested in clinical events.

In psychiatric practice this tendency is compounded by the emotional nature of the disorders being dealt with, but this should not blind perception of rational points which the patient might be making, or of emotional behaviour which is not in fact part of the disorder.

A further complication arises when patients are being detained and/or treated compulsorily. This may greatly affect the presentation of need for adjuvant therapy.

In mental health practice generally, adjuvant treatment is required (a) when a patient has to be told of the diagnosis of their illness, (b) when the implications of a psychiatric diagnosis (which may be of great personal and family import, e.g. in cases of schizophrenia or dementia) have to be explained to the patient's relatives, and (c) when patients are to be given psychotropic medication with important side-effects whose nature must be explained in detail.

TREATMENTS: SPECIFIC MEASURES

General points

When the formulation of the patient's difficulties has led to the decision that a specific psychological treatment is needed, this should entail saying *for what* the treatment is needed. From this should follow a statement of *the goals* of treatment, which involve relating current problems to their proposed solutions. The next question is about the best way of achieving these goals.

To answer this, it is helpful to judge the extent to which *specific* procedures are available to deal with the problems as formulated. There are some important instances when this is so (see below). In the many instances where several different approaches may have some chance of being helpful, the choice should depend on (a) consumer preference, (b) provider preference, (c) availability, (d) practicalities and (e) economics. Commonly, a patient is offered what happens to be available in the setting that they 'happen' to have attended, rather than a fully informed choice between various possibilities. Of course, referral agents may effectively choose the treatment as a result of their decision to refer to one centre or individual rather than to another, but in many services this choice is constrained, which makes choosing between treatment possibilities even more difficult.

Levels of therapy

Each form of psychological treatment has some degree of complexity, and can be thought of as being on one of three levels of conceptual and procedural sophistication. Roughly, levels approximate to the need for human, general professional and specific professional expertise, respectively.

Level One methods are summarized as Attentive Listening, Level Two methods include Problem Solving and Support, and the most important Level Three methods are Cognitive-Behavioural and Psychodynamic approaches.

Level One: attentive listening

Self-disclosure in the presence of an attentive and friendly person tends to reduce distress. The professional task is to attend to what is being said, indicating by words (e.g. clarifying enquiries or making sympathetic comments) or non-verbal signals, such as nods, grunts and smiles, that what is being said is being registered and understood, and to invite the person to continue the process (within practical limits) until they feel that the task is complete.

As already indicated, this 'therapy' is applied to some degree in the course of many clinical conversations aimed at 'history taking', etc. As a *specific therapy* it is the first-line treatment for acute distress or trauma, e.g. immediately following bereavement, assault or a life-threatening crisis. The method often involves face-to-face contact, but may be applied by telephone (e.g. as in helplines run by the Samaritans, the Gay Switchboard, the Rape Crisis Helpline, etc.).

The art of attentive listening is required in more complex specific treatments, as well as forming part of adjuvant therapies.

Level Two: problem solving

In practice, 'Attentive Listening' often includes some elements of problem solving, to the extent that the listener feels competent to suggest what the help-seeker might do. On other occasions, Problem Solving is the main measure used. This is appropriate in two main types of situation: when the patient has a conflict which for some reason they have been unable to solve without external help, and when the patient's problem-solving capacities have become generally impaired. The commonest reason for the first is when the patient experiences competing pressures concerning an important issue as irreconcilable, while a general problem-solving problem is usually associated with multiple pressures, and often with significant depression of mood.

The principles of this intervention are (a) information about alternative courses of action should be obtained and set out in an orderly fashion in writing; (b) the pros and cons, including the practical consequences, of each possible course of action are reviewed, and again set out in writing; (c) the steps required to make a decision are reviewed and set out in writing; and (d) the decision is made and its effects followed.

Writing is important because a characteristic component of the helplessness which accompanies a sense of inability to solve a problem is the experience of inchoate, anxious thoughts which intrude into consciousness but not in the reasoned sequence required for considered decision making. Writing points down as they present themselves is a way of 'catching thoughts' before they move out of the mind to be replaced by more unprofitable ideas.

Time is also important in decision making. This is because problem solving is enhanced when emotional tone is relatively calm, and high-intensity emotions tend to decrease with time. 'Sleeping on it' is sound advice.

Common clinical situations involving the need for problem solving therapy include marital conflicts where one partner is having an affair and a decision to leave the partnership (never easy) is in question; parenting difficulties concerning children's education, leaving home, teenage behaviour, etc.; deciding to become attached to a sexual partner to whom one is attracted; occupational situations involving change or loss of job. In short, conflicts in any of the important areas of life may present for clinical help and be amenable to this type of therapy.

When, as a clinician, one is consulted about a problem of this type, it is good practice to enquire whether the patient appears to be repeating a pattern of maladaptive difficulty in a particular area. For example, a person may with difficulty extricate themselves from a brutal and abusive relationship, only to 'somehow' become involved in another one of the same type. In such cases there is usually some learned problem deriving from early life, e.g. certain kinds of abuse or deprivation in childhood, and a third-level intervention may be indicated.

Level Two: support

'Supportive therapy' is sometimes spoken of as a simple business which anyone can do easily. This is misleading. It is true that anyone should be able to do it, or at least anyone who deals with the same patients over relatively long periods of time, but it is not always easy. One reason for this is the elusive term 'support'. When it means something specific, and not what is here described as 'attentive listening', it refers to procedures which make a person feel better about their lot, even though this remains unchanged or becomes worse.

'Support' can be understood by citing specific examples. The relative who cares on a day by day basis for an elderly person with Alzheimer's disease is dealing with a difficult coping problem for which 'support' is necessary, including various forms of practical assistance and emotional sharing and 'respite'. Support means 'helping someone cope with' a situation. Hence it may be needed to cope with dying, or to cope with a dying relative, or with caring for someone with schizophrenia, learning disability, chronic medical illness, HIV infection, etc. In its most demanding form, support means sharing emotional and life stress with someone *even though* it is not possible to do anything substantial to ameliorate the realities of the situation.

Difficulties for clinicians in providing support often arise either because sharing someone else's traumatic feelings is in itself painful, or from a general sense in clinicians that they must always be 'doing something', the equation of hope with action. Often this amounts to a denial of the realities of disability or death. Support does *not* imply that nothing can be done; support means agreeing that while 'cure' may not be possible, meaningful benefit can be obtained and described in terms of 'care' rather than 'cure'.

Note *that supportive therapy, and also problem-solving, can be provided in various therapy modes, i.e. as individual therapy or in groups.* The victims of particular illnesses, or their carers or families, often find membership of groups of fellow-sufferers of great value. The style and ethos is variable; the 'quasi-religious' approach of Alcoholics Anonymous, and its congeners in the fields of

Drug Dependence and other addiction disorders, is very effective in 'supporting' abstinence for many people, but is quite different from the approach of self-help groups set up in the UK by the Alzheimer's Disease Society, or the Schizophrenia Fellowship, to name only two such organizations. The general points to note are that group membership can have supportive effects, and that patients can provide support for themselves, often with some involvement with professionals.

Level Three: cognitive-behavioural approaches

Cognitive and behavioural *principles* and methods offer a general approach to a wide range of problems, and include specific techniques applicable to symptoms, problems or (sometimes) the patient's condition as a whole.

THE GENERAL APPROACH

This is based on the 'ABC' (the *Antecedents* of *Behaviour*, and its *Consequences*). The process begins with the description of current behaviour, going beyond the generalities so often used, such as 'he is always angry with me' or 'I never go out anywhere', to *detailed* accounts of exactly what has been happening. Descriptions are often usefully supplemented by measurements of one or more of the quantifiable aspects of behaviour, namely frequency, intensity, duration and latency.

Assessment of current behaviour can be evaluated as more or less frequent than is desired, or as quantitatively undesirable, or the problem may involve behaviour which does not at present occur at all. So the current assessment leads to a value judgement of behavioural excesses and deficits which inform treatment goals, which themselves should be described in detail.

Identifying the antecedents and consequences of current behaviour helps to delineate the processes involved in sustaining the present state of affairs. This can often usefully be done in terms of the notion of *reinforcement*, a learning theory concept which applies to influences which make specifiable behaviours more (positive reinforcement) or less (negative reinforcement) likely. Reinforcers are often social in nature, e.g. praise (usually positive) or criticism (often negative), or appetitive, as when behaviours become linked to rewarding or aversive aspects of eating, drinking, sex or sleep.

The next task is to discuss with the patient possible ways of bridging the now explicit gap between current behaviour and desired goals. The key here is to divide the gap into a sufficient number of small steps to ensure that the patient succeeds, thereby reversing the experience of continued behavioural failure which is almost universal among patients. Self-monitoring through detailed diary keeping, and sufficient relevant practice, are the main means of achieving the goals. The therapist's task is to advise the practice and review the patient's monitoring data, on which the next set of exercises will probably be based. The reader will appreciate that this resembles an educational role system more than a medical one.

Although the above comments are framed in terms of 'behaviour', the principles apply equally to 'cognitive' approaches, for the idea of behaviour includes 'internal variables such as thoughts or feelings, including thoughts about, or constructions of, what is happening externally'. 'Cognitive therapy' often facilitates the achievement of desired *external behavioural* goals, because the problem often lies in the meaning of event or behaviour as much as in the behaviour itself. Cognitive therapy is also applicable when *thought processes* are troubled, which most commonly occurs when thinking is systematically distorted in association with mood problems. For example, a generally negative way of thinking is common in depression, and thinking is often generally interrupted in anxiety. Cognitive deficits tend to interfere with problem solving, decision making and the capacity adaptively to intend acts (shown, for example, in many cases of self-poisoning).

Thought processes may be interfered with by arousal, emotion, or pain of high intensity, reduction of which may alone be sufficient for normal cognition to be re-established. Hence arousal reduction techniques may be a helpful first phase of intervention; they usually involve relaxation training, e.g. by inviting the subject to contract and relax various muscle groups deliberately in sequence, in a slow rhythm in time with the phases of respiration, using a calm and relaxed voice.

Relaxation *alone* is usually insufficient, and specific behavioural advice is needed in most cases. Maladaptive high levels of arousal often occur when people with particular cognitive 'styles', notably a tendency to view themselves as relatively worthless and the future as relatively hopeless, encounter stressful life events which produce a sense of helplessness in the absence of adequate coping responses. *Imitation* is a powerful stimulus to behavioural change and encouragement by the therapist to try specified new behaviours, perhaps practised in the imagination or in reality during therapeutic sessions, is a potent source of therapeutic change.

Level Three: dynamic approaches

The term 'dynamic' can be understood as implicating to aspects of experience and functioning of which the subject is unaware. Defined in this way, cognitive therapy is dynamic, because much cognitive activity occurs outside conscious awareness, and because the meanings attached to behaviours are often unrealized. Dynamic notions, however, helpfully draw attention to distortions of appraisal, volition and experience arising from internal processes evolved from earlier life problems. Adverse childhood experiences broadly include *deprivation* (of protection, control, affection, nurturance or mutuality required by the developing individual), *separation* from or *loss* of care-givers or others to whom the person was closely emotionally attached; or *abuse* (exposure to violent or sexual actions of others, especially damaging when the abusers are putative care-givers).

The effects of adverse experiences vary with the phase of development at which they occur. The most profound effects follow the earliest experiences, and may lead to profound difficulties in trusting others in close relationships, in behaving as a secure, autonomous individual, or in emotional control or the ability to plan and execute adaptive sequences of actions.

Children learn their interpersonal behaviour repertoires from their experience or relationships as they develop, and problems in adulthood can often be traced to earlier troubled patterns of relationship. A common pattern is that of early attachment to a care-giver within a relationship which has been predominantly negative through abuse, deprivation or inconsistency. For example, a son exposed to a violent father may grow up afraid of violence, and yet be violent towards his own son, or the daughter of a hated violent drunkard father may later become attached to a partner with similar characteristics.

The nature of such links can often be clarified by enquiry into the individual's experiences of 'falling in love', because the characteristics of the individuals to whom one becomes strongly attached in adulthood are inevitably framed by the characteristics of one's early care-givers.

Commonly, aversive childhood experiences at a vulnerable age are coped with by psychological processes which have the effect of separating various parts of the developing personality, e.g. sets of thoughts, impulses, feelings or memories, which for health should be connected together. Dynamic therapy involves trying to enable the patient to reconnect what has been so split. For example, in health an individual grows up with a view of each parent which is generally positive but may include some elements of 'fault' or 'inadequacy'. For a patient, the parent may sometimes be thought of as 'perfect' and at other times regarded as totally negative, and therapy would seek to integrate these contrasting sentiments.

Dynamic therapeutic approaches involve detecting relationship patterns of current significance to the patient, and exploring these in awareness to facilitate improved function. This can often appropriately involve an intense time-limited therapy where issues of attachment, separation and loss can be re-created in terms of the patient's experience of the relationship with his or her therapist. At other times, the exploration cannot be hurried, and may take a considerable time. In general, the therapist–patient relationship is an important vehicle for change because, as previously noted, intimate self-disclosure facilitates the emergence of emotions and thoughts with childhood qualities.

Level Three: therapy contexts

Every therapy has a context, defined by the number, length and interval between sessions, the mode of therapy (individual, group, etc.), the situation in which therapy takes place, the service contractual background (e.g. private or public health system), and the therapeutic aims and objectives, whether these are set out explicitly or not. All of these variables shape what happens during therapy, and may contribute to outcome, either positively or negatively. Thus the evidence suggests that the outcome is better when the session number is pre-determined than when the treatment is open-ended, and treatment which appears to be endless and aimless may make patients worse. Therapy modes generate their own momentum from the social systems formed by the therapeutic arrangement, i.e. processes occur in

therapy simply because therapy is taking place with a couple or in a group rather than with an individual patient. These processes may make important contributions to outcome (see, for example, Yalom (1985) on group therapy).

Level Three: indications

Treatment choice may depend on factors concerning (a) the problem for which treatment is sought, (b) the therapy, (c) the patient and (d) the therapist.

THE PROBLEM

In some instances there is clear evidence for the superiority of certain therapies in achieving particular goals. This evidence chiefly relates to cognitive-behavioural methods, in which the treatment content is defined. Important examples of *disorders* which may be expected to respond to treatment are (a) phobias (which respond to methods which emphasize approach rather than avoidance, in reality and/or in imagination), (b) psychogenic sexual dysfunctions (such as premature ejaculation, erectile failure and orgasmic failure in the female), (c) obsessive-compulsive disorders (especially when rituals are dominant) and (d) many cases of depression, especially of mild to moderate intensity.

In addition, cognitive-behavioural methods are often applicable to *symptoms* as part of an overall treatment package. This principle applies to many behavioural deficits and excesses, including eating, drinking and drug problems, social skills deficits, violence and other emotion control difficulties, self-care problems arising, for example, in the context of schizophrenia, dementia or severe learning difficulties, and deliberate self-harm.

Behaviour is a 'final common path' resulting from the interplay of many factors. Hence it may often be modifiable by influences impinging on it via different routes. Hence with many problems different approaches may have beneficial effects that are achieved by different means. It is in the above instances that the evidence for specificity is strongest.

THE THERAPY

The point here is that psychological treatment requires a 'contract' or 'deal' between patient and therapist. The patient needs to know what is being proposed, and its rationale. Cognitive-behavioural methods are relatively easy to describe, but may not appeal to patients who regard them as 'only superficial', or whose anxiety about confronting problems directly is very great. Dynamic treatments often appear ineffable, but need not be so because, like any other therapy, a dynamic therapy should have goals which are realistic and definable. Group therapies of all kinds are usually relatively hard to 'sell', because patients usually experience problems as personal and often as a matter of embarrassment or shame, not easily shared with others, and naturally they begin by thinking of therapy as an individual matter.

THE PATIENT

As noted above, the patient must find the treatment acceptable. In addition, he or she needs to consider the treatment as explained to be hopeful and something in which he or she wishes to participate. This is a function partly of therapist 'sales talk', and partly of pre-determined views about therapies which many people nowadays develop from the lay press and elsewhere.

The patient's personality and social circumstances may also contribute to the choice of therapy. For instance, time constraints derived from work responsibilities may make a brief intervention preferable to a longer one. Furthermore, some personality variables may make group membership extremely difficult, even when a group format might on other grounds be the chosen method.

THE THERAPIST

The impact of hope and enthusiasm on therapy is a two-edged sword, emerging from both therapist and patient. *Other things being equal*, what the therapist believes in and is enthusiastic about is preferable. To the extent that the therapist needs skills related to particular methods, the choice of therapy will obviously be limited if relevant skills are unavailable.

Discussion of many currently available psychological treatments, e.g. couple and family methods, psychodrama, transactional analysis, or Gestalt therapy, to mention only three, is beyond the scope of this chapter. In evaluating the claims of any therapy, the enquirer should ask what types of gain may be expected from what types of input,

using which kinds of procedure which must be ethical as well as potentially beneficial.

WHAT THE STUDENT SHOULD KNOW

The reader is reminded of the concept of psychotherapy levels outlined at the beginning of this chapter, namely that the simpler levels of influence are mediated through ordinary human interaction rather than via expert professional processes, and that treatment decisions should follow adequate assessment and formulation. Accordingly, some aspects of psychotherapy assessment and provision may properly be dealt with by students or relatively junior staff.

As a guide, the student *should* be able by the end of training to:

- do in 'attentive listening';
- provide simple 'problem solving' advice;
- make a behavioural assessment using the 'ABC';
- understand the principles of formulation and treatment allocation decisions;
- understand the main activities of cognitive-behavioural and dynamic approaches, and the general indications for their use.

In addition, the interested student *may* also:

- learn particular therapeutic techniques, e.g. relaxation; and/or
- see one or more sessions of particular expert (Level 3) activities, e.g. a session of family, group, couple or sex therapy.

Further reading

Beck, A.T., Rush, A.J., Shaw, B.E. and Emery, G. 1979: *Cognitive therapy of depression*. New York: Guilford Press.

Cleese, J. and Skynner, A.C.R. 1984: *Families and how to survive them*. London: Methuen.

Crowe, M.J. and Ridley, J. 1990: *Therapy with couples*. Oxford: Blackwell.

Hobson, R.F. 1985: *The heart of psychotherapy*. London: Tavistock.

Horowitz, M.J. 1988: *Introduction to psychodynamics*. London: Routledge.

Ryle, A. 1990: *Cognitive-analytic therapy: active participation in change*. London: Wiley.

Yalom, I.D. 1985: *The theory and practice of group psychotherapy*. New York: Basic Books.

17 CHILD AND ADOLESCENT PSYCHIATRY

INTRODUCTION

Child psychiatry is a medical discipline that deals with children and adolescents with emotional, behavioural and developmental disorders. Importantly, child psychiatry takes account of the following:

- clinical presentations vary with age, as the subjects are immature and developing;
- disorders are mostly multifactorially determined; family and schools are very important influences;
- certain disorders arise from delays or abnormal development;
- behavioural disorders are of importance.

COMMON PRESENTATIONS

Childhood

EMOTIONAL DISORDERS

These include anxiety, fearfulness, sadness, depression and somatization. School refusal may be part of an emotional disorder, particularly phobic avoidance.

CONDUCT DISORDERS

These include lying, stealing, destructiveness and fighting, and are associated with relationship difficulties.

DEVELOPMENTAL DISORDERS

These include the following:

- failure of normal development: encopresis, enuresis, language delay, clumsiness;
- hyperkinetic syndrome: restlessness, overactivity and inattentive behaviours;
- pervasive developmental disorders including autism and Asperger's syndrome.

Adolescence

Presentation is the same as for childhood, but the disorders are more differentiated. More 'adult type' disorders are seen with older adolescents.

EMOTIONAL DISORDERS

These include depression, phobias, anxiety states, obsessional neurosis, school refusal, deliberate self-harm, and eating disorders, i.e. anorexia nervosa, bulimia nervosa and obesity.

CONDUCT DISORDERS

These include stealing, aggression and truancy.

ALCOHOL AND SUBSTANCE ABUSE

PERSONALITY DISORDERS

Antisocial, borderline, etc.

PSYCHOSES

These include brief reactive psychosis, drug-induced psychosis, manic-depressive psychosis and schizophrenia.

EPIDEMIOLOGY OF CHILD PSYCHIATRIC DISORDERS

The epidemiological surveys carried out by Rutter and his colleagues of the entire population of 9–11 year olds on the Isle of Wight, followed up at age 14–15 years, were a landmark for child psychiatry. Psychiatric disorder was considered to be present if 'abnormalities of behaviour, emotions or relationships were sufficiently marked and sufficiently prolonged to be causing persistent suffering or handicap in a child him or herself, or distress or disturbance in the family or community'. The findings from this and other studies have led to the following conclusions.

- The prevalence in rural communities of child psychiatric disorder among 10–11 year olds is 6.8 per cent. This rate is almost doubled in urban areas. Conduct disorder is the most common disorder (60 per cent), followed by emotional disorders (40 per cent).
- Conduct disorder, and inattentive and overactive behaviours are more common in boys, accounting for the male excess in childhood. Emotional disorders are equally prevalent between the sexes in childhood, but show a female preponderance in adolescence.
- Childhood conduct disorder is strongly associated with family discord and specific reading retardation (SRR).
- Children with chronic illness have twice the incidence of psychiatric illness (11 per cent). Brain injury is a risk factor for child psychiatric disorder. Children with active epilepsy have a much higher rate of psychiatric disorder, at 35 per cent.

- The prevalence of psychiatric disorder amongst 14–15 year olds is 13 per cent when only parental interviews are taken into account. This increases to 21 per cent based upon interviews with the adolescents themselves.
- Depressive feelings and disorders increase after puberty; 40 per cent of teenagers report feelings of misery and depression, 20 per cent report feelings of self-deprecation and 7 per cent report suicidal feelings.

Pre-school children

Richman's study of a London borough suggests that:

- seven per cent of 3-year-olds have moderate to severe behaviour problems; 15 per cent have mild behaviour problems;
- disorders in this group are not necessarily transient; 60 per cent of disorders at 3 years persist over the next 5 years;
- psychosocial adversity is associated with psychiatric disorder; maternal depression and family discord predict disorder at 8 years;
- speech and language delay at the age of 3 years predicts the development of psychiatric disorder over the next 5 years.

AETIOLOGY OF CHILD PSYCHIATRIC DISORDERS

The aetiology of child psychiatric disorder is complex and often multifactorial. The development of a disorder depends not only upon the presence of risk factors and how these interact, but also upon the presence or absence of protective factors. The presence of one risk factor does not necessarily imply an increased likelihood of psychiatric disorder, but the combination of, say, two factors increases the risk by between two and four times. Likewise, some children remain well adjusted in the most adverse circumstances, as a consequence of protective factors, such as a close confiding relationship with an adult.

Risk factors

CONSTITUTIONAL FACTORS

- Genetic
- Chromosomal abnormalities

PHYSICAL FACTORS

- Intra-uterine infections
- Prematurity
- Injury, particularly brain injury

TEMPERAMENTAL FACTORS

- Irregularity
- Negative moods
- Poor adaptability

FAMILY FACTORS

- Family discord, separations and divorce
- Family violence

ENVIRONMENTAL AND SOCIAL FACTORS

- Stressful life events
- School – poor organization

Protective factors

CHILD FACTORS

- Positive temperament
- Above-average intelligence
- Social competence

FAMILY FACTORS

- Family closeness
- Adequate role setting
- Good relationships

COMMUNITY AND SOCIAL FACTORS

- Positive supportive friendships
- Continuing education
- Non-deviant partner

These factors will now be considered in more detail.

CONSTITUTIONAL FACTORS

Genetic factors

Polygenic influences are thought to be important in traits of intelligence, temperament, personality and specific disorders such as infantile autism, depression, hyperkinetic syndrome and reading disabilities.

Chromosomal factors

Psychiatric disorders are found at higher rates than would be predicted solely from impairment of intelligence, i.e. in Down's syndrome (trisomy 21), Kleinfelter's syndrome, Fragile X.

PHYSICAL FACTORS

Intra-uterine infections/toxins

These include rubella, toxoplasmosis, AIDS, alcohol and drugs.

Premature birth

Behavioural and developmental abnormalities are more often associated with very low birth weight in boys than in girls. This is not just a function of low IQ.

Injury

This refers particularly to brain injury. The incidence of psychiatric disorder in neuro-epileptic children is 35 per cent. Children with chronic physical disease have twice the rate of psychiatric disorders, and three times the rate if associated with physical handicap.

TEMPERAMENTAL FACTORS

Children vary in temperament along nine proposed axes: activity level, rhythmicity (regularity), approach, withdrawal, adaptability, threshold of responsiveness, intensity of reaction, quality of mood, distractibility, attention span and persistence. Difficult children, at risk of developing psychiatric disorder, are characterized by irregularity of biological functions, negative and withdrawal responses, non-adaptability, and intense mood expression, which is frequently negative.

The child's temperament is an important aspect of the 'goodness of fit' of the interaction between the child and the mother. A bad fit increases the likelihood of psychiatric disorder, while supportive family functioning largely mitigates difficult temperament.

FAMILY FACTORS

Chronic family discord and violence are strongly associated with the development of conduct disorder. Maternal depression is a risk factor for psychiatric disorder. Parental mental illness, particularly if both parents suffer, is a serious risk factor. Large family size is associated with specific reading retardation and conduct disorder.

ENVIRONMENTAL AND SOCIAL FACTORS

Life events

Life events, such as losses, death of a parent or relative, illnesses, birth of a sibling, moving house, etc., have been shown to be risk factors for the development of psychiatric illness. Moderate to serious undesirable life events have been noted to occur in up to 60 per cent of new onset psychiatric cases, independent of diagnosis. Life events increase the relative risk of developing a psychiatric disorder by between 3 and 6 times. Exit events, such as losses, appear to be important in the genesis of severe emotional disorders such as anxiety, depression and somatization. In the case of emotional disorders, two measures of maternal adversity – poor confiding relationships and the presence of maternal distress – appear to interact with life events, increasing the risk up to 96 times.

School

Major differences are found in scholastic achievement and rates of behavioural disturbance between secondary schools with a similar intake of pupils. Poorly organized schools have an adverse effect.

Urban environment

The rate of psychiatric disorders is almost doubled in urban areas. It is difficult to disentangle specific effects of urban life. The adverse effects of urban life may be largely explicable in terms of the higher concentration and greater frequency of family discord, social disadvantage and disorganization. Delinquent activities often decrease when a youth moves from an urban to a rural area.

Protective factors

Protective factors act in the presence of adversity to modify or ameliorate maladaptive responses; they do not necessarily foster normal development in the absence of risk factors. They include the following.

CHILD FACTORS

Positive temperament; social competence; academic achievement; high self-esteem.

FAMILY FACTORS

Supportive parents; family closeness; adequate rule setting; good relation with one parent, even in a severely discordant, unhappy home.

COMMUNITY AND SOCIAL FACTORS

Positive and supportive friendships; continuing further education; planned marriage or partnership with non-deviant spouse.

ASSESSMENT

The assessment procedure can vary according to the orientation of the child psychiatrist. However, it broadly consists of the following stages.

Introductory stage The whole family is seen together and information gathered. A clear behavioural account of the problem with chronology, etc., is obtained. Older adolescents may wish to be seen alone.

This is followed by either

Individual interviews These are often essential as the parents may not be fully aware of the child's emotional difficulties. For younger children, observation of play and drawings are informative. With verbal techniques, account must be taken of the child's maturity.

with

Parental interviews In addition to the information obtained directly from the parents, it is useful to observe how the child separates from the parents, and the quality of the parents' relationship. It is important to identify any parental distress or mental illness.

or

Whole family interview Family interactions, including communication, alliances, and repetitive patterns of behaviour become the focus of interest. The child's symptomatic behaviour may appear to be related to maladaptive family behaviour or beliefs.

Further investigations In cases of eating disorders and neuropsychiatric disorders, physical examination is necessary with particular reference to the central nervous system (CNS). Measurement of weight, height and head circumference is important. Psychological testing may be helpful, i.e. IQ testing using the Wechsler Intelligence Scale for Children.

Further information is often required from the child's school, social workers, paediatricians, etc. If it is a school-based problem it may be best to conduct the interview at school, or if it is a medical problem on the paediatric ward conjointly with the paediatrician.

In primary care settings it is wise for the general practitioner or health visitor to see the child outside school hours, and also to see the child separately from the parents.

FORMULATION

Formulation consists of a concise summary of presenting problems and a description of the case as understood by the clinician with regard to four areas:

- predisposing factors
- precipitating factors
- perpetuating factors
- protective factors

Treatment plans and contingencies should be outlined with a likely prognosis.

CLASSIFICATION

Classification of child psychiatric disorders in the UK is based upon a multi-axial diagnostic system which provides information about the following:

- Axis I – psychiatric diagnosis (ICD-10)
- Axis II – specific developmental delays
- Axis III – intelligence level
- Axis IV – medical conditions
- Axis V – psychosocial circumstances

Delivery of child psychiatric services

In each District Health Authority there should be one child psychiatrist for every 120 000 members of the population. Traditionally, child psychiatric services are community based in child guidance clinics. Psychiatric assessments and treatments are delivered by multidisciplinary teams consisting of a child psychiatrist, psychologist, psychotherapist, social worker and community psychiatric nurse, with links from education via educational social workers and educational psychologists.

Children and adolescents may be assessed and treated individually or with their families, but an increasingly important component of mental health services is indirect, via *consultation* to the professionals working directly with children and adolescents. For example:

Health
GPs, health visitors, paediatricians. Consultation or joint work is especially important for children with chronic disease, e.g. diabetes, asthma or terminal illnesses, and in cases of child abuse.

Education
Teachers, educational social workers and educational psychologists. For behavioural and emotional problems manifest at school, and for school refusal and truancy.

Social services
Social workers, residential social workers. For children from 'problem' families where children have been 'accommodated' or 'looked after' (old terminology, 'received into care') because of family disharmony, abuse, criminal activity or being out of control (Children Act, 1989).

Courts
Civil: Family Court, High Court, for decisions regarding parental access, custody, etc.

Criminal: Youth Court, Crown Court For forensic opinions, assessment of criminal responsibility, influence of psychiatric states upon offending behaviour, treatments and disposal.

A child psychiatrist is not only an expert on child mental health, but has knowledge of child development, family life and adult mental illness.

Most child psychiatry is delivered on an outpatient basis, or via a day-service with groups for particular disorders, i.e. sexual abuse, anxiety, school refusal, etc. Residential or in-patient services are based regionally for the few severely disturbed children and adolescents with, for example, psychoses, serious self-harm, risk of suicide, or severe eating disorders.

Local policies vary. However, behaviourally disturbed adolescents may be best accommodated by social services and treatment provided jointly by social services and psychiatric services.

SPECIFIC CLINICAL SYNDROMES

Conduct disorders

Conduct disorder refers to children presenting with abnormalities of behaviour characterized by persistence of severe aggression, stealing, lying, destructiveness and, more rarely, arson. The child or adolescent may have associated relationship difficulties.

Conduct disorder is the most common psychiatric disorder in older children and teenagers, and is up to three times more common in boys than in girls. Conduct disorder is frequently longstanding, and referral often occurs when the family and the school raise concerns. Conduct disorder is associated with family and environmental factors – in particular, marital discord, family violence and poor parental supervision. In the younger onset, specific reading delays are commonly found, and may form an important factor in the overall picture of school failure and later truancy.

Comorbidity is frequent. Conduct-disordered boys often present with overactive, inattentive and distractible behaviours, cardinal features of the hyperkinetic syndrome. Emotional symptoms are seen, in particular depression and anxiety. Mixed disorders of emotion and conduct are common. The prognosis depends upon the persistence and severity of the behaviour disorder, with a better outcome for brief disorders. Related adult outcomes include, for the severely affected, personality disorders, drug and alcohol abuse, and later delinquency and adult criminality.

It is important to differentiate between delinquency and conduct disorder. Delinquency is a socio-legal term and refers to law-breaking activities in anyone below the age of 17 years. Many delinquents are not psychiatrically disordered, and only some conduct-disordered children become delinquent.

Emotional disorders

Symptoms of emotional disorder vary across the age span and include anxiety, fearfulness, phobias, panic and later depression. Early-onset emotional disorders are less differentiated and often mixed in their presentation. Common emotional disorders include stress reactions, anxiety states (including school refusal), depression, eating disorders, obsessional neurosis and hysteria.

STRESS REACTIONS

These are characterized by an acute presentation of anxiety and depressive symptoms. Stress reactions can result in serious disruption of social and school life. These reactions often follow life events, i.e. loss, such as the death of a relative, hospitalization, break-up of friendships in adolescence, moving house, birth of a sibling. Often they are self-limiting and best dealt with in the school or primary health care setting.

ANXIETY STATES

Separation anxiety with excessive dependency and fearfulness resulting in withdrawal is seen in infancy and throughout childhood, and can recur in late adolescence. It is often associated with maternal anxiety and depression. Generalized anxiety occurs in school-age children alongside specific fears and phobias. Animal phobias are common within this age group. Later in adolescence social phobias are seen. Anxiety states in adolescence are often associated with significant social withdrawal and disruption of social relationships. Common somatic presentations of anxiety include headache, vomiting, palpitations and abdominal pain.

SCHOOL REFUSAL

This may be a presentation of an emotional disorder, and needs to be differentiated from truancy – which is an intentional school non-attendance, often associated with conduct problems. School refusal peaks at the age of 5 years and in early adolescence. Early-onset school refusal often presents as an acute situational anxiety and, if treated promptly, has a good prognosis. School refusal in adolescence is often associated with anxiety and depressive symptomatology and marked social difficulties, including withdrawal. Family difficulties and neurotic disorders are common, and the outcome in this age group is much more mixed. Liaison with the school is necessary to ascertain whether particular school factors, i.e. bullying or educational failure, are implicated in the aetiology.

DEPRESSION

It is now recognized that children can suffer from major depressive illnesses. Pre-pubertal depressive disorders occur more frequently in boys and are often secondary and associated with a family history of alcoholism or antisocial behaviour. Post-pubertal depressive disorders differ in several significant ways: they are often primary, more common in girls, and more often associated with a family history of major affective disorder. An increase in depressive disorders is seen after puberty. Pooled conservative estimates suggest that the prevalence rate of major depressive disorders is about 4 per cent.

There is some agreement that the essential symptom pattern of major depressive illness is similar in children, adolescents and adults, although age-specific features do occur. The core features are a persistent abnormality of mood, with depression, loss of interest or loss of pleasure. Associated symptoms include agitation, restlessness, inability to concentrate, and recurrent thoughts about death. Psychosocial impairment is substantial, with social withdrawal, school refusal, suicide attempts and substance and alcohol abuse. In males, antisocial behaviours are common. In adolescent males, for example, bereavement problems can present as a mixed depressive/conduct disorder.

Major depressive disorders in adolescence are associated with ongoing family difficulties, low self-esteem and stressful life events. Comorbidity with anxiety states and behavioural disorders is frequent; indeed, pure presentations of depression are not common.

OBSESSIVE-COMPULSIVE DISORDER

This needs to be distinguished from the relatively common and normal ritualistic behaviour seen in 6-year-olds of walking on cracks in the pavement, touching lamp posts, etc. Obsessive-compulsive disorder occurs in up to 0.3–1 per cent of adolescents. The picture of obsessive thoughts and compulsions is similar to that seen in adulthood. There is a strong continuity into adult life, with a correspondingly poor prognosis for severe forms

of the disorder. Comorbidity is shared with depressive disorders, anorexia nervosa and Gilles de la Tourette's syndrome.

ANOREXIA NERVOSA

This is a severe eating disorder commonly occurring in adolescence, but pre-pubertal presentations do occur. Females outnumber males by a ratio of 9:1. The characteristic symptomatology includes avoidance of carbohydrate-rich foods, distortion of body image, fear of fatness, and excessive self-induced weight loss (more than 15 per cent of ideal weight), or a failure to gain weight, with a resultant decrease in the percentile charts. Denial is frequent. Amenorrhoea in post-pubertal cases is invariably present, while in pre-pubertal cases delayed puberty, with resultant stunting of growth, is seen. With increasing weight loss a lowering of mood and obsessional features can become prominent.

Pre-morbid histories often include early eating difficulties and occasional neurotic traits. The aetiology is multifactorial and includes genetic, familial and sociocultural pressures which emphasize the pursuit and achievement of thinness for women. The girl is often a high achiever and a perfectionist, but one who has low self-esteem and a profound sense of ineffectiveness. Familial attitudes may restrain the growth of autonomy and independence.

BULIMIA NERVOSA

This occurs in late adolescence, but presentation for referral for help may be delayed because of associated secrecy (see Chapter 10 for further information on eating disorders).

Developmental disorders

Specific developmental delays in reading or mathematical skills can present as failure at school, with associated emotional problems and conduct disorder.

Enuresis

Functional enuresis (i.e. enuresis in the absence of demonstrable organic causes) is arbitrarily defined as the involuntary voiding of urine day or night at least twice per month between the ages of 5 and 6 years. As a rule of thumb, 10 per cent of 5-year-olds and 1 to 2 per cent of teenagers are enuretic. Enuresis can be nocturnal or daytime, and it may be primary (lifelong) or secondary (occurring after a period of continence). Uncomplicated enuresis is not necessarily associated with, or an indicator of, psychiatric disorder. Familial histories of enuresis are common. It is associated with social disadvantage.

Treatment, in the form of reassurance and advice about toilet training, may be all that is required. For more complicated cases, behavioural methods, including a star chart or bell and pad, are useful. Other successful behavioural methods include operant techniques with tangible rewards and fading. Rarely, tricyclic antidepressants may be useful as a short-term measure for emergencies, e.g. holidays. In resistant cases, an antidiuretic hormone, desmopressin (DDAVP), administered intra-nasally, has proved to be effective. Associated psychiatric problems may respond to individual psychotherapy or family therapy.

Encopresis

This is the passing of normal faeces in abnormal places. Children usually acquire faecal continence by the age of 4 years. This may be delayed in those with mental impairment. Physical causes of faecal retention, including painful anal fissures, etc., and Hirschsprung's disease, need to be excluded. Encopresis may be associated with anxiety and anger in a child, and often arises in the context of a disturbed parent–child relationship. A coercive, angry parenting style may result in a negativistic refusal by the child to defecate.

Encopresis may be retentive, regressive or aggressive. For those with retention, treatment often includes toilet re-training, the use of laxatives to soften stools and, in severe cases, enemas. Toilet re-training using behavioural techniques with rewards may often be all that is required. Actively involving the parents in trying to address relationship difficulties is the mainstay of treatment in moderate to severe cases.

Hyperkinetic syndrome

This is a neurodevelopmental disorder of pervasive, disinhibited, poorly organized and poorly regulated, extreme over-activity associated with a short attention span and distractibility (ICD-10). There has been vigorous debate about the existence of a distinct disorder separate from conduct disorder, with which it is often associated. Differences in diagnostic criteria have accounted for a 20-fold difference in prevalence rates between the USA and the UK, with a strict and probably under-inclusive ICD-9 criterion giving an estimated prevalence of 0.1 per cent. Males are more often affected, by a ratio of 3:1, and have a history of neurodevelopmental delays. Onset is before the age of 3 years.

Short attention span and overactivity can result in school difficulties and educational failure. Often this is compounded by behavioural problems. With increasing age, overactivity tends to diminish; however, the attentional problems remain.

In moderate and severe cases, educational failure, impulsivity and behavioural difficulties can herald a poor prognosis, with 25 per cent of cases presenting with relationship difficulties and antisocial behaviour in adulthood.

Treatment studies suggest parental counselling, and intervention at school, with behavioural modification, including rewarding of on-task behaviours, can be useful. The hyperkinetic syndrome is one of the disorders in child psychiatry that responds to medication, such as CNS stimulants, e.g. amphetamines, methylphenidate and pemoline, or tricyclic antidepressants, e.g. imipramine. A child psychiatrist should be involved in a decision to treat, which should ideally be based on a single case-control design with placebo, using ratings, follow-up and drug-free holidays.

With medication, task orientated behaviours increase, and over-activity levels tend to diminish, with a resultant improvement in mother–child interactions. Unfortunately, educational improvement does not necessarily follow. Interestingly, children with a mixed picture of hyperactivity and an emotional presentation of anxiety or misery do not show such improvement. Manipulation of diet, e.g. exclusion of food additives, is controversial, but may be beneficial in a few selected cases.

Autism

'Nuclear' autism is a rare condition (4.5/10 000 children) characterized by a specific pattern of

- abnormal development of cognition, language and socialization;
- abnormal style of functioning with rigidity, stereotypy and inflexibility;
- non-specific behavioural problems such as overactivity and temper tantrums.

Onset is usually before the age of 3 years, with males more commonly affected.

Development of verbal and non-verbal language is aberrant, not just delayed. There is a failure to communicate by gesture, body movement or facial expression. Speech is delayed or not acquired at all. It is often non-reciprocal, with monotonous phrases, echolalia and pronomial reversal.

Social abnormalities tend to be profound, with a pattern of lack of responsiveness as an infant to cuddles or being picked up, late development of social smiles, gaze avoidance and failure to make eye contact during conversations. Commonly, there is a lack of differentiation of social response to approaches by parents and strangers. These children are often described as being 'aloof'. Autism has been conceptualized by some as an impairment of the capacity for empathy.

Many children are mentally impaired with associated specific cognitive abnormalities. Rote memory and visuo-spatial skills may be excellent, but symbolization and abstract reasoning are generally poor. A child may be interested in mechanical things, and have a detailed knowledge of train timetables or the workings of gears, etc., but display no creative thinking.

Autistic children resist change and become preoccupied with routines, e.g. the same clothes and rituals. Play tends to be rigid and stereotyped, and lacks symbolic representation. Non-specific problems such as overactivity and destructive behaviours, e.g. head-banging, can be very problematic. In adolescence a proportion of autistics develop epilepsy, and some experience a regression of skills, with associated behavioural problems, particularly violence.

The aetiology is multifold. The disorder is not homogeneous, and there may be many routes, including genetic and brain damage. In about 50 per cent of the cases there are specific associated syndromes, e.g. tuberose sclerosis, phenylketonuria (PKU). To date, there is little convincing evidence for the involvement of environmental factors.

Treatment is complex and best supervised by an experienced team consisting of a child psychiatrist, psychologist, educationalist, speech therapist, etc. Parental counselling is necessary. The mainstay of treatment is a specific educational programme, using behavioural principles. The outcome is variable, with a poor prognosis in those with lower IQ and those who fail to acquire language of any sort by the age of 5 years.

CHILD MALTREATMENT

Child abuse forms an increasingly important aspect of child psychiatry. Children who have been abused or neglected appear to be at risk of developing emotional and behavioural disorders. Those who have been sexually abused are at particular risk of later psychosexual maladjustment, anxiety, depression, suicidal behaviour and possibly borderline personality disorder. Child sexual abuse also appears to be a risk factor for the later development of sexual abusive behaviour, particularly in males, thereby completing a vicious cycle.

Neglect, and emotional, physical and sexual abuse are not mutually exclusive. There is overlap, e.g. children who are neglected are also at risk of physical and sexual abuse.

Presentation

Children who have been neglected appear to have chronic low self-esteem, to be hungry for attention, social and peer approval and to have non-discriminatory friendships, attaching themselves to strangers. Failure to thrive, with a reduction in height and weight percentiles, which is corrected upon hospitalization, is characteristic.

Emotionally abused children present as anxious, depressed and withdrawn. Younger children are noted to have frozen watchfulness or developmental delay as a result of rejection, deprivation, excessive scapegoating or chronic exposure to domestic violence and disharmony.

Non-accidental injury (NAI) is an important presentation of physical abuse, and paediatricians, general practitioners, health visitors, etc., need to be alert to this.

The presentation of child sexual abuse is multifaceted. Sexual abuse may be suspected when a child presents with precocious sexual behaviour or knowledge or, less specifically, with emotional and behavioural problems, particularly running away, deliberate self-harm, hysterical states and eating disorders.

Prevalence

Emotional abuse and neglect may be widespread, and the prevalence depends upon the criteria used for definition. Sexual abuse is often defined after Schechter and Roberge (1976) as 'the involvement of dependent, developmentally immature children and adolescents in sexual activities they do not truly comprehend, and to which they are unable to give informed consent, and that violate the sexual taboos of family roles'.

Reports from the National Society for the Prevention of Cruelty to Children (NSPCC) in 1991 suggested that 42 500 children under 18 years of age were on the Child Protection Registers in England and Wales, a rate of 4.2 per 1000 children, of whom 23 per cent had been physically abused, 15 per cent neglected, 13 per cent sexually abused and 6 per cent emotionally abused; 47 per cent were registered with the indicator of grave concern. Pooled conservative estimates of child sexual abuse suggest that 10 per cent of girls and 2 per cent of boys have been sexually abused, with 47 per cent of cases involving familial contacts and 40 per cent acquaintances.

Assessment procedures

Whenever a child or adolescent discloses abuse he or she should be taken seriously and the disclosure evaluated by an experienced clinician or social worker. Specific techniques may be necessary including, for young children, the use of anatomically correct dolls, drawing materials, and dolls' houses showing sleeping arrangements, etc. It is most important that a complete psychiatric assessment of the child, circumstances, family relationships, etc., be undertaken, and attention is not solely or singlemindedly focused upon the abuse. Child Protection issues need to be addressed, and this should involve collaboration with the local Social Services Department or the National Society for the Prevention of Cruelty to Children (NSPCC), according to the principles of the Children Act 1989 (Department of Health, 1989), and the practice of multi-agency work (Home Office, 1991). Abuse within institutions and abuse rings involving prostitution of boys and girls occur, and child psychiatrists may be involved in the investigation and subsequent treatment.

Legal interventions, including removal of the abuser from home and Emergency Protection Orders, are made by the Courts. A child psychiatrist may be involved in the assessment of the child and family, and later offering therapy. Ideally, treatment should also be available for the perpetrator(s).

OTHER SYNDROMES

Munchausen by proxy (Meadow's syndrome)

This is factitious illness in a baby or young child caused by maternal abuse of the child through falsification of an illness, administration of drugs or poisons. Warning signs include:

- inexplicable recurrent illnesses;
- serious symptoms that reflect no known medical syndrome;
- illness that does not occur when the child is separated from the mother.

Often the mother is over-attentive and refuses to leave the child throughout the hospital admission, but nevertheless appears to display a lack of concern, despite serious symptoms.

The most common illnesses include bleeding, neurological symptoms, fever, rashes, biochemical abnormalities and persistent seizures – seemingly resistant to carefully administered anticonvulsants. This is an extremely serious syndrome with the death of the child being by no means uncommon. The mothers are often discovered to have personality disorders and show remarkable denial and dissociation. Legal interventions designed to protect the child are essential. Careful assessment and a treatment programme, including close liaison with paediatricians, child psychiatrists and social services, are necessary.

Deliberate self-harm

This is rare below the age of 12 years, and rates rise until the mid-teens (400 per 100 000). It is more common in females. Not all cases are referred to hospital. Ninety per cent of recorded hospital cases involve self-poisoning, particularly by means of paracetamol. Self-poisoning increased spectacularly in the 1970s, accounting for up to 10 per cent of general medical admissions. The cause of this rise is unknown, but various factors were blamed, including stresses arising from sexual liberation, a rise in the number of broken homes and a proliferation in the prescribing of tranquillizers. The most common self-injurious behaviour is wrist-cutting, which can often be multiple and difficult to treat.

In Oxford, the most common background characteristics to deliberate self-harm include broken homes, family psychiatric disorder, family suicidal behaviour and physical and sexual abuse. A precipitant is often the breakdown of a relationship with parents or boyfriend. The motivation underlying the overdose is often reported as being to die or to escape from an intolerable situation. However, clinicians rarely judge the act to involve a high degree of suicidal intent. The act is often impulsive; in one study, two thirds of cases considered self-poisoning for less than an hour beforehand. Many adolescent self-poisoners report depressive symptoms.

Assessment, especially for younger adolescents, should involve the family. Particular issues to be addressed include the circumstances surrounding the overdose, including motivation, degree of suicidal intent, presence of psychiatric disorder, current personal and family problems and suicidal behaviour as well as resources and support.

The outcome is variable, with those with acute presentation often settling within a month, while one third remain unchanged, particularly if associated with chronic behavioural and family problems. The risk of repetition is about 10 per cent.

Assessment should be undertaken by a trained counsellor or child and adolescent psychiatrist. Assessment and treatment issues should be based upon a crisis intervention model, using problem-solving techniques, for both the individual and their family.

Suicide

Although rare in adolescence (3 per 100 000), suicide rates in western societies have shown a disturbing increase, particularly in older male teenagers, aged 15–19 years. In the UK, the most common methods include hanging and self-poisoning. The precipitants are largely unknown. However, background factors include broken homes, psychiatric disorder and suicidal behaviour in the family, and psychiatric disorder in the teenager, particularly depression, angry and impulsive conduct disorder, and drug and alcohol abuse. Prevention is problematic because of the rarity and impulsiveness of the act and the ubiquitous nature of the precipitants.

Alcohol and substance abuse

Among teenagers alcohol is increasingly abused, although reliable estimates of the prevalence are not available. Problematic drinking is often seen in response to unpleasant dysphoric affects and the belief that alcohol enhances social prowess. Most of the small number of adolescents who progress to regular or heavy substance abuse have coexistent psychiatric disorders, such as mood disorder, conduct disorder, anxiety states, etc. Other risk factors for substance abuse include being a victim of physical or sexual abuse, having substance-abusing or alcoholic parents and social problems, e.g. broken home, unemployment. Adolescents increasingly appear to be using so-called recreational drugs such as cannabis, 'Ecstasy' and cocaine. Physical and psychological dependence is seen.

Psychoses

Psychoses are rare in early adolescence, becoming more common in later adolescence and early adulthood. The presentation and symptomatology are not markedly different from adult types, although up to one third of cases are undifferentiated or short-lived reactive psychoses. Schizophrenia occurring in adolescence has a poor prognosis. Manic-depressive psychosis is seen after puberty. Drug-induced psychoses are seen in up to 20 per cent of presentations.

Treatment, in particular pharmacotherapy, needs to be undertaken by specialists in child and adolescent psychiatry.

TREATMENT ISSUES

Treatment should follow a thorough assessment of the child and adolescent, their family and, where necessary, school or other factors. In child psychiatry, treatment often involves a multidisciplinary team consisting of a child psychiatrist, psychologist, child psychotherapist or family therapist. The child psychiatrist may be involved in assessing the child's mental state, formulating a treatment plan and liaising with other members of the team. A necessary prerequisite is a *formulation* with a clear description of the problem, and the aims and goals of treatment, with reference to the most appropriate treatment model. Treatment must take account of the issues surrounding consent, the emotional and cognitive maturity of the subject and the appropriate life cycle of the family.

Consent

Consent can only be considered to be valid if it is informed and freely given. Following the case of Gillett versus West Norfolk and Wisbeck Area Health Authority, children under 16 years of age can legally give effective consent to medical treatment, independently of their parents' wishes, provided that they have sufficient understanding and intelligence. This statement, although enshrined in the Children Act (1989), was partially reversed in 1992 in the case of *Re W*, an orphan girl in a children's home who refused to eat. In a ruling, Lord Donaldson stated that no one under 18 years of age has an absolute right to make his or her own decisions about medical treatment, especially when that decision is a refusal.

There is a requirement for practitioners to obtain the consent of parents and of the minor to treatment, if the adolescent is of sufficient age and cognitive maturity. The clinician must explain the treatment, benefits and risks, and also the consequences of not receiving the treatment.

In order to judge whether an adolescent can understand and therefore be in a position to consent to treatment or to refuse it, the clinician must take account of the following:

- age;
- level of intelligence, cognitive, emotional and language development;
- psychiatric condition and whether this interferes with his or her judgement;
- parent–child relationships.

If, following assessment, the adolescent is deemed not to be in a position to give informed consent, the latter may be sought from those who exercise parental authority (Children Act, 1989). Should the adolescent be competent but refuse treatment there should be further attempts at persuasion and review, including consideration of a second opinion. The legal procedures for overriding a minor's refusal to consent to treatment involve either:

1. exercising parental authority (Children Act, 1989); or
2. the High Court via:
   (a) inherent jurisdiction of the Court Section 100 Children Act (1989); or
3. Mental Health Act (1983) – there is no lower age limit.

Legal advice may be necessary.

Collaborative work

Treatment in child psychiatry often includes collaborative work with statutory agencies, such as Social Services. For example, in a case of child sexual abuse (CSA), Social Services may be involved in child protection issues (e.g. Emergency Protection Orders) and disclosure work, while a child psychiatrist may be asked for an assessment or treatment of the child and their family and to make recommendations for the perpetrator.

CONSULTATION

Consultation to professionals dealing directly with children and adolescents, such as teachers and social workers, forms an increasingly important element of the work of a child psychiatric service. The aim is to enhance the professionals' understanding of a child's dilemma and thereby allow them to deal directly with the child without involving face-to-face psychiatric contact. Consultation has the advantages of promoting professional skills, avoiding stigmatization and being cost-effective.

INDIVIDUAL BEHAVIOURAL TREATMENT

This is particularly useful in younger children, and in those with specific disorders, such as enuresis and sleep disorders. For older children, cognitive behavioural techniques are applicable, as in cases of anxiety, anger management, obsessive-compulsive disorder, phobias, depression and above all bulimia nervosa.

DYNAMIC PSYCHOTHERAPY

This usually involves weekly sessions concentrating on the expression of emotional problems and gaining insight, using play therapy for younger children, and art therapy and verbal insight therapies for older children and adolescents. Insight therapies such as these may need to be longer term. Child analysis is reserved for a small proportion of cases, usually along the lines suggested by Anna Freud or Melanie Klein. Parents are seen separately.

FAMILY THERAPY

Usually this involves the whole family. Symptomatic behaviour is thought to be related to communication and hierarchical problems and dysfunctional alliances within the family. Behavioural and structural family therapy is useful for younger onset anorexia nervosa, cases of abuse and cases involving deliberate self-harm. Active involvement of the child is necessary, with the use of drawing and play material.

GROUP THERAPY

In cases of child sexual abuse, group work is increasingly used for both victims and juvenile perpetrators.

PARENTAL COUNSELLING AND EDUCATION

Advice and education are useful for the parents of children and adolescents with conduct disorders. Dysfunctional parent–child interactions, which escalate into problem behaviours, are illustrated using role play, real-life situations and videos. This is combined with an education programme. Teaching packages, which may be therapist-aided or self-instructional, using a video, have proved beneficial at least for younger children.

Teaching problem-solving skills is useful for both parents and adolescents within a crisis intervention model in cases of adolescent self-harm. As for adults, psychoeducation combined with family measures, aimed at reducing high levels of expressed emotion (EE), is used to reduce relapse rates in schizophrenia and other psychoses.

SPECIAL EDUCATION

Special education, often involving behavioural elements, is an important aspect of the treatment of the pervasive developmental disorders (PDD) such as Asperger's syndrome and autism.

DRUGS

Pharmacotherapy is indicated in a few specific disorders, e.g. haloperidol and clonidine for Gilles de la Tourette, stimulants and antidepressants for hyperkinesis, neuroleptics for psychosis, and lithium for manic-depressive psychosis. Antidepressants are used in cases of severe depression, although to date evidence for their efficacy in childhood and adolescence is lacking. In contrast, serotonergic antidepressants (SSRIs) are effective in treating moderate to severe obsessive-compulsive disorder.

For enuresis, behavioural treatments are indicated. Tricyclic antidepressants (TCA) should only be used as a short-term measure, while desmopressin (DDAVP) is reserved for resistant cases.

RESIDENTIAL TREATMENT

This is only sparingly used in child psychiatry. Some children may need temporary placement in foster homes because of adverse family circumstances. Adolescents with self-harming and dangerous behaviour, psychoses and life-threatening eating disorders may require admission to a specialized adolescent unit.

OUTCOME OF CHILDHOOD PSYCHIATRIC DISORDERS

This is an active area of research interest, particularly for depression. As yet only a few definitive statements can be made. In general, acute disorders, a stable family, good problem-solving ability and higher IQ augur a better outcome. Developmental disorders, e.g. enuresis, generally have a good prognosis. However, intractable cases associated with multiple problems continue into adolescence. The hyperkinetic syndrome has a poor prognosis and may presage conduct disorder, drug abuse and adult antisocial criminality and alcoholism. Conduct disorder, particularly when associated with aggression, shows strong continuity into adulthood, with an increased risk of all psychiatric disorders. Severe conduct disorder is associated in 25 per cent of cases with antisocial personality disorder. Milder cases may have a better outcome.

Recovery from adolescent depression occurs in 90 per cent of cases, although for some this is delayed by up to 24 months. A third or more cases experience recurrence of depression with significant psychosocial impairment. Depression is a risk factor for suicide in 2 to 4 per cent of out-patient samples of depressed children and adolescents.

Schizophrenia in adolescence has a poor outcome, while manic-depressive psychoses may not necessarily have a worse outcome than adult forms, continuing to present a fluctuating, periodic picture into adulthood.

Further reading

Barker, P. 1995: *Basic child psychiatry*, 6th edn. Oxford: Blackwell Scientific Publications.

Graham, P. 1992: *Child psychiatry: a developmental approach*, 2nd edn. Oxford: Oxford University Press.

Rutter, M., Taylor E. and Hersor, L. 1994: *Child and adolescent psychiatry, modern approaches*, 3rd edn. Oxford: Blackwell Scientific Publications.

Steinberg, D. 1987: *Basic adolescent psychiatry*. Oxford: Blackwell Scientific Publications.

LEARNING DISABILITY

INTRODUCTION

Learning disability is the term currently used in the UK to describe people with impaired social functioning due to intellectual deficits. It has recently replaced the term 'mental handicap'. The international term remains 'mental retardation' which is synonymous with learning disability. Different professions describe this population in different ways depending on the needs that they present. Thus the population of people with learning difficulties as defined by educational authorities overlaps with the group of people with learning difficulties as defined by social service planners and those with learning disability as defined by medicine. Although these groups overlap, they are not completely synonymous.

The borderline between learning disability and normality is not sharp. As in most conditions, such as dementia, alcoholism or even diabetes, the way in which people are diagnosed as having learning disability depends as much upon social events which lead them to contact with medical staff as upon their intellectual deficits. This is most noticeable at the borderline, where few people reach psychiatric services, and those who do usually reach them because of behavioural or emotional difficulties.

The diagnosis of learning disability requires

- a reduced level of intellectual functioning (IQ less than about 70);
- resulting in impaired adaptive behaviour;
- occurring before the age of 18 years.

Further subdivision on the basis of IQ is as follows:

- mild (IQ 50–70) – prevalence 3 per cent;
- moderate (IQ 35–40) ⎫
- severe (IQ 20–35)   ⎬ prevalence 0.3 per cent;
- profound (IQ less than 20) – prevalence 0.05 per cent.

The diagnosis of learning disability requires subnormality of intelligence. People think of someone as being intellectually disabled because they display social incompetence in critical situations. However, this idea of social incompetence has been incorporated into definitions of mental retardation only incompletely using the idea of 'adaptive behaviour'. The main way in which intelligence is statistically described to define learning disability is through the Intelligence Quotient (IQ). This apparently innocuous number has become such a topic of criticism with regard to its assessment and calculation that its definition is now a statistical one, based on relative performance in an age-matched group. However, its original definition is still useful as a working concept; most psychological tests produce a measure of a person's ability in terms of mental age. For children, IQ is the ratio of mental age divided by chronological age (multiplied by 100); for adults, IQ is best considered as the ratio of mental age divided by a chronological age of 16 (multiplied by 100). A person's IQ is usually the result of a formal test which cannot fully reflect the complete range of physical, cognitive, emotional and social ability. However, it is still used as the

TABLE 18.1 Proposed multi-axial classification for mental retardation (learning disability) under ICD-10 (World Health Organization, 1993)

Axis	Content	ICD-10 codes
Axis 1	Psychiatric disorders (including personality disorders)	F00-69; F90-99
Axis 2	Disorders of psychological development (e.g. language disorder, autism)	F80-89
Axis 3	Mental retardation (learning disability) (can add coding to show presence of impairment of behaviour)	F70-74
Axis 4	Organic causes of mental retardation and associated physical impairments	A-E; G-Y
Axis 5	Abnormal psychosocial factors	Z55-65

main guide to subdivide learning disability into mild, moderate, severe and profound types. The deficits and skills of a person with learning disability are best described using a multi-axial diagnostic system. One such system is ICD-10 (Table 18.1).

Adults with mild learning disability can be expected to acquire independence in most self-care and domestic activities, as well as being able to earn money by unskilled work. The main difficulties can be expected in reading, writing and monetary skills, in emotional and social immaturity and in ability to adapt readily to social expectations or external stressors.

Adults with moderate learning disability usually have more obvious impairments and rarely achieve more than simple literary or monetary skills. Most need some level of supervision and close support to participate in domestic activities.

Adults with severe learning disability frequently have additional disabilities such as epilepsy, or physical or sensory disabilities. Most need supervision with their self-care.

Adults with profound learning disability usually need close supervision and care for their entire life. Many are able to feed themselves with a spoon. Most can understand and make simple statements and requests. Most have multiple disabilities.

AETIOLOGY

In discussing the aetiology of learning disability, one needs to take the medical model used when discussing disease one stage further. The medical model has a primary cause, usually a physical cause (e.g. a cerebral haemorrhage) producing secondary effects, or signs and symptoms (e.g. memory loss or hemiplegia). The third stage that should always be considered is that of the social disability caused by the signs and symptoms. This is little discussed in most branches of medicine, but is now gaining increasing emphasis, especially in the rehabilitation of people with chronic illness. Equally, it must be recognized that even in acute medicine it is social disability that causes people to seek medical help. For example, a person with diabetes often finally decides to go to their doctor because of the social problems being caused by their physical symptoms, and not just because of the symptoms themselves. Because of the multiple stages in producing 'disability', it is usually a gross simplification to speak of one cause for the aetiology of a person's learning disability. Similarly, it is very difficult to predict accurately the degree of learning disability that will be produced by a specific organic cause.

Discussion of the aetiology of learning disability is further complicated by the fact that several 'causes', such as cerebral palsy or hypothyroidism, are in fact not primary causes, but secondary effects of several known or unknown primary causes.

Table 18.2 shows the ascribed origin of learning disability in a survey of Swedish school children. Similar surveys exist for other populations, but the categories of analysis differ, making comparisons difficult. All surveys are flawed; in this survey there was a smaller number of mildly learning disabled (0.4 per cent) identified than statistically predicted, and Fragile X syndrome was not recognized.

TABLE 18.2 Presumed origin of learning disability in a group of Swedish children aged 8–12 years. (Reproduced with permission, Hagberg, B., Hagberg, G., Lewerth, A. and Lindberg, U. (1981) Mild mental retardation in Swedish school children: II. Etiological and pathogenetic aspects. *Acta Paediatrica Scandinavica* **70**, 445–52).

Origin	IQ < 50 (%)	IQ 50–70 (%)	IQ 70–75 (%)
Genetic	47	15	23
Abnormal chromosomes	29	4	3
Abnormal genes	5	1	6
Probable genetic*	12	10	14
Acquired as fetus	8	8	3
Alcohol	—	8	3
Infection	7	—	—
Acquired perinatally	15	18	3
Anoxia-related	12	17	—
Infection	3	1	3
Acquired postnatally	11	2	—
Childhood psychosis	1	2	—
Unknown	18	55	71
Family history of LD	4	29	46
No family history	14	26	26

*Children with multiple congenital anomalies and those with syndromes of uncertain genetic origin (includes Fragile X).

Mild learning disability

People with mild learning disabilities usually do not have a clear aetiological diagnosis for their disabilities. Most have a family history of low measured IQ, but it is unclear whether this reflects a polygenetic influence, the effects of environment, or the effects of undocumented specific causes. In the past it has been assumed that the majority of cases were due to polygenetic or sociocultural effects, but the recognition of the Fragile X and Fetal Alcohol Syndromes has suggested that more specific causes will be discovered. However, it is worth noting that at present it is rare for a child from a family of high socio-economic class to have either a mild or a severe learning disability, without a medical cause being apparent.

Severe and profound learning disability

Studies of people with at least severe learning disabilities reveal a higher incidence of identified primary causes, and most of these are genetic, reflecting the severity of effects needed to produce severe disability. Estimates of the frequency of specific causations vary greatly between studies and probably reflect the variety of populations studied and methods employed. However, in all studies the causation of a substantial proportion remains unknown.

Chromosomal and genetic primary causes

The fertilized human egg frequently fails to develop into an infant. At least 15 per cent of conceptions are spontaneously aborted by mid-pregnancy. This proportion may well be much higher if eggs that fail in the first few days and are not noticed as being a miscarriage are included. Studies of spontaneous abortions show that at least 60 per cent have chromosomal abnormalities and estimates of chromosomal abnormalities at conception range between 10 and 50 per cent. Most embryos with abnormal chromosomes appear to abort spontaneously and few reach full term.

The two most common and important genetic causes of learning disability are those found in Down's syndrome and Fragile X. Down's syndrome is the most common autosomal chromosome abnormality causing intellectual impairment. Other autosomal chromosome abnormalities are much rarer and usually lead to death in infancy.

Learning disability is about 15 per cent more common in males than in females in the community. This is partially due to recessive genes on the X-chromosome being unopposed in males, who by definition do not have a second X-chromosome. Fragile X is the most common gross abnormality of the sex chromosomes that leads to intellectual impairment. Although an abnormal number of sex chromosomes is more common, such as Turner's syndrome (X0), Klinefelter's syndrome (XXY) and the 'super male' (XYY), it is unusual for these syndromes to produce marked learning disabilities.

There is a very large number of single genes known to cause learning disability, but almost all are extremely rare, and unlikely to be met in clinical practice. We shall confine ourselves to describing one of the more common autosomal dominant conditions, Tuberose Sclerosis, and the most common autosomal recessive metabolic disease, Phenylketonuria. For further details of rarer syndromes a more specialist textbook should be consulted.

DOWN'S SYNDROME

Down's syndrome is the most common cause of severe learning disability known, being diagnosed in one third of people with an IQ of less than 50. It was first well described by Dr John Langdon Down in 1865, who labelled it mongolism, a label whose use is now discouraged.

The majority of people with Down's syndrome (95 per cent) have an additional chromosome 21 (trisomy 21). This additional chromosome is normally of maternal origin (probably more than 90 per cent of cases) and the risk of occurrence increases 50-fold with increasing parental age. About 3 to 4 per cent of people with Down's syndrome have additional material from chromosome 21 due to an unbalanced translocation of chromosomes which attaches part of a third chromosome 21 to another chromosome. About half of these are fresh mutations, but the remainder occur because a parent has a balanced translocation. Such a parent has a high risk of having further children with Down's syndrome. A further 1 to 2 per cent of people have Down's syndrome due to mosaicism, with only part of their cells having trisomy 21. From studies of people with only part of an additional chromosome 21 (as a translocation) it is possible to say that it is the distal segment of the long arm of chromosome 21 whose triplication is vital for Down's syndrome.

Down's syndrome occurs in about 100 in 100 000 live births. Of these, in the UK a third are diagnosed prenatally. A further 15 in 100 000 pregnancies are probably currently medically terminated because of Down's syndrome.

A diagnosis of Down's syndrome can be confirmed prenatally by culturing and examining fetal cells obtained through amniocentesis. This procedure carries a risk of miscarriage and should only be offered to high-risk pregnancies where the pregnancy will be terminated if the result is abnormal. This risk can now be predicted more accurately after sampling maternal blood for alpha-fetoprotein, unconjugated oestriol and human chorionic gonadotrophin. At later stages of the pregnancy, Down's syndrome can be detected by skilled ultrasound examination. Most infants with Down's syndrome are recognized immediately after birth upon routine paediatric examination. A few suffer from heart or gut abnormalities which require rapid intervention if they are to survive infancy, but most who survive the first 5 years can expect to live until at least middle age.

People with Down's syndrome are usually severely intellectually disabled, and in addition suffer from a wide range of physical abnormalities which require monitoring, including heart and gut abnormalities, eye and teeth problems, recurrent respiratory infections, obesity and sleep apnoea, dry skin, hypotonia, joint laxity and atlanto-axial instability, deafness and epilepsy. In addition, after the age of 30 years they have an increasing risk of hypothyroidism and an Alzheimer-type dementia (55 per cent of cases by the age of 50 years). They need regular medical reviews to ensure maximal physical and mental health. Fertility in women with Down's syndrome is low and in men it is almost non-existent, although most are sexually active.

FRAGILE X SYNDROME

Although people with the Fragile X phenotype have been clinically described since 1943, the chromosomal abnormality causing the syndrome was not discovered until 1977 and is still being elucidated. Recent DNA analysis has shown that the syndrome is caused by abnormal duplications of the DNA code for argine (CGG) at a specific site (q27.3) on the long arm of the X-chromosome. Probably 3 per cent of the population have a small number of these duplications and are therefore carriers. The abnormality increases with each generation, and the number of replications determines the severity of effect, people needing at least 150 copies to develop the full syndrome. The abnormality can now be demonstrated by DNA probes, but the original method of diagnosing Fragile X involved culturing cells in a folate-deficient medium whilst under chemical stress. This older test produces a constriction in the distal arm of the X-chromosome of affected individuals (giving the name Fragile X), but only a few cells show it, despite the elaborate cell culture, and the test is not infallible, making it difficult to establish the epidemiology of this syndrome accurately.

It is estimated that up to 60 in 100 000 of all

births and 100 in 100 000 male births may have Fragile X syndrome, but no studies have been made of 'normal' children in order to establish its full incidence and phenotype. Up to 9 per cent of people known to have a learning disability probably have Fragile X syndrome, but estimates have ranged up to 30 per cent.

Many children with Fragile X syndrome are not identified until they are older. They are usually male, tend to have a distinctive long face with prominent forehead and large simple ears and almost all males have large testes postpubertally. There is usually a family history of males with learning disability, although some females may also be affected. About one third of people with Fragile X are either severely or profoundly intellectually disabled, but a significant number pass their initial milestones well and only fall behind after the time of speech development.

Several physical problems are common in the group, with excessive joint laxity, flat feet, sight abnormalities and mitral valve prolapse reported. Most suffer from hyperactivity and attention deficits as children and benefit from the usual treatment for hyperactivity. Autism may be more common in this group, but they are usually keen to be sociable, although when greeting people they often avert their gaze, turning the top half of the body to do so. They are often stressed by many things occurring around them, and when so stressed many characteristically bite themselves, developing calluses on their wrists. They sometimes need treatment for anxiety. Speech and language development is always retarded, and the more vocal often repeat themselves in order to maintain the pace and flow of conversation. This problem can benefit from speech therapy.

It is intriguing that a known specific genetic abnormality can produce such behavioural characteristics in a person. How this occurs demands further research.

TUBEROSE SCLEROSIS

The frequency of Tuberose Sclerosis, or Epiloia, is generally estimated to be 10 in 100 000, but it will prove to be much more common once less severely affected people are more routinely diagnosed. This is an autosomal dominant condition, although 60 per cent of cases are due to fresh mutations. It usually appears to be due to a gene on the long arm of chromosome 9 (9q34), but families with evidence of other chromosomal abnormalities have been found. Its expression is highly variable, and

many people are found to have it only after they have been examined closely because a relative has a more severe form.

A child with Tuberose Sclerosis appears normal at birth, but as time progresses, 60 per cent of cases develop seizures, often within the first year of life, at the time of vaccination, which can increase anxiety about vaccine damage. There is then increasing mental impairment. Many later develop a classical butterfly distribution of flesh-coloured nodules (angiofibromas) on the face. In addition to the facial nodules, other skin abnormalities may occur, such as *café-au-lait* spots, shagreen patches, fibrous patches and nail-bed fibromas. Nodules occur elsewhere, as hamartomas in the brain and rectum, as rhabdomyomas in the heart, as phakomas in the retina and as angiomyolipomas in the kidneys. Most lumps are asymptomatic. Many people with mild forms of Tuberose Sclerosis are not mentally impaired, but 40 per cent have learning disability, and many of these have poorly controlled seizures. Some people with multiple brain tumours have autistic traits and hyperactivity. Some die young as a result of fits, but most mildly affected people have a normal life span, although some die early as a result of brain tumours or kidney problems.

PHENYLKETONURIA (PKU)

This is the most common single-gene recessive defect that is well documented, with an incidence of 12 in 100 000. Three different forms of defect have been identified, all of which result in the build-up of the amino acid phenylalanine in the body, which at high levels is toxic to the nervous system. Half of all cases are due to classical phenylketonuria, in which there is a defect in the enzyme that breaks down phenylalanine, namely phenylalanine hydroxylase. Untreated sufferers typically start as 'normal' infants with blue eyes and blond hair, but after a few months they become irritable, hypertonic, develop seizures and become increasingly retarded. A special phenylalanine-restricted diet from birth prevents this from occurring. Such a diet can be suspended in adolescence, although doing so often results in an irritable person. In non-classical phenylketonuria, the enzyme defects cause a wider disruption of metabolism and treatment is less successful. It is cost-effective to test for PKU at birth and it is universally tested for in the UK, but an appreciable minority still do not start the special diet within 3 weeks of birth.

Other congenital causes

The three most common congenital 'causes' of severe learning disability, other than genetic factors, are Cerebral Palsy, Neural Tube Defects and Hypothyroidism. These are syndromes produced by a range of known and unknown causes, and are thus secondary and not primary causes of learning disability. Alcohol is a relatively common cause of mild learning disability, and will also be discussed as an example of toxins causing disability.

HYPOTHYROIDISM

Congenital hypothyroidism has a variable incidence of about 25 in 100 000. Severe hypothyroidism, or 'cretinism' as it used to be called, has long been recognized as a cause of learning disability, and some of the earliest colonies for learning disabilities were those for cretins at Abendberg in Switzerland, opened in 1839.

Congenital hypothyroidism is not clearly of genetic origin, and probably has many causes, like cerebral palsy. It is cost-effective to test biochemically for hypothyroidism at birth and most areas now do so. Treatment with thyroxine is then simple, and adequate treatment starting before 3 months of age will prevent intellectual disability. However, many children with hypothyroidism have other abnormalities, especially deafness, which can impair intellectual development.

CEREBRAL PALSY

Cerebral palsy is a disorder of posture or movement but it commonly causes learning difficulties, and people with cerebral palsy often display intellectual impairment. As well as having congenital causes it can also be the result of postnatal events which cause its prevalence to increase with age, and by the age of 5 years it occurs in about 250 in 100 000 children. About 30 per cent of the infants with cerebral palsy who were born at full term have severe learning disabilities. Although only 20 per cent of low-birth-weight babies with cerebral palsy have severe learning disabilities, cerebral palsy itself is much more common in these babies, being ten times more frequent in infants weighing under 2500 g at birth, compared with those born heavier.

Cerebral palsy is not a single entity. Probably less than 10 per cent of cases are caused by perinatal factors. Birth asphyxia is rarely the cause of either cerebral palsy or learning disability. Much more common causes are vascular and haemorrhagic lesions, many of which occur prenatally, but both of which are very difficult to prevent. Genetic abnormalities and congenital infections are also causes of cerebral palsy. Better obstetric practice is therefore unlikely to reduce the incidence of cerebral palsy significantly, and better neonatal care may indeed raise it by increasing the number of low-birth-weight babies who survive.

CONGENITAL INFECTIONS

These infections by Cytomegalovirus, Rubella, and Toxoplasma Gondii are most dangerous to a fetus when they occur before 16 weeks, but currently they are not a common cause of learning disability, with all congenital infections probably causing severe learning disability in less than 3 in 100 000 births. All of these people would have cerebral palsy in addition.

The most common infection is Cytomegalovirus, with an incidence of 300 in 100 000 live births, but most infected infants appear to be unaffected, and only 10 per cent develop neonatal problems and display neurological damage. This includes the 6 per cent of cases who develop hearing loss. Neurological problems occur when the mother is infected during the first 16 weeks of pregnancy and are most severe in earlier infections.

Congenital Rubella is well known for causing cerebral palsy, microcephaly, deafness, blindness and heart disease, but is now rare due to the national immunization programme. Nationally, about 20 infants with congenital rubella are reported annually. Toxoplasmosis is even rarer, with only six cases being reported nationally each year.

The natural history of Human Immunodeficiency Virus infections in infants is still poorly documented.

NEURAL TUBE ABNORMALITIES

These are defects in the closure of the neural tube. The less severe form, Spina Bifida, is compatible with early life and has a variable incidence of between 70 and 150 in 100 000 live births. The causes are unknown, but must act before 30 days of gestation, when the neural tube usually closes.

Much research has been expended on causation, revealing many associations but no clear cause. The most hopeful advice at present appears to be a combination of folate-rich diets before and during pregnancy, combined with fetal screening, although only the more severe forms produce significantly elevated maternal serum alpha-fetoprotein levels.

Due to the very poor outcome of any treatment in severely affected infants, many centres restrict intervention to certain groups, closing any spinal defects and later, if necessary, preventing hydrocephalus by inserting a cerebral shunt to drain off any cerebral fluid which is not being properly reabsorbed. People with Spina Bifida can have a wide range of orthopaedic, urinary, bowel, endocrine and visual problems, as well as seizures and intellectual disability. Up to 10 per cent of cases will have learning disability, and almost all of these will be multiply handicapped.

FETAL ALCOHOL EFFECTS

Estimates of the frequency of Fetal Alcohol Syndrome vary immensely, but it probably occurs in more than 100 in 100 000 births. However, people with fetal alcohol syndrome are not necessarily learning disabled.

Alcohol is a toxin. Drinking 2 units of alcohol per day in early pregnancy reduces birth weight, and more serious effects are observed if more than 4 units are consumed each day. The effects are variable, but often include microcephaly, a smooth philtrum with a thin smooth upper lip, heart abnormalities, hyperactivity and poor fine co-ordination. Measured intelligence is not usually profoundly impaired and the average IQ is in the mid 60s. Many people with this syndrome do well in mainstream education.

Postnatal causes

Very few people with learning disability can attribute their disability directly to a single postnatal event. The most common direct postnatal causes of severe learning disability are abuse, injury, infection and toxins, but the incidence of these appears to vary widely and the data for them is of little use. Other postnatal causative factors in learning disability include epilepsy, superimposed psychiatric illness and autism, which will be discussed below.

Children with mild learning disability usually have at least one parent with a low IQ and are nine times more likely to come from a family of lower socio-economic class. It is impossible to dissect the reasons for this and allocate relative risk values to congenital causes, postnatal events or socio-economic influences. Low socio-economic class is associated with low birth weight, higher perinatal morbidity, poor housing, large families and poor education, all of which are also associated with mild learning disability.

EPILEPSY

Epilepsy is a symptom whose effects can worsen learning disabilities and which is more common in learning disability. In the UK about 0.5 per cent of the population will have epilepsy at any one time, although probably 6 per cent of people have a seizure at some time in their life. Epilepsy occurs in 30 per cent of people with an IQ below 50, and in almost all profoundly and multiply handicapped people. This is because of the high incidence of seizure-provoking neurological abnormalities in this population. Temporal (and probably frontal) lobe seizures are common, and should be suspected of causing any behavioural disorder. Seizures provoke disability both directly and indirectly. For example, they interfere with concentration, learning and memory; only severe seizures can cause further damage. People with seizures often become anxious about the social embarrassment of having a seizure and so lose their self-confidence and avoid social activities.

Control of seizures involves the correct diagnosis of the presence and type of seizure and a balancing of the beneficial and adverse effects of drugs. It is almost always beneficial to reduce the frequency of a person's seizures. Very few people with learning disability need to have total fit control for social reasons (e.g. because they drive), and to achieve this many need to be on doses or combinations of drugs which cause unpleasant side-effects. Drugs such as phenobarbitone and phenytoin, which in themselves impair cognitive functioning, should only be used if more modern anticonvulsants are not effective. Reducing seizure frequency will usually decrease the severity of behavioural disorders, especially if the latter occur around the time of seizures. However, in a few people a reduction in seizure frequency can increase behavioural disorder, both as a result of drug side-effects and also sometimes as a direct result of the reduced frequency of seizures.

SENSORY DEFICITS

Sight and hearing deficits are very frequently associated with learning disability. Subtle deficits can easily be missed by carers and are often not looked for in the psychiatric examination. However, they are a potent cause of further handicap and they both cause and worsen learning disability, as well as causing frustration and behavioural disorders.

All people with learning disability should have their eyesight carefully checked. Eye pathology, such as cataracts, squints, and long or short sight, is common in many congenital syndromes, and about one third of people with learning disability either need spectacles or are registered as blind or partially sighted. Crude estimates of visual acuity can be misleading; people with quite blurred vision can still see a small object on the floor if it contrasts strongly with the background and will often go around picking up bits of fluff to find out what they are. People with a slight squint, or a squint corrected too late for stereoscopic vision, will be able to see clearly, but be unable to judge depth and will be uneasy with stairs and kerbs. An ophthalmologist can test visual acuity fairly well in quite uncommunicative and uncooperative people, if necessary using such techniques as revolving drums with differing thickness of stripe. Stereoscopic vision in the more disabled person is best detected by careful observation. Eyesight deficits should be corrected where possible, allowing for the increased risks associated with surgery in the disabled.

Population surveys suggest that up to one third of people with a learning disability have impaired hearing. A minority of these are recognized by the carers (the clinician becomes accustomed to the statement 'he can hear if he wants to'). Formal audiometry tests can be carried out on most people if the testers are used to working with people with a learning disability, but some of the more profound cases need brain-stem responses measured under general anaesthetic in order to establish the hearing profile, although more recent specialist techniques can measure these responses without the need for a general anaesthetic. People who do have hearing impairment benefit from an environment which caters for this, i.e. one where people use sign language as well as speaking, people look directly at each other when speaking, and loop systems are installed to improve the usefulness of hearing aids. Hearing aids are useful in the more severely deaf, but need perseverance

and enthusiasm by all concerned to ensure that they do not become a further handicap.

DIAGNOSIS AND PREVENTION

There are many important points at which learning disability can be reduced or prevented.

Before conception

- Genetic counselling – should be offered to parents with:
    - recurrent miscarriages;
    - family history of genetic abnormality.
- Good diet, with vitamin E and folate prior to conception (to avoid neural-tube defects).
- Ensuring that the mother is immune to rubella prior to conception.

During pregnancy

- Avoidance of alcohol and smoking during pregnancy (to avoid low birth weight and fetal alcohol syndrome).
- Avoidance of drugs during pregnancy.
- Good diet with added iron and folate.
- Good obstetric monitoring and care – termination of abnormal fetuses:
    - screening maternal blood for Down's syndrome and neural-tube defects using
        - alpha-fetoprotein,
        - unconjugated oestriol,
        - human chorionic gonadotrophin;
    - chorion biopsy/amniocentesis if there is a high risk of chromosome abnormalities;
    - ultrasound screening.

At birth

- Good monitoring of birth, and intervention if needed.
- Use of anti-D antibody for mother if there is rhesus incompatibility.
- Treatment of jaundice.
- Infant blood screening for hypothyroidism, phenylketonuria, homocystinuria (and others as judged useful and cost-effective).
- Physical examination by paediatrician for abnormalities.

After birth

- Screening for sensory impairment and developmental delay at 8 weeks, 18 months and 3½ years.

- Medical and educational monitoring whilst at school.
- Immunization and vaccination.
- Prevention of child abuse.
- Avoidance of social deprivation and malnutrition.
- Support of families and help with psychological effects of disability.
- Treatment of mental illness.

Most measures taken before pregnancy involve primary prevention. Screening during pregnancy carries the risks of false-positive results and of terminating a normal pregnancy. If an abnormal pregnancy is detected, all that can be offered at present is termination, rather than cure, but modern genetic research may discover forms of treatment for genetic disorders. However, the incidence of most genetic disorders is so low that it is unlikely that it will be commercially viable to develop any treatment, and termination is likely to remain the mainstay of 'curing' genetic disorders. New screening techniques do not appear to have had a gross effect on the general incidence of learning disability in children in the developed world. Good obstetric care is the prime means of preventing perinatal causes of disability, but recent advances in care do not appear to have further reduced the incidence of perinatal causes, partially due to the increasing survival of babies with a very low birth weight, without a corresponding improvement in the prognosis of these infants.

It has become more universal for infants to be screened at birth for hypothyroidism, PKU and homocystinuria, as it is cost-effective to screen for and treat these infants. Immediate paediatric examination also picks up some of the obvious causes of learning disability, such as Down's syndrome, and enables early intervention to ensure that the child does not underachieve due to additional handicaps.

TABLE 18.3 Normal infant milestones as reported by parents

6 weeks:	Smiling at people
6 months:	Sitting with support, responds to own name, laughs
1 year:	Walking with support, speaks three or more words
1½ years:	Climbs up stairs
2½ years:	Usually dry day and night

As children develop, mothers are usually the first to notice that the progress of their child is falling behind that of others, but may well decide that this does not need mentioning to professionals. However, one should know the normal milestones which parents are likely to remember and to report (Table 18.3).

Once it is suspected that a child has developmental delay, then he or she and the family should be assessed in detail by a multidisciplinary team, including a paediatrician, speech and language therapist, audiometrist, psychologist, physiotherapist, social worker and community nurse. A plan of action is drawn up which aims to prevent further handicaps developing and which supports the family adequately. This usually occurs in Child Development Centres in the UK.

Even in developed countries, reducing poverty and environmental deprivation is more likely to achieve significant further decreases in the prevalence of learning disability than are further advances in obstetric and neonatal care.

PSYCHOLOGICAL EFFECT OF LEARNING DISABILITY

All families in which disability occurs are different. For each family and person affected, the disability has a different meaning and impact. A couple's ability to cope with their child's disability depends as much on their personal past experiences, their personal relationship, support and lifestyle, as on the exact disability of their child.

Having said this, the feelings engendered by having a disabled child occur at many levels and in many directions. Guilt, embarrassment and fear, as well as bereavement and grief at the loss of a normal child, are all common. This ocean of interacting emotions can produce a large number of reactions that significantly handicap the development of the child and result in a parent 'burying' the family situation by helping others or becoming involved in campaigns, and neglecting other relationships within the family (Table 18.4).

The clinician who tells parents of their child's impairments, or who has to deal with the families of disabled people, needs to be sensitive to the emotions of the family members, all of whom should be given the opportunity to speak, to express their feelings and to ask questions.

TABLE 18.4 Common reactions of parents to birth of an abnormal child (based on MacKeith, 1975)

Feelings	Manifestations
Shock	Disbelief of diagnosis; emotional refrigeration
Guilt	Depression; overprotection
Biological reaction 　Protection of the helpless 　Revulsion at the abnormal	 Overprotection Rejection; care without warmth; lavish care
Bereavement 　Anger 　Grief	 Anger at self, and at others; rejection of help Depression
Feelings of inadequacy in rearing	Loss of confidence; inconsistent care
Embarrassment	Withdrawal from social contact
Fear of the unknown/future	Inactivity; procrastination

Information should not be forced upon them, but given honestly when it is requested and repeated as often as needed. Continued support and guidance should be offered but not forced – and are unlikely to be accepted until the parents have been able to express and deal with some of their own feelings and to absorb some of the facts about their child. The clinician must also be aware that each major stage of a child's development – for example, going to school, adolescence, leaving school, or moving away from home – will create a further surge of feelings in a parent, making it even more difficult for that stage to be dealt with successfully. Through all of this the clinician must also be aware of any siblings and try to ensure that their needs are not neglected.

Few people care to imagine what a person with learning disability experiences as he or she develops socially. However, these people are normally aware of their social failings throughout their lives. Awareness of one's own disability is a continuous process. For example, as an infant you are treated differently, you attend a different school, your younger siblings overtake you in ability and their friends no longer play with you, you then cannot find a girlfriend, and you discover that you will be unable to have the job, car, house or spouse that the media lead you to expect. In addition, you are often stigmatized and ridiculed. Your relationships with other disabled people are devalued and you are likely to be abused sexually and physically.

Not surprisingly, many people with disability react adversely to these experiences, further handicapping themselves, for example, by insisting on behaving like an infant, avoiding new situations or social events, refusing to take responsibility for their own behaviour, using violence or tantrums to control the world around them, or becoming extremely self-centred and retreating into a fantasy world.

PSYCHIATRY OF LEARNING DISABILITY

The psychiatry of learning disability is a relatively new specialty, although doctors have been involved in the care of the learning disabled for many years. This area of psychiatry grew out of a need to understand and treat disturbed behaviour in this group of people.

Behaviour disturbance is more common in the learning disabled than in a non-disabled population, occurring in 60 per cent of cases in some surveys. Behavioural changes are now often labelled 'challenging behaviour' which is itself defined as 'behaviour of such an intensity, frequency or duration that the physical safety of the person or others is likely to be placed in serious jeopardy, or behaviour which is likely to seriously limit or deny access to and use of ordinary community facilities' (Special Development Team, University of Kent). This definition includes all behaviours that limit interaction, both active and passive. However, the term is now often used more restrictively as a euphemism for aggression.

The assessment of behavioural changes requires a full social history and physical examination, as they can be caused by various factors, including environmental stress, physical disorders and psychiatric illness, and because planning an approach to improve the behaviours usually requires a good knowledge of the person's characteristics.

Assessment should aim to determine:

- current developmental level
- social skills
- any changes in skills in the last few years
- personality
- usual reactions to stress
- recent life changes and environmental stresses
- current environmental support
- evidence of psychiatric disorders
- evidence of physical disorders

Environmental stress

Growing up is not easy for someone with learning disability. The environment is usually unpredictable, with few routines which often change. There is little security and little opportunity for activities that boost one's confidence and self-esteem (such as useful work or valued relationships). Relationships with carers or others are often terminated with little warning or opportunity to grieve appropriately.

The living conditions of a person should be examined, and modified if necessary with the consent of that person. He or she will often feel more comfortable with a more sheltered, structured environment as a base from which to explore the world, especially if he or she feels valued in this modified environment. Conflicts and uncertainties in the person's life should be addressed, and they should be given the opportunity to express their concerns and feelings and to discuss their past adverse experiences, including those of abuse if they feel able to do so.

Physical disorders

Physical illness is more common in people with learning disabilities than in the general population. Many of the disorders which cause learning disability are associated with physical illness. In addition, most have problems communicating and cannot describe their bodily sensations well. Few can describe accurately the site and nature of any pain they experience.

All clinicians should seriously consider whether a behavioural change is due to physical illness, especially if it is due to constipation, infections of the upper or lower respiratory tract, ears or urinary tract, or due to the pain of dental disease, peptic ulcers or oesophageal reflux. They should also check for physical abnormalities such as sensory impairment, epilepsy or cardiovascular disease that might be further impairing a person's ability to adapt to stressors. In addition, they should consider the possibility of drug side-effects as the cause of any changes.

Psychiatric illness

Although mental handicap is often confused with mental illness in popular attitudes, they are quite different, as the newer term learning disability makes clear. However, mental illness is more common in people with a learning disability than in the abler population, and major depression is probably twice as common. This probably reflects the level of stress to which such people are exposed.

Mental illness may be more common, but it is often more difficult to diagnose as it cannot be communicated as well, and as it presents differently to mental illness in the general population. If he or she can communicate at all, a person with learning disability has a smaller vocabulary with which to describe their feelings and experiences. They will find describing personal emotions difficult, and will often deal with psychic stress by regressing and returning to old, well-learnt methods of coping with stress, such as self-injury or violence to others. Altered moods often have to be deduced from several behavioural changes, each of which could itself could be due to several different causes. Altered mood states or psychosis will often be evident, mainly because the disruption of concentration makes the person lose personal skills such as continence.

Hallucinations and delusions are often difficult to diagnose. Like young children, adults with severe learning disability often blur fact and fantasy, thought and reality. They can report imaginary things as though they are fact, but be clearly in control of these imaginings. This 'delusion' often has an ego-strengthening function, and only becomes pathological when the person appears to be unable to control what is imagined or when the 'hallucinations' intrude on their concentration. However, the hallucinations and delusions are usually much simpler than in a more able person and they often help to indicate the person's mood.

The physical treatment of mental illness is similar to that in the general population, except that there is an increased sensitivity to side-effects, coupled with difficulty in reporting them. Neuroleptics are often needed in much smaller doses to control psychoses and should be introduced gradually if possible. Non-physical treatments, such as counselling and environmental manipulation to reduce stress, can obviate the need for drug treatment. These non-drug therapies are a very important adjunct to all physical treatments and should always be included in the treatment plan.

DEPRESSION

Depression is common, especially grief reactions. It frequently leads to regression in behaviour, with previously abandoned behaviours returning. The person will often withdraw, losing interest in socializing or joining in tasks. They can be tearful, and appear sad, and they may become incontinent. In severe depression they can display the usual biological signs of depression and hallucinations may occur. They often appear irritable as they are reluctant to be disturbed and may resist having to join in activities (including talking to others) by using violence. While withdrawn in this way they may become obsessed with bodily sensations and constantly complain of pain. They can also become very anxious. Treatment with counselling, environmental manipulation (reducing stress) and antidepressants is usually effective, although care must be taken not to worsen any seizures with the antidepressant, which is usually needed in standard doses. Electroconvulsive therapy is rarely necessary, but is as effective as in the general population.

MANIA

Mania rarely presents as euphoria and almost always presents as irritability and disinhibition. The disinhibition can involve sexual matters. The person's thoughts become pressured in more extreme states and they may be unable to sleep or settle, or even to eat, as they become increasingly active. In the more able, pressure of speech can be notable. The person will often appear confused, and paranoia and hallucinations can occur.

SCHIZOPHRENIA

Schizophrenia is rarely diagnosed in the more disabled population, as they do not have an adequate vocabulary to describe their experiences clearly enough to meet the diagnostic standards for schizophrenia, and because epilepsy and autism frequently complicate the clear diagnosis. However, schizophrenia-like psychoses are more common than in the normal population. They respond to standard treatments for schizophrenia, although neuroleptics are usually needed in smaller doses than are commonly used. People with learning disability and schizophrenia (once labelled *pfropfschizophrenie*) have a poor prognosis, because they start with a less resilient personality and poorer social competence.

DEMENTIA

Dementia frequently occurs in people with Down's syndrome as they age. It is similar to, if not identical with, Alzheimer dementia. People with Down's syndrome almost universally show histological changes of dementia in the brain by the age of 35 years, and 55 per cent display clinical evidence of dementia by the age of 50 years, but some live for up to 70 years with minimal signs of dementia. As dementia advances in Down's syndrome it is often associated with epilepsy.

As a group, people with learning disability who do not have Down's syndrome do not appear to suffer from senile dementia significantly more frequently than members of the general population.

OBSESSIVE-COMPULSIVE STATES

These are difficult to diagnose in the learning disabled, as they are rarely able to communicate their experiences well enough for a diagnosis to be made. Many have routines which keep their life ordered and reduce anxiety, and others have stereotypies which usually act either to comfort or to stimulate the person. These should not be diagnosed as obsessional states unless they are new, constitute a ritual and require completion for satisfaction. More typical obsessional rituals such as hand-washing are the forms of obsession usually diagnosed.

PHOBIA

Probably the most common phobias in people with learning disability are animal phobias, which occur in about 10 per cent of residents of institutions. The most common type is a dog phobia. These phobias can usually be treated by modelling, relaxation and graded exposure.

ANXIETY STATES

These are common, but probably underdiagnosed, and frequently neglected, again because of communication difficulties. Panic disorder does occur and treatment is the same as in the general population. Relaxation exercises, modified for understanding and associated with other cues, such as relaxing music, can be as effective as in a more able group.

ATTENTION DEFICIT DISORDERS/HYPERACTIVITY

These are also more common. They can be a serious source of stress to carers as well as impairing a person's ability to learn. Treatment is the same as in the general population and they usually improve with age.

PERSONALITY DISORDERS

Personality disorders are rarely considered when people with a learning disability are psychiatrically assessed, but there is evidence that they can be diagnosed and that they occur more frequently in this population. The most commonly diagnosed type is sociopathic personality disorder.

AUTISM

Classic autism occurs in about 20 in 100 000 children, but a further 50 cases will display many of the characteristics of autism. Autism is described elsewhere in this book (Chapter 17), but it is worth noting here that 75 per cent of people with autism are sufficiently impaired to have learning disability. It is a puzzling and stressful disorder both for the person affected by it and for the carers involved. In adult life, many people with this disorder improve as they are taught how to handle anxiety and stress and how to function despite their impairments, but the underlying impairments do not disappear. This is a pervasive developmental disorder for which no effective treatment has been found other than a highly structured style of education and living, combined with treatment, where necessary, of hyperactivity, anxiety, mood disorders and any psychosis that occurs.

ETHICS

The way in which our society treats people with a learning disability raises many ethical dilemmas. The core dilemma is how we balance our respect for all people as humans beings, of inherent value and with inherent rights, whilst we also act in a way that makes it clear that we consider that abnormality should be avoided.

Fetal screening implies a decision to terminate abnormal fetuses. The dilemma concerns precisely which abnormalities justify termination. This is often decided on the basis of expected quality of life, but the way in which quality of life is judged provokes much debate. Economics of care are sometimes raised to justify decisions, but this is a highly dubious approach, unless an equal monetary value is placed on all people.

Similarly, the neonatal period often raises the dilemma of how energetically an infant should be treated. Nowadays infants with spina bifida are often not treated if they have multiple or severe problems associated with their spinal abnormality. It is still debated how aggressively people with Down's syndrome should be treated, but it is usually agreed that potentially fatal abnormalities that occur in Down's syndrome should be treated no less aggressively than in other infants. Of more debate is whether or not people with a physically abnormal appearance should have their appearance surgically changed. Should people with Down's syndrome have their tongues reduced in size for cosmetic reasons or to help their speech?

A different dilemma arises later on when people with learning disability require treatment. As with any person, physical treatment without consent is technically assault. Parents or guardians can only consent on a child's behalf and not on behalf of an adult. Any treatment should be discussed with the person and his or her consent sought. However, it must be decided beforehand if the person can give consent that is meaningful. If it is meaningful, then the person can *refuse* as validly as they can *give* consent and their refusal must be respected. It is the personal responsibility of the treating clinician to decide whether the person can give or withhold consent with validity. What constitutes valid consent must depend in part on the nature of the treatment. Simple treatments such as having a bath, and its consequences, are probably more easily understood than, say, radiotherapy for cancer. People who are severely learning disabled are unlikely to be able to think ahead and to appreciate fully the future consequences of their treatment. If a person cannot consent, then it is the responsibility of the treating clinician to consult with family, carers, and other doctors, in order to establish that there is general agreement that the treatment is necessary and in the person's best interests. In general, all treatment should be appropriate and in the best interests of the person. Experimental treatments are unethical.

The most debated treatment is probably sterilization, which in England can only occur with the consent of a judge. However, a judge's consent does not appear to be considered necessary for hysterectomies for hygiene reasons, and these occur much more frequently than sterilizations *per se*.

There are several doctrinal campaigns relating to how people with learning disability are treated by others. The most popular of these is 'normalization', which stresses that people with learning disability have the same value as normal people, and should be fully integrated into society, being treated with the same socially valued devices with which others expect to be treated. Ethically this movement carries at its heart the conundrum of how to encourage disabled people to prefer to mix with more able people, without implying that relationships with disabled people are of less value than those with the non-disabled.

Most people with a disability engage in some form of sexual activity, although people with temporal lobe epilepsy seem to have a reduced sexual drive. Carers and parents often have great difficulty in accepting this adult activity, and by not addressing it and educating the person, increase any inability of that person to behave in a socially appropriate way. Fortunately, most learning disability services have now developed a local public policy document on how their employees should react to sexual activity in their clients. The children reared by mentally disabled parents provoke much concern in the caring agencies. There is little valid research to support most of the reactions of professionals to these couples raising children, but they justify the provision of high-quality support and education for these parents.

LEARNING DISABILITY AND THE LAW

The Mental Health Act (1983) for England and Wales recognizes learning disability in two ways. First, learning disability itself is included in the term 'mental disorder', for which detention for assessment under Section 2 for 28 days can apply. Second, learning disability with abnormally aggressive or seriously irresponsible conduct is included in the terms 'mental impairment' and 'severe mental impairment', for which treatment and guardianship orders can apply.

Despite popular folklore, there is little systematic evidence that people with mild learning disability have a higher likelihood of committing criminal acts, once the tests used are able to differentiate between low intelligence and lack of education. The effect of learning disability in making someone a criminal may prove to be even smaller once studies have also taken the effects of social class into account. Obviously, people with a learning disability are not sophisticated criminals. Recently, the Mansell and Reed reports have highlighted the increasing pressure on health services to readmit a larger number of criminals with a learning disability, as their incarceration in prison is of little long-term benefit.

SERVICES

Services for people with a learning disability are never designed by the people who they serve. As a result, the services created are more often based on local ideology than on need, and vary immensely both between countries and within the UK. Services in England are the result of a chain of events. The 1913 Mental Deficiency Act inaugurated the growth of mental deficiency colonies, run by local authorities and charities, whilst others were supported at home. The National Health Service Act removed the colonies (along with the poor law infirmaries) into the Health Service. Institutional care of the mentally handicapped then became increasingly medicalized, with doctors recruited to work in the newly labelled hospitals, whilst care in the community continued to be dominated by local authority social services staff. The last 20 years have seen the difficult transfer of care back to the local authorities and a growth of the model of 'care in the community'. The recent 'Community Care Act' has now made the assessment of and provision for the needs of people with a learning disability the prime responsibility of local authorities, with an obligation on health services to co-operate with assessments and agreed care plans.

Care in the community has been a national preoccupation since the 1960s. The Kings Fund Centre (1980) popularized the concept of 'an ordinary life', with everybody living as far as possible in ordinary accommodation indistinguishable from other houses in the street. The closure of hospitals saw the transfer of people to such houses. Recently there has been increasing concern about the issues of isolation within the community and of the mini-institutions now in the community. The Department of Health has become more pragmatic, permitting the development of long-term residential health care if it is financially justified.

The variation in local service provision reflects the local outcome of several national dilemmas. First, there is the dilemma of where the division between health and social service care should be. This is most noticeable in the services for people with aggressive behaviour and for those with profound and multiple handicaps. It has been further complicated by the growth of privately run establishments which can provide care for these people and which take people financed by either health or local authorities. The other dilemmas are whether the person will receive his or her service from a specialist or generic service and how much money can be spent on care. The most important issue with all these dilemmas is that the people in need do receive a service. Divisions between services must not cause gaps in the services available, although this is often the case.

The following are components of a good service for adults with a learning disability.

Support services

- Financial support for person and carers
- Support workers and families.

Community assessment and therapy

- General practitioner
- Community Learning Disability Team care co-ordinator.

Residential services

- Respite care
- Board and lodging scheme
- Assessment and therapy units (health)

- Long-stay residential units
  with physical security
  with 24-hour nursing staff
  with 24-hour care staff
  with visiting care staff.

Day-care services

- Resource and activity centre
- Adult education service
- Sheltered employment
- Supported open employment.

In adults with learning disability, care is usually co-ordinated through the GP and Community Learning Disability Team, although the team's name differs across the country. The team should consist of staff employed by both health and social services, and usually involves a learning disability nurse, a social worker, an occupational therapist, a psychologist, a psychiatrist, a speech and language therapist and a physiotherapist, although some teams include others, such as support workers. Team approaches to care bring with them the problem of co-ordination of care, and most teams, encouraged by the Community Care Act, now operate a system of prime workers for each client who co-ordinate care provided by the team and other sources. The name of this post changes with time, and is now becoming the 'care coordinator'. In addition, this team usually contains the main local expertise for assessing and treating behavioural changes, including aggression, and is capable of assessing most behaviours without removing the person from his or her usual settings.

For children with learning disability, health care is potentially more fragmented, with medical input from GPs, community paediatricians and specialist paediatric services, including child psychiatry and learning disability psychiatric services. In the past, almost everyone with a learning disability went to a specialist school, for the 'educationally subnormal (moderate or severe)', now often relabelled schools for 'learning difficulties (moderate or severe)'. These were often useful sources of co-ordination of care for the attending children. It has recently become more popular to advocate 'mainstreaming' for the child with learning disability, whereby he or she is integrated into the mainstream schools, with individual support. Recent financial constraints on education appear to be encouraging this trend, although it will often encourage increased isolation for the family and child, and make the co-ordination of care more difficult.

The role of the health service itself in the care of people with a learning disability is as vigorously debated as its role in the care of the elderly. Having a learning disability does not in itself mean that the person requires health services, but equally health services should not be denied to such people just because they have learning disability. Whilst the person should have full access to generic health facilities (such as general medicine and surgery), he or she appears to benefit from the attention of a more specialist service for psychiatric care, as do the elderly. Part of this is usually a specialist assessment and treatment unit, although several are usually needed to allow for the varying behaviours and vulnerabilities of the people admitted to them. The psychiatrist in learning disability is a vital component in the assessment and treatment of behavioural changes and health needs, working with the community team and hospital staff, and liaising with other medical staff to ensure that the person with learning disability obtains the best service possible and increases his or her social competence as quickly as possible.

Further reading

Craft, A. (ed.) 1994: *Practice issues in sexuality and learning disabilities*. London: Routledge.

Craft, M., Bicknell, J. and Hollins, S. 1985: *Mental handicap*. London: Bailliére Tindall.

Howells, G.J.R. 1989: Down's syndrome and the general practitioner. *Journal of the Royal College of General Practitioners* **39**, 470–5.

Kings Fund Centre 1980: *An ordinary life: comprehensive locally based services for mentally handicapped people.* Project paper no. 24. London: Kings Fund Centre.

MacKeith, R. 1973: The feelings and behaviour of parents of handicapped children. *Developmental Medicine and Child Neurology* **15**, 524–7.

Russell, O. 1985: *Mental handicap*. London: Churchill Livingstone.

19 PERSONALITY AND ITS DISORDERS

Definition

Personality can be defined as the enduring patterns of thinking, feeling and behaviour which make one individual distinguishable from another.

The personality of any person is what makes it possible to recognize them, i.e. what gives them a distinctive identity (in a psychological sense) over a period of time, and to predict how they are likely to react to given circumstances.

ELEMENTS OF PERSONALITY

- Present since teenage years
- Consistent over time
- Recognized by friends and relatives
- Stable in different situations.

The elements of personality are important for psychiatrists because, under the stresses (social, psychological and biological) that induce mental disorder, the response to the stressors will be coloured by the personality of the person. On recovery from the illness the personal resources of the person play a vital role in restoring him or her back to a place in the community.

Normally shy and suspicious people are unlikely to engage in group therapy or the day hospital. People with an easy ability to make friends can quickly re-establish social contacts following a bout of illness.

Despite the importance of personality, psychiatrists often rely on the person's own description of the type of person they were before they were unwell (pre-morbid personality). Medical notes often contain only a few non-specific lines which are not helpful. There is a need to explore this issue with someone who knows the person well and can explain the person's habitual ways of behaving, responses to stress, ability to make relationships, etc.

Questions to ask when assessing personality

- Do they make friends easily?
- Can they sustain relationships?
- Are they usually happy/miserable/worrying?
- Are they very tidy/punctual/exacting?
- Do they ever lose control or behave violently?
- How do they react to frustration?
- Do they stand up for themselves?
- Have they talked about the future and what they wish for it?
- Are they able to express feelings?
- How do they respond to difficult situations?
- Do they behave impulsively?
- Are they prone to mood swings?

ABNORMAL PERSONALITIES

DEFINITIONS

Personality disorders are characterized by deeply ingrained maladaptive patterns of behaviour that are recognizable from adolescence and continue into adult life. The abnormality may be in the balance of personality elements, their quality or expression, or in its total aspect. The person and/or society suffer as a result (World Health Organization, 1978).

Personality can be conceptualized according to two major models:

- Trait Model (e.g. Eysenck's personality model); The person is scored on a number of different traits (neuroticism, introversion/extraversion, etc.);
- Categorical Model.

A number of criteria are used to define the personality type and a person either fulfils these or does not. The current major diagnostic systems (ICD-10 and DSM-IV) use a categorical model.

Relationship between psychiatric illness and personality disorder

'All people with a psychiatric disorder have a personality disorder'

This would seem to be manifestly untrue, although some personality disorders merge into psychiatric disorders with no clear break. Some people have their personalities damaged by a chronic psychiatric illness, e.g. schizophrenia.

'Personality disorders are mental illnesses'

This position has a number of implications. In some respects it sees the behaviour of individuals with personality disorders as a proper target for therapeutic medical activity. It also suggests that some antisocial behaviours are due to illness, and this removes them from the sphere of the law to that of medicine. Moreover, it suggests that the responsibility for such acts no longer lies with the perpetrator.

'Any relationship is purely coincidental'

Some people with psychiatric disorders also have personality disorders and some do not. This is probably the most practical position to adopt, but one must be careful to give people adequate treatment (both psychological and physical) and not to leave symptoms distorted by the personality disorder untreated. The tendency is to blame the personality disorder for any unresolved symptoms. This is particularly true of depression in those with antisocial or histrionic personalities.

Determinants of personality

- genetic determinants – an excess of personality disorders is seen in the probands of people with schizophrenia and those with antisocial personality disorder
- neuropsychological determinants – subtle changes in cognitive functioning have been shown in some types of personality disorder
- family environment (childhood deprivation and abuse)
- social factors (poverty, housing, culture)

The development of personality involves a complex interaction of factors which come together in late adolescence/early adulthood. Adoption studies suggest that genetics are important (especially in the antisocial personality), but that factors relating to the type of parenting and social milieu can override these biological factors.

SPECIFIC PERSONALITY DISORDERS

The description of personality disorders in this section follows the DSM-IV classification, which presents the clearest typology available.

Paranoid personality disorder

Features of paranoid personality disorder

- Sense of exploitation
- Preoccupied with mistrust
- No confidants
- Sensitivity to insult.

People with paranoid personality disorder suspect that others are taking advantage of or harming them. They are consistently preoccupied with ideas of mistrust or doubt about the loyalty of their acquaintances. Consequently they do not confide in people and they develop grudges as a result of insults which are read into innocent remarks or actions.

In clinical practice they are difficult to interview, as they do not disclose much information and are suspicious of our motives for collecting information.

Prevalence

- 0.5–2.5 per cent in the general population
- 10–30 per cent in in-patient units
- 2–10 per cent in out-patient populations

There is an increase of this disorder among the probands of people with chronic schizophrenia.

Schizoid personality disorder

People with this disorder rarely come into contact with services during the early part of their life. Later, when they become more frail and unable to look after themselves it is difficult to engage them in services, especially those which require any type of communal activity.

They keep at a distance from social relationships including family ones, and they spend almost all of their time alone, lacking close friends or confidants. They have few interests and take little pleasure in any aspect of life, tending to be emotionally cold or 'flat'.

Features of schizoid personality disorder

- keep a distance from social relationships
- few intersts and pleasures in life
- emotionally cold and flat

Schizotypal personality disorder

People with schizotypal personalities also have difficulties with personal relationships involving any degree of closeness. However, they are also rather eccentric people. They have odd beliefs in mystical influences or magic that control behaviour and which are not the norm for their culture, and they speak in vague, elaborate, circumstantial ways. They are suspicious of others and have ideas but not delusions of reference.

People with schizotypal personality disorder may seek treatment for anxiety or depression, which develop as a result of their interpersonal difficulties. In a clinical setting many of these people are found to have major depressive disorders, but under stress some can develop a schizophrenia-like illness, usually of short duration.

There is an excess of this disorder among the relatives of patients suffering from schizophrenia.

Features of schizotypal personality disorder

- suspicious
- eccentric
- have unusual beliefs
- speaks in unusual vague and circumstantial ways
- problems with close personal relationships

Antisocial personality disorder

This is the term currently used to describe the person who repeatedly acts with a disregard for and transgresses the rights of others.

They do not conform to social norms, and frequently break the law of the land. They are irritable and reckless, getting into fights, unconcerned about the effects of their actions on themselves or others. They have little ability to plan ahead and they act impulsively. People with this disorder cannot tolerate frustration and demand instant gratification of their wishes. This pattern is repeated without remorse and with little ability to learn from experience.

Antisocial personality disorder has a long and complex history and should not be equated purely with criminality. Any assessment needs to be made in the light of the cultural, social and

Features of antisocial personality disorder

- they violate and have little regard for the rights of others
- do not conform to social norms, breaking the law
- impulsive and do not learn from their behaviour
- high rates of substance abuse
- can die young and violently

economic circumstances in which the person lives. Such individuals have multiple relationships and wreak havoc in the lives of those with whom they come into contact. Their ability to lie and give glib reassurances can make them quite seductive, but in time problems with relationships develop, and these are damaging to partners and children.

People with this disorder have high rates of substance abuse, which complicates the picture and they tend to die prematurely, often by violent means (e.g. as a result of accidents or suicide).

Prevalence

- 3 per cent in males
- 1 per cent in females
- in clinical population the prevalence varies hugely depending upon the setting (3–30 per cent)

Antisocial personality disorder is more common in the first-degree relatives of those who have the disorder. Adopted-away children also have higher rates, although the new family environment does ameliorate the situation.

Course

The antisocial personality tends to burn out over time, especially by the fifth decade. Some social relationships can keep the problem in check until it is disrupted.

CASE 19.1

A 68-year-old man had a history of drunkenness, violence and theft in his early years, but after marrying at the age of 34 years he got into no more trouble with the police. The relationship was turbulent and ended with his wife's death of chronic obstructive airway disease. He was unable to look after himself and moved to a residential home for the elderly, where he stabbed a care assistant following an altercation over his breakfast.

Borderline personality disorder

'Borderlines', as they have rather inelegantly become known, have a pattern of very unstable personal relationships which result from intense fears about real or imagined abandonment. They are very sensitive to environmental cues and can

rapidly alternate between different 'self states', plunging into sudden rages or even psychotic episodes (borderline with psychosis) when they feel that they are being left. The abandonment is perceived as implying that they are bad. Under such circumstances they indulge in impulsive actions such as self-mutilation or suicidal gestures (8 to 10 per cent complete their suicide, and this or repeated self-mutilation are common reasons for presenting to the mental health services), as desperate attempts to ensure that they are not left alone. These acts also assuage the chronic sense of emptiness and boredom which they feel. Prison or the police cell provoke particularly bad reactions in such people. Substance abuse is common.

Their personal relationships move rapidly from intense idealization of their partner to a sense that the person does not care about or value them. These shifts in viewpoint make it difficult for the partner to cope with the relationship, which soon dissolves in a predictable manner.

Features of borderline personality disorder

- a fear of rejection and loss
- suicidal and self-mutilating behaviour
- rapidly changing moods and behaviour ('self states')
- feelings of emptiness and boredom
- brief psychotic episodes
- many have a history of childhood sexual abuse
- 75 per cent are female
- 2 per cent of the general population
- 10 per cent in out-patients
- 20 per cent amongst in-patients
- 30 to 60 per cent of all personality disorders
- five times more common in first-degree relatives
- in their thirties or forties they usually gain more stability

Histrionic personality disorder

People with this disorder wear their hearts on their sleeve in no uncertain terms. They display excesses of emotion and indulge in attention seeking behaviour. When they are not the centre of attention they feel uncomfortable and have to wrest the spotlight back on to themselves. They display provocative sexual behaviour in inappropriate situations, using physical appearance to attract attention and approbation. They tend to be mercurial, changing rapidly, moving on to the next interest very quickly, and unable to sustain attention over a long period.

About 2 per cent of the population have this type of disorder. It is more commonly diagnosed in women than in men.

Features of histrionic personality

- centre of attention
- excessive display of emotion
- inappropriate sexual behaviour
- attention seeking behaviour

Narcissistic personality disorder

People with this disorder sustain an inflated sense of their own importance, making out their abilities to be greater than they really are. This makes them boastful and blind to others' perceptions of them, believing that they will be seen as very impressive. They will wonder about a world which does not seem to appreciate their values, and they attempt to associate only with people who they perceive to be as important as themselves. The community prevalence of this disorder is less than 1 per cent, and 50 to 75 per cent of the patients are male.

Features of narcissistic personality disorder

- inflated sense of their own importance
- boastful
- unable to see that others may not appreciate them
- attempts to associate only with people as important as they perceive themselves to be

Avoidant personality disorder

People with this disorder avoid situations in which any criticism might be forthcoming. They have chronic feelings of inadequacy, and so do not take promotion at work. They do not become involved with new people unless they are certain of being liked. They are shy, restrained and often forgotten people.

Features of avoidant personality disorder

- avoid situations in which criticism may be given
- chronic sense of inadequacy
- shy and restrained
- only involved if sure of praise

Dependent personality

These people are unable to manage their day-to-day affairs without the help of others. They cannot assume responsibility for decisions for fear of disapproval and seek a great deal of reassurance before any task is undertaken. They experience fears of being left alone and unable to cope, and have a low opinion of their own abilities.

Features of dependent personality

- difficulty making decisions without loss of support
- fear of disapproval
- fears of being alone and being unable to cope
- low opinion of their own abilities

Obsessive-compulsive personality disorder

For this group of people things have to be just so. A place for everything and everything in its place is their motto. This excessive adherence to rules and details diverts them from the very activity that they are trying to achieve. They will work to excess, not for the money but for its own sake, and feel uncomfortable with time on their hands. Leisure activities become 'projects' to be organized down to the nth degree and carried in a perfect manner. Their houses become full of objects that cannot be thrown out because 'they may be useful one day'. These people are rigid and inflexible about money and moral issues. This sense that there is only one way to do things means that they have trouble fitting in with others, and they can be very frustrating to work with.

It is sometimes difficult to distinguish this disorder from an obsessive-compulsive disorder (see Chapter 9 on anxiety disorders), but careful evaluation of the phenomena involved should identify the differences.

> **Features of obsessive-compulsive personality disorder**
>
> - inflexibility
> - a sense of there being only one way to do things
> - failure to appreciate creative solutions
> - over-meticulous attention to the system and details
> - failure to get things done as a result of excessive attention to detail
> - a tendency to check and re-check

The disorder is present in twice as many males as females and has a prevalence of 1 per cent in the community.

MANAGEMENT OF PERSONALITY DISORDERS

Views about the management of personality disorders vary greatly within the psychiatric profession. For some they are not regarded as psychiatric disorders at all, and unless there is comorbidity (e.g. a person with obsessive-compulsive personality disorder who develops a depressive illness), they are not seen to be the responsibility of psychiatry. Repeated acts of deliberate self-harm and offending bring personality-disordered people into frequent contact with psychiatrists.

Medication

Medication can be used in certain circumstances (e.g. neuroleptics can be used to treat the transient psychotic phenomena of a patient with borderline personality disorder) or if there is comorbidity (e.g. a depressive illness in a person with histrionic personality disorder).

Psychotherapy

Psychotherapy with this group can be very difficult, time-consuming and, at times, unrewarding. Attempts to get the person to examine their feelings and behaviours and the consequences of these are fraught with problems. These elements have been present for long periods of time and are often not even seen as problems by the putative patient. Their ability to learn from their experiences may also be limited.

A wide range of therapies, from short focused therapies involving just a few sessions through to long-term individual support and even long-term group-living with a psychotherapeutic input (therapeutic communities), have been employed with varying degrees of success. Behavioural methods such as social skills and assertiveness training can be of great value in some cases (e.g. avoidant personality disorder). Behavioural methods are combined with a cognitive element. For people with antisocial personality disorder, society often deems that punishment rather than therapy is required. This may be short sighted, and a combination of the two approaches is required to rehabilitate the person to a more constructive way of life. Important components of rehabilitation include vocational training, relationship skills and anger management training.

Issues in the management of personality disorders

- Should personality disorders be treated as a medical problem (i.e. as an illness)?
- Should punishment be the only management when the law is transgressed?
- Medication is of limited use in certain circumstances.
- Which form of psychotherapy should be used, and for how long?
- What elements are required for rehabilitation?

Further reading

Dolan, M. 1994: Psychopathy – a neurobiological approach. *British Journal of Psychiatry* **165**, 151–9.

Stein, G. 1992: Drug treatment of personality disorders. *British Journal of Psychiatry* **161**, 167–84.

Tyrer, P., Casey, P. and Ferguson, B. 1991: Personality disorder in perspective. *British Journal of Psychiatry* **159**, 463–71.

20 ADDICTION

It is important to start by clarifying the language used when talking about addiction.

DEFINITIONS

Intoxication

Short-term psychological and physiological changes caused by a psychoactive substance.

Abuse

Long-term effects of psychoactive substances.

Hazardous use
Consumption of psychoactive substances that carries a high risk of long-term damage to health.

Harmful use
Consumption of drugs or alcohol that is already causing detectable damage to health.

Dependence syndrome

A psychophysiological phenomenon caused by repeated administration of a psychoactive substance (i.e. not all drug users are drug-dependent).

Withdrawal state

This can be physiological and/or psychological, and refers to disturbed physical and mental functioning when the psychoactive substance is abruptly discontinued.

Tolerance

The need for increasing doses in order to produce the same effect.

Craving

An overwhelming desire to consume the psychoactive substance.

ALCOHOL ABUSE

Introduction

Recent evidence suggests that the levels of harm caused by alcohol consumption in some developed countries are actually declining, but alcohol abuse still represents an important source of ill health and economic loss.

Alcohol problems continue to increase in the developing world.

Alcohol dependence syndrome

The alcohol dependence syndrome consists of the following elements:

- compulsion to drink, with loss of control after a few drinks, and craving when alcohol is not available;
- withdrawal symptoms, which after several years of high alcohol intake start to occur when the blood alcohol level falls, typically on waking in the morning. Withdrawal symptoms include 'shakes' (tremulousness), anxiety, dry heaves (nausea and retching) and sweating. The patient may go on to develop delirium tremens. Withdrawal symptoms are suppressed by 'relief drinking', which is often surreptitious;
- priority is given to alcohol drinking, with neglect of family, career and health;
- there is increased tolerance, although in advanced alcohol dependence tolerance may actually decrease;
- reinstatement ('rekindling'), i.e. loss of control with a return to heavy drinking after a period of abstinence.

The elements of the alcohol dependence syndrome can thus be summarized as compulsion, withdrawal, priority given to drinking, tolerance and reinstatement.

Recognizing and assessing the problem drinker

CASE 20.1

A 54-year-old teacher was admitted for bilateral inguinal hernia repair the evening before his operation. The following evening, when most of the other patients on the list were lying quietly or moving very gingerly, he was stomping up and down the ward, sweating heavily, and demanding to be allowed home. He was disorientated in time and place, and information obtained from a visitor revealed him to be a regular heavy drinker, although he had only admitted to consuming a few units of alcohol per week.

Be aware of the social damage asociated with excessive alcohol consumption, including violence, deterioration of relationships, money problems, and difficulties at work because of impaired productivity, absenteeism and accidents. High-risk occupations include catering and the licensed trade, the entertainment industry, travelling salesmen, journalists, the armed services, merchant seamen and, of course, the medical profession.

Be aware of associated medical problems – these include digestive tract disorders, liver disease, memory impairment, neuropathy (presenting as tingling in the legs), convulsions, depression, anxiety and impotence. Deliberate self-harm is also commonly associated with alcohol abuse, especially in men.

Take a detailed account of the amount of alcohol consumed on a typical day, starting in the morning. Is there 'relief' drinking or surreptitious drinking?

Use the CAGE questionnaire:

C Have you ever thought that you should Cut down on your drinking?
A Have people ever Annoyed you by criticizing your drinking?
G Have you ever felt Guilty about your drinking?
E Do you ever have an Eye-opener (i.e. a drink first thing in the morning to steady your nerves)?

Review the systems and organs most commonly affected, namely the upper gastrointestinal tract, the liver and the nervous system.

Arrange laboratory tests. The γ-GT is raised in 80 per cent of problem drinkers, and the MCV in 60 per cent.

EPIDEMIOLOGY

- 5 in 1000 members of the general population are alcohol dependent
- 25 in 1000 are problem drinkers
- Alcohol dependence syndrome is most common in middle age (40–55 years)
- The male:female ratio is 2.5:1
- The middle classes are the least affected.

AETIOLOGICAL FACTORS

Genetic factors

Twin studies show a high concordance rate for alcoholism, with 70 per cent for monozygotic twins and half this value for dizygotic twins. If a sibling or parent is alcoholic, the child is 2.5 times more likely to develop alcoholism than a member of the general population. Adoptee studies also support the notion of some genetic effect.

Psychological factors

There may be modelling in which the pattern exhibited by the parents is imitated by the children. In some cases a classical operant reinforcement may occur as withdrawal symptoms are reduced by further drinking.

Social and cultural pressures

The high incidence in certain occupations suggests that the combination of peer-group pressure and the ready availability of alcohol, combined with boredom and a lack of female company, are important factors. In some cultures alcohol consumption is prohibited, whilst in others it is regarded as a sign of virility and manliness.

Damage caused by alcohol abuse

The damage caused by alcohol abuse can be physical, psychological and social in nature.

PHYSICAL DAMAGE

Direct toxic effects of alcohol

- hepatitis and cirrhosis
- neuropsychiatric syndromes and peripheral neuropathy
- anaemia
- cardiomyopathy
- pancreatitis
- haemochromatosis
- low-birth-weight babies and fetal alcohol syndrome with facial deformities, low intelligence, low birth weight and small stature

Neuropsychiatric syndromes

These include:

- memory blackouts or amnesia for events when drunk;
- delirium tremens (DTs).

CASE 20.2

A 42-year-old nurse had been drinking heavily over the previous 5 years since the breakup of a relationship. She had stopped drinking, for reasons that were unclear. When her friend brought her to hospital, she was highly aroused, sweaty, flushed and had a tachycardia. She was extremely frightened of the small animals that she thought she could see darting about the room. When briefly left alone she attempted to kill herself by hurling herself off the chair on which she had been sitting.

Features of delirium tremens

- clouding of consciousness
- disorientation
- impairment of recent memory
- disorders of perception with illusions and hallucinations, frequently of a visual nature
- agitation and fearfulness
- sleeplessness
- sweating, fever, tachycardia and raised blood pressure
- electrolyte abnormalities
- risk of chest infections

Delirium tremens occurs during withdrawal after several years of heavy drinking. It develops within 24 hours after withdrawal, can last for 3 or 4 days, and is worse at nights. If left untreated it has a significant mortality, not only from physical problems but also from suicide.

Withdrawal fits

Generalized convulsions can occur between 1 and 14 days after stopping alcohol consumption. Carbamazepine can be used as prophylaxis if seizures are known to have occurred previously.

Malnutrition

Malnutrition occurs for several reasons:

- diversion of money away from food to alcohol;
- gastritis with loss of appetite;
- impaired absorption from the small intestine;
- reliance on alcohol for calorie intake.

TOXIC NUTRITIONAL DISORDERS

Wernicke's encephalopathy (acute)

This occurs when the heavy drinker has had an inadequate food intake for several months or more.

Features of Wernicke's encephalopathy

- drowsiness
- concentration and short-term memory deficits
- disorientation and misidentifications
- ataxia
- ophthalmoplegia (6th nerve palsy and nystagmus)
- peripheral neuropathy (classically present but not invariable)

Korsakoff's syndrome

This is a permanent state which can occur in those who survive Wernicke's encephalopathy.

Features of Korsakoff's syndrome

- marked loss of recent memory and the inability to learn new material
- disorientation in time
- confabulation – filling in memory gaps with old memories or imagined events

Both Wernicke's encephalopathy and Korsakoff's syndrome are associated with haemorrhage in the mamillary bodies and medial dorsal nucleus of the thalamus. The pathogenesis is thiamine deficiency, usually combined with the direct toxic effect of alcohol on the brain.

ALCOHOLIC DEMENTIA

Cerebral and cerebellar atrophy are seen on CT scan in patients who present with global impairment of cognition, rather than the profound memory problems with otherwise relatively well preserved functions that are seen in Korsakoff's syndrome.

In alcoholics who are not cognitively impaired, large ventricles and sulcal widening are seen in 50 per cent of cases.

ALCOHOLIC HALLUCINOSIS

CASE 20.3

A 50-year-old man with a long history of heavy drinking went to his local police station to complain about 'men threatening to hang him'. His complaint was dismissed, so he went to a nearby jeweller's, smashed the window with a brick, and then returned to the police station asking to be arrested, as a way of obtaining sanctuary from the menacing voices.

Auditory hallucinations of a threatening or abusive nature occur in clear consciousness. The voices may talk directly to the person, or talk about him or her in a running commentary. The voices can be so vivid that the patient repeatedly moves residence in order to try to escape, or else reports innocent neighbours to the police. The voices may persist for weeks or even months after withdrawal. Conversely, alcoholic hallucinosis can also occur while the person continues to drink heavily.

LONG-TERM PSYCHOLOGICAL AND SOCIAL CONSEQUENCES OF ALCOHOL ABUSE

These include deterioration of the personality, depressed mood with an increased risk of suicide, anxiety, erectile impotence and morbid jealousy. Alcoholism is associated with marital conflict, violence, job loss and road traffic accidents.

Treatment of alcoholism

Total abstinence is recommended:

■ for those over 40 years of age;
■ for those with evidence of physical damage;
■ for those for whom a controlled drinking programme has failed.

Controlled drinking is recommended:

■ for those under 40 years of age;
■ for those with no signs of physical damage.

Despite intensive treatment, about 50 per cent of cases will continue to have an alcohol-related problem.

WITHDRAWAL FROM ALCOHOL

Controlled withdrawal from alcohol can be carried out on a domiciliary basis provided that:

■ the problem drinker lives with a capable adult;
■ he or she can be reviewed daily by a health professional (a general practitioner or community nurse);
■ there is no history of delirium tremens or fits.

DRUGS USED IN DETOXIFICATION TO PREVENT DELIRIUM TREMENS AND FITS

Carbamazepine

This is given in an initial dose of 200 mg three times a day for 3 days. The dose is then reduced by 100 mg daily over the next 6 days. This may be supplemented by a hypnotic such as temazepam (10–20 mg) for insomnia during the first few days only.

Chlordiazepoxide

This long-acting benzodiazepine is used in a dose of 80–100 mg daily for 3 days and is then phased out over 7 days. The long half-life allows for a smooth reduction in blood levels of the drug.

Chlormethiazole (Hemineverin)

Chlormethiazole, despite its long history of use in the field, is not recommended because:

■ it has a marked euphoriant effect which leads to rapid psychological dependence;
■ in combination with alcohol it can cause a lethal respiratory depression. It can also cause this

alone when used in the form of an intravenous drip;

■ it has been widely misprescribed as a supposed long-term treatment for alcohol abuse.

Thiamine

Thiamine in a dose of 300 mg three times a day for 9 days will compensate for deficiency of this vitamin, preventing Wernicke's encephalopathy or Korsakoff's syndrome.

ADDITIONAL TREATMENTS FOR ALCOHOL ABUSE

Education

Providing information to the problem drinker about the consequences of continued abuse of alcohol is an important part of any treatment. This should include not only the physical effects but also the psychological and social consequences of drinking.

Alcohol Damage Inventory

Completing this inventory highlights the range and extent of the damage caused by alcohol abuse, and provides a starting point from which therapy can begin.

> **Headings used to assess damage caused by alcohol abuse**
>
> ■ relationships – violence, moodiness, impotence
> ■ work – absenteeism, low productivity, accidents
> ■ financial aspects – calculation of the weekly outgoings on alcohol consumption and related activities (e.g. minicabs home, loss of income)
> ■ legal aspects – debts, fines, driving offences

Cognitive-behavioural therapy

The patient is asked to monitor the moods, situations or activities that were previously associated with drinking, and alternative ways of dealing with these are worked out and practised (e.g. instead of visiting the pub on the way home from work, find another route home; instead of using alcohol in social situations to reduce anxiety, learn anxiety management and assertiveness techniques).

Group therapy

Self-deception is commonly found amongst regular heavy drinkers. Group therapy provides an opportunity for frank and accurate feedback from other members of the group concerning the problems that the patient faces.

Self-help groups

Alcoholics Anonymous

This self-help organization makes problem drinkers feel welcome and offers its members a great deal of support. While it can be life-saving to some problem drinkers, others are deterred by its religiose style.

Alanon

This is a sister group for the partners of alcoholics. It fosters a challenging and confrontational approach which can be invaluable for family members who have inadvertently 'colluded' with their alcoholic relative by treating them as a helpless victim and tolerating physical and psychological abuse.

Chemical deterrents

Disulfiram

Disulfiram blocks the oxidation of alcohol so that it accumulates as acetaldehyde.

When a person takes disulfiram regularly, the ingestion of alcohol causes:

■ flushing;
■ headache;
■ rapid pulse (with the danger of cardiac dysrhythmias);
■ nausea.

Disulfiram treatment must not be started within 24 hours of drinking alcohol. Some people find this 'chemical crutch' helpful in the short term as a way of learning to live without alcohol. Its main disadvantages are as follows:

■ side-effects (nausea, halitosis and loss of libido);
■ the hazards of interaction with alcohol;
■ it encourages a passive attitude in the problem drinker, who simply relies on a 'chemical solution' rather than reappraising and restructuring their attitudes and regimes.

Psychotropic drugs

Treatment with benzodiazepines after detoxification is to be avoided, as it only leads to further chemical dependence. For those who also have depressive illnesses, treatment with antidepressants or prophylaxis with lithium or carbamazepine are indicated.

ADDITIONAL PSYCHOTHERAPEUTIC INPUT

This is often required, e.g. in the form of marital therapy or other forms of counselling.

CONTROLLED DRINKING

Controlled drinking programmes are suitable for young problem drinkers who have no history of severe dependence or withdrawal symptoms.

Aspects of drinking taught in controlled driking programme

- the damage caused by heavy drinking (see above)
- the unit system (i.e. how much they are drinking: 1 unit is equivalent to a glass of wine or half a pint of beer)
- how to control intake

Guidelines for controlling intake:

- never drink alcohol to slake your thirst
- alternate alcohol with a non-alcoholic drink
- do not participate in 'round' drinking
- switch to low-alcohol drinks
- pace the speed of your drinking
- avoid drinking in response to mood, e.g. anger, depression or boredom

COMMON DRUGS OF MISUSE

Despite a requirement that medical practitioners in the UK report all people known to be or suspected of being addicted to opiates or cocaine to the Chief Medical Officer, the official statistics on drug use have always been unreliable. The problem is described as having reached epidemic proportions since the explosion of drug use in the 1960s. Issues

such as HIV infection, drug-related crime and the widespread use of 'Ecstasy' have highlighted substance abuse in recent years.

The following drugs are the most commonly misused, either alone or in combination:

- sedatives/hypnotics, e.g. benzodiazepines (especially temazepam), alcohol;
- stimulants, e.g. amphetamines, cocaine, 'Ecstasy' (MDMA);
- opioids, e.g. heroin, methadone;
- others, e.g. cannabis, solvents.

Assessment of the drug abuser

Areas to cover

- the reasons for the request for medical help, and the person's hopes for the future
- the drugs that the user claims to be taking
- the amount of each drug taken (it may be easier to estimate this from the amount of money spent on the drugs)
- the damaging effects of these drugs upon the person and those around them
- what happens if they do not take the drug (withdrawal symptoms)
- what they do in order to obtain the drug (theft, prostitution, etc.)
- the history and patterns (what makes them start, what makes them stop) of the abuse
- evidence of psychiatric comorbidity (e.g. depression)
- the personal and social strengths that the user can employ for the future

PHYSICAL ASSESSMENT

Assessment of the general physical state

- puncture marks, scars or abscesses (evidence of intravenous injection greatly increases the possibility of HIV infection);
- cardiovascular status (the risk of subacute bacterial endocarditis with intravenous injection);
- marked constriction or dilatation of the pupils;
- jaundice (hepatitis B).

STEREOTYPES

Drug users do not all conform to the stereotype of the unemployed intravenous heroin user living in a squat, supplementing his or her income by stealing car radios and small-time dealing. Drug misusers include schoolboy solvent sniffers, adolescent experimenters, weekend ravers, stable long-term methadone users, and those who are dependent upon prescribed drugs, especially tranquillizers.

Opioids

These include the following:

- heroin;
- diamorphine;
- methadone;
- pethidine;
- Temgesic;
- Diconal;
- DF118.

CASE 20.4

A 22-year-old man attended casualty late on a Saturday night. He had run out of money the previous day and had been unable to obtain any more heroin from his dealer. He was highly aroused, his pupils were dilated, his eyes were running, and he complained of severe stomach cramps. He was given Lomotil and thioridazine, which relieved many of his symptoms. He was advised to go to a voluntary agency for further care.

Opioids can be taken intravenously, smoked, swallowed or, in the case of heroin, 'snorted' (i.e. absorbed through the lining of the nasal passages).

The main positive effect of opioids is euphoria, with an initial 'rush' or 'buzz'.

Negative effects of opioids

- respiratory depression
- constipation
- loss of appetite
- loss of libido

Tolerance to the drug develops quite rapidly, and increasing doses are therefore required. Tolerance is also lost rapidly, and this is a partic-ular danger if the person goes back to using the drug at the same level after a period of abstinence. Accidental overdosage may occur.

WITHDRAWAL SYMPTOMS

Withdrawal symptoms develop after about 6 hours

- craving for the drug
- restlessness and insomnia
- pain (in joints, bones and muscles)
- running nose and eyes
- sweating
- abdominal cramps and diarrhoea
- dilated pupils
- tachycardia

The symptoms reach a peak at 36–48 hours. They are rarely fatal, but are intensely unpleasant. The effects of methadone withdrawal are delayed and less intense.

EPIDEMIOLOGY

The data for the number of addicts are unreliable, but figures of around 20 000 in the UK have been proposed. The usual age of presentation is between 20 and 30 years with a male:female ratio of about 4:1. All social classes are involved in the use of these drugs.

AETIOLOGY

No single clear factor explains the use of these drugs in any individual.

There appears to be no genetic component to drug dependence. As with alcohol, 'modelling' is a potent explanation. Living in a group in which such behaviour is usual and encouraged makes it more likely that drug use will be taken up.

Positive reinforcement following the taking of the drug makes repeated use likely. The availability of the drug is also important. Much higher levels of use are observed in areas such as Hong Kong where opiates have been readily available.

DETOXIFICATION FROM OPIATES

Methadone

The initial dose of methadone is equivalent to the person's intake of opioid drug. This can be a difficult calculation to make because:

- addicts may exaggerate their daily consumption (in contrast to alcoholics, who tend to underestimate it);
- street heroin has no standard potency.

The range is usually 20–60 mg daily, and the dose is reduced by 25 per cent every 3 days.

Clonidine

Clonidine, an alpha-noradrenergic agent, is used in some centres, but in such cases the patient's blood pressure must be monitored closely.

LONG-TERM MANAGEMENT OF OPIATE ABUSE

By the early 1980s, the long-term prescribing of methadone to addicts (methadone maintenance) was beginning to be questioned in terms of both its efficiency and the message it conveyed to addicts. However, with the advent of HIV infection, 'harm minimization' has been given priority, with the dispensing of injecting equipment and condoms to intravenous addicts in 'needle exchange' schemes. This is combined with an attempt to persuade intravenous users to substitute oral methadone for parenteral heroin, so reducing the risk of transmission of blood-borne viruses (HIV and hepatitis B).

About 30 to 40 per cent of opioid misusers become abstinent in the long term.

Harm minimization

Aims of harm minimization

- to stop or reduce the use and sharing of injecting equipment
- to reduce drug use
- to reduce unsafe sex

Methods employed

- education about the hazards of sharing equipment and of unsafe sex
- education about the sterilization of equipment
- offering needles (25-gauge orange) and syringes (2 ml), preferably in exchange for used ones
- providing condoms
- prescribing oral methadone
- offering support

Stimulants

CASE 20.5

A 34-year-old man was admitted to hospital via casualty. He was highly aroused and frightened, and believed that a large stretch of south-east London had been re-created somewhere in Asia by his drug dealer, who was trying to harm him. He knew this to be so because many of the cars only had one person in them. He absconded shortly after admission, but when seen later he spoke of the 'bad' batch of speed he had been sold just prior to his admission.

The most commonly abused psychostimulants are 'Ecstasy' (MDMA, a mixture of an amphetamine-like substance and a mescaline-like substance), amphetamines (sulphate, 'Speed') and cocaine. 'Crack' is an especially potent preparation of cocaine, made by 'cooking' cocaine with baking powder and water. It is easily carried and distributed, and it produces a rapid 'high' when inhaled. Cocaine can be injected or 'snorted'.

EFFECTS OF STIMULANTS

Main effects of stimulants

- a rapid 'high'
- euphoria
- disinhibition
- overactivity
- insomnia
- garrulousness

Side-effects of cocaine and amphetamines (less marked)

- excited overactivity
- dilated pupils and shakiness
- tachycardia and an increase in blood pressure
- seizures and cardiac arrest
- sensation of insects crawling under the skin (formication or the 'cocaine bug')
- paranoid psychosis (see Chapter 7 on schizophrenia)

No physical withdrawal syndrome is experienced in association with these drugs, but the psychological withdrawal can be very intense, with craving, depression and lack of energy.

Both amphetamines and cocaine are excreted from the body relatively quickly, and can only be identified in the urine for a short period.

TREATMENT

The drugs can be stopped abruptly, and the withdrawal problems of rebound depression and lack of energy can be treated with a tricyclic antidepressant.

Hallucinogens

The most commonly used hallucinogens in the UK and Eire are:

- LSD (lysergic acid diethylamide);
- psilocybin (found in 'magic mushrooms').

Hallucinogens can cause distortion or intensification of sensory perceptions. This can include the sense that sounds have colours or that actions are music (synaesthesia). These drugs can also distort the body image and the passage of time. The user may find these experiences elating or intensely frightening (a 'bad trip'). The treatment for the panic and anxiety induced by a bad trip consists largely of reassurance and nursing the patient in a comforting environment. This can be supplemented by a benzodiazepine or a neuroleptic if required.

There are no physical or psychological withdrawal symptoms, but some LSD users have 'flashbacks', consisting of an intense and distressing recurrence of sensory distortion occurring weeks or even months after taking the hallucinogen.

Solvent abuse

This is mainly a group activity engaged in by boys and youths aged between 8 and 19 years. The solvents used are found in household and industrial preparations, including glue (toluene and acetone), petrol, lighter fluid (butane), aerosols and fire-extinguisher contents.

Intoxication starts within minutes of inhaling the substance and lasts for up to 2 hours, causing euphoria, disorientation, blurred vision and speech, ataxia, nausea and vomiting. Forty per cent of solvent abusers experience visual hallucinations. Some solvents have irreversible neurotoxic effects.

Causes of death through solvent abuse

- cardiac dysrhythmias
- respiratory depression
- trauma
- asphyxia
- inhalation of vomit

Solvent abuse is a dangerous recreation. There is no physical withdrawal syndrome (although craving can occur), so it is best to discontinue solvents abruptly.

Cannabis

This drug is smoked either as 'grass' or marijuana (*Cannabis sativa* leaves) or as a resin made from the flowering heads of the plant. The psychoactive constituent is delta-L-tetrahydrocannabinol.

The desired effect is euphoria, and sometimes distortion of time and space. Ingestion of high doses leads to a delirium which resolves without the need to prescribe medication.

There are no physical withdrawal symptoms, but regular users develop cravings. The drug can be identified in the urine over a long period of time, as it is absorbed by the body fat and only excreted slowly.

CANNABIS PSYCHOSIS

It is unlikely that cannabis can cause a chronic psychosis in its own right. It appears that large doses taken by a vulnerable individual may result in an acute organic confusional state (delirium) or a transient psychotic illness with a labile mood. For those who have schizophrenia, the use of cannabis may adversely influence the prognosis.

Further reading

Edwards, G. and Peters, T.J. (eds) 1994: *Alcohol and alcohol problems*. London: Churchill Livingstone.

Ghodse, A.H. 1995: *Drugs and addictive behaviour: a guide to treatment*, 2nd edn. Oxford: Blackwell Science.

21 OLD AGE PSYCHIATRY

Why is this chapter in the book? Why are there old age psychiatrists? These questions may be answered under three headings:

- population demographics;
- epidemiology of mental disorders;
- special needs.

DEMOGRAPHICS

People are living longer and there is a huge increase in the population of the so-called 'oldest old' (aged 85 years or older) (see Figure 21.1). The elderly are among some of the most disadvantaged members of the community. Deprived of work and

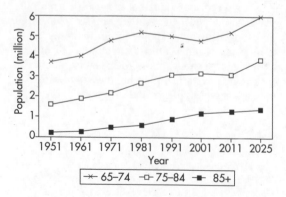

FIG 21.1 Projected increase in the population aged over 65 years in the UK.

status they are regarded as a burden by many people, and their care has been neglected for many years. Problems of how to provide for this group are very much to the fore in many industrialized nations.

What is it like being old? Everybody wants to live for ever but no one wants to get old. Even if you ask the elderly what it is like to be old, many will give a negative response but tell you that for them it is not too bad, better than they expected. They will also tell you that they are the lucky ones and that for others it must be terrible.

Negative stereotypes of the old persist, especially in cultures where the elderly are not respected for their wisdom or as repositories of traditions.

EPIDEMIOLOGY OF PSYCHIATRIC DISORDERS IN THE ELDERLY

The other main reason for there being old age psychiatry services is the epidemiology of psychiatric disorders in the community.

The number of people under the age of 65 years suffering from dementing illnesses is small. Over the age of 65 years dementia becomes much more common, but it important to realize that 8 out of 10 people at the age 80 years do not have any problems of this nature.

TABLE 21.1 Epidemiology of psychiatric disorders in old age expressed as a percentage of the total population

Disorder	Percentage of the population
Depression	10
Severe depression	3
Phobic disorders	10
Generalized anxiety	4
Dementia	
Over 65 years of age	5
Over 80 years of age	20
Psychosis	1

As can be seen from Table 21.1, other disorders, depression and psychotic illnesses also present in old age.

SPECIAL NEEDS

The complex mix of social, medical and psychological problems that some elders experience requires special attention. The elderly frequently present with multiple problems in each of these areas.

Assessment

CASE 21.1

A 75-year-old woman was referred to the service by her home help because she was becoming increasingly miserable. She was now housebound because of her osteoarthrosis and she sees few people since she was widowed 3 years ago. Her family had moved away. She suffered from glaucoma and hypertension, and was on a huge cocktail of medication to relieve her pain and treat her blood pressure. Her house was rented and there had been no repairs for many years. She could not get into her lavatory because her Zimmer frame was too wide, and she could no longer get up the stairs to bed. There were steps down to her kitchen with no handrail, and the carpet consisted of small mats on a linoleum floor.

When assessing elderly people it is rare that one professional alone can carry out a full assessment or implement an integrated care package.

Elderly people who present with psychiatric disorders frequently have general medical disorders which need to be taken into account. The above case is typical of referrals to old age services and requires the assessment and integration of care from a wide range of professionals and agencies.

The ideal multidisciplinary team for the assessment of elderly mentally ill includes the following:

- occupational therapists;
- community psychiatric nurses;
- psychologist;
- social worker;
- psychiatrist;
- physiotherapist.

The other important issue is liaison with other services (inter-agency working). Case 21.1 illustrates the need for input from elderly medicine, social services and possibly also the voluntary sector to develop a plan of care which will require careful co-ordination. Involvement of the person themselves, regardless of their apparent capabilities, and also of their carers and relatives, is vital.

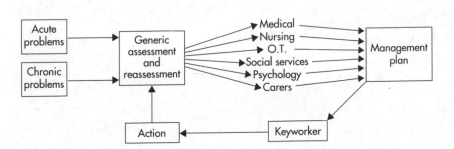

FIG 21.2 Multidisciplinary assessment in the elderly.

Groups to be considered when developing a care plan

- the elderly person
- old age psychiatry team
- elderly medicine
- primary care teams
- social services
- voluntary agencies
- carers and relatives

Services for the elderly

PROVISION OF SERVICES

The provision of services for the elderly with mental health problems needs to take account of the following issues:

- knowledge of the local population and the epidemiology of psychiatric disorders in the elderly, so that the levels of service required to meet these needs can be provided;
- user friendliness – access to the service must be easy. The service must go to the client in the first instance, and there must be as few hurdles as possible before an assessment can take place;
- service integration – the services must be integrated with those providing care to other groups of elders, e.g. health care of the elderly services and social services departments (see above list of groups to be considered when developing a care plan);
- quality assurance – programmes must be in place to ensure that the services delivered are of a good standard.

Requirements of Mental Health in the Elderly Services

- services must be user friendly
- ease of access
- adequate provision
- integration of services
- quality assurance

SOME SPECIFIC DISORDERS

Dementia

This is a chronic, acquired and usually progressive impairment of a wide range of cognitive areas, sufficient to interfere with the day-to-day life of the sufferer. Dementia is not an inevitable consequence of ageing.

PRESENTATION

It is often difficult to identify the precise time when a dementing illness starts. It is often insidious, and only when a crisis erupts and people look back do they realize that there have been problems for some time.

CASE 21.2

An 82-year-old woman was found wandering the streets in the middle of the night with no coat on. She was taken to hospital where no physical illness was identified, but she was found to be disorientated in place and time, and to be suffering difficulties with her memory. She was admitted to a social services home. Her relatives later gave a history of problems dating back some 3 years with increasing difficulties in self-care and memory, which they had put down to her age.

It is possible to divide the illness into several broad stages. No particular symptoms (except memory problems) are inevitable at any one stage, and the clinical picture will vary greatly from one person to another.

Symptoms of the early stages

- mild confusion over day-to-day matters
- odd behaviours (e.g. putting slippers in the refrigerator)
- concern about losing control of one's affairs
- depression
- agitation
- loss of interest in the wider aspects of life

Symptoms of the middle stages

- increasing forgetfulness
- wandering at night
- repeated questions
- neglect of personal care
- needing help with dressing
- difficulty in expressing oneself
- irritability
- hallucinations and delusions

Symptoms of the late stages

- severe confusion
- inability to recognize people
- needing help with all day-to-day tasks
- incontinence
- personality change
- physical decline and death

Basic investigations

- full blood count (FBC)
- erythrocyte sedimentation rate (ESR)
- blood sugar (BS)
- thyroid
- vitamin B_{12} and folate
- urine analysis
- urea and electrolytes (U & Es)
- liver function test (LFT)
- calcium and phosphate
- syphilis serology
- chest X-ray

Indications for further investigation

- early onset
- atypical picture
- need to diagnose more accurately

Further investigations

- computerized tomography (CT) scan
- electroencephalogram (EEG)
- magnetic resonance imaging (MRI) scan
- dynamic imaging (SPECT or PET)
- lumbar puncture

ASSESSMENT

A history taken from the person suffering with dementia may not be very revealing. The importance of obtaining a history from an informant cannot be stressed too highly.

Assessment of cognitive state is dealt with elsewhere (see schema for recording mental state). A standardized form of assessment (e.g. the Mini Mental State Examination) is useful because it can measure the rate of change in the person and assess the impact of any therapeutic strategies.

Assessment from all disciplines is vital (see above). The ability to manage everyday tasks and the development of appropriate care packages is essential.

Physical examination, with particular attention to the central nervous system and the cardiovascular system, must be performed.

INVESTIGATIONS (DEMENTIA SCREEN)

Reversible dementias are rare, but a basic physical screen for them must be performed. Exactly who should have more extensive investigations is unclear. People who develop their dementia when very young or who do not fit the usual clinical picture should have a more detailed investigation. When specific treatments become available, detailed investigation of the type of dementia will be required.

MANAGEMENT

Drug therapies

There are no products licensed for the treatment of dementia in the UK (see below).

Non-specific therapies
The balance between the treatment of physical problems and side-effects caused by the medication must be carefully judged. Iatrogenic complications may make life worse for the sufferer.

Depression

If depression is present it must be treated in its own right. In view of the anticholinergic properties of the tricyclic antidepressants, serotonin selective reuptake inhibitors are the drugs of choice (e.g. paroxetine).

Psychotic symptoms

People who suffer disabling psychotic symptoms (delusions and hallucinations) should have these treated with antipsychotic medication.

Behavioural disturbances (e.g. agitation or aggression)

Thioridazine is a popular choice for treating behavioural disturbances, but it has no special merits over most other neuroleptics. Chlorpromazine is not recommended because of its adverse side-effect profile. These major tranquillizers act in a non-specific manner.

Other drugs

A wide range of other drugs has been used to treat behavioural disturbances, but none seems to work in a consistent and reliable way (e.g. trazodone, buspirone).

MANAGEMENT AT HOME

Most people with dementia live at home. Usually this is a familiar environment where the person is able to function for much longer than if they are moved to a new and unfamiliar environment. To facilitate care in the home, services may be arranged, including home helps, meals-on-wheels, nurses to check medication, befrienders, put-to-bed services, etc.

Isolation may be combated by day centres and clubs where social interaction can be facilitated.

Adaptions to the home can make it much more user-friendly for the demented person.

Carers

The burden of looking after a person with dementia can be very severe. Many of the pleasurable expectations that you have of your retirement disappear if your partner develops dementia. It is especially difficult if the sufferer is agitated, sleeps poorly, and is incontinent or aggressive.

Strategies to relieve carer burden

Giving the carer information about the illness, what to expect and what services are available is important. Carers' groups provide a vital point of contact for many people. Sharing the problems and realizing that one is not alone can make life bearable. Longer courses of 'education' have proved effective in training carers how to approach the problems presented by the person with dementia.

For some carers, respite and sitting services which give them the opportunity to get other things done goes some way towards easing the stress which they experience.

Money and dementia

It can be difficult for the person with dementia to manage their finances. Many entrust others to take care of these affairs in an informal way, but this can lead to problems, both for the sufferer who is at risk of exploitation and for the carer who may be accused of misconduct.

More formal arrangements can be made. The sufferer may make over Enduring Power of Attorney to a trusted carer who will then manage their finances. This is usually done at an early stage in the illness when they are able make the decision.

If they are not deemed capable of making the decision, then they can be referred to the Court of Protection who will appoint a person to take control of their finances and who will be accountable to the court.

Making a will

The ability to make a valid will is judged by 'testamentary capacity'. General practitioners may well be asked to judge whether a person is of 'sound disposing mind and memory', the criteria for which are as follows:

- understanding the purpose and nature of the will;
- knowing what property and possessions the person owns;
- knowing who might have justifiable claims on the property and possessions; this requires them to know the names of their nearest relatives;
- ability to judge the relative strengths of the claims that might be made by the nearest relatives, without distortion due to paranoid beliefs or severe memory impairment.

SOME SPECIFIC DEMENTIAS

Alzheimer's disease (AD)

CASE 21.3

A 73-year-old man was referred by his family doctor. He was reported to have experienced a gradual worsening of memory problems over the last 5 years, and was now having increasing difficulties communicating with his wife. He needed more help with day-to-day activities, and was often up at night. He frequently did not recognize his wife. Examination showed him to have difficulties in all areas of cognition. A diagnosis of probable Alzheimer's disease was made.

The five A's of Alzheimer's disease (after Burns, Howard and Petit, 1995)

- amnesia
- aphasia
- apraxia
- agnosia
- associated symptoms: psychiatric symptoms (depression, delusions, hallucinations) and behavioural symptoms (aggression, wandering, sexual disinhibition, sleep disturbance)

DIAGNOSIS

No definitive clinical diagnosis can be made for AD. A definitive diagnosis can only be made at autopsy or on brain biopsy (rarely performed), when the characteristic neuropathology can be identified (see below).

RISK FACTORS FOR ALZHEIMER'S DISEASE

The cause of AD is not known, but a number of risk factors have been identified.

Age
The incidence of AD increases with age.

Genetic factors

Clues from Down's syndrome
All sufferers from Down's syndrome (trisomy 21) develop dementia. This has similarities to AD at a microscopic level. Some workers have found an association with chromosome 21, but only a few early-onset cases can be explained by this abnormality.

Other genetic clues
Other early-onset cases have been linked to chromosome 14. Some late-onset cases have been linked to chromosome 19. More recently, people who were homozygous for the E_4 allele which produces apolipoprotein E (itself linked to chromosome 19) have been shown to have a 90 per cent chance of developing late-onset AD. Apolipoprotein E may act to make the deposition of amyloid more likely.

Risk factors for Alzheimer's disease

- age
- genetic (especially being homozygous for E_4 allele)
- head injury
- aluminium exposure

BRAIN ABNORMALITIES IN ALZHEIMER'S DISEASE

Gross abnormalities (see Figures 21.3 and 21.4)
These include the following:

- enlargement of the sulci and shrinkage of the gyri;
- enlargement of the ventricles.

Neuropathology
There is neuronal loss, which is most marked in the frontal and temporal lobes.

Senile plaques (Figure 21.5)

- are extracellular
- have an amyloid core (composed of the amyloid precursor protein)
- have aluminium at the centre
- have paired helical filaments (made of tau protein) around the core
- are found in the hippocampus and neocortex
- have been correlated with the degree of dementia in life

Tangles (Figure 21.6)

- are intracellular
- consist of paired helical filaments

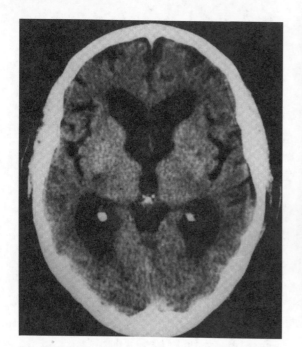
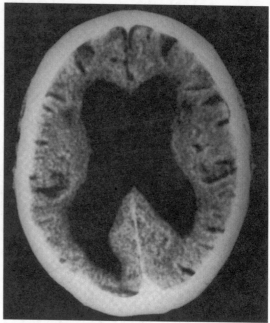

FIG 21.3 CT scan showing cerebral atrophy and ventricular enlargement in Alzheimer's disease.

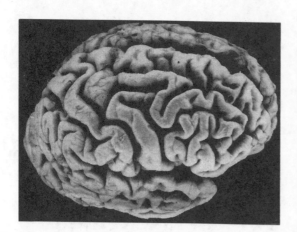
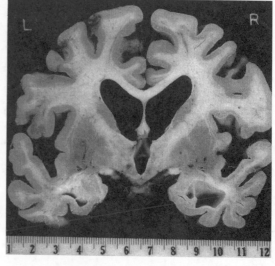

FIG 21.4 Sections of the brain in Alzheimer's disease showing gross atrophy and enlargement of the ventricles.

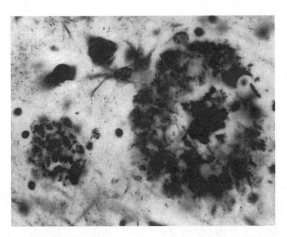

FIG 21.5 Senile plaques.

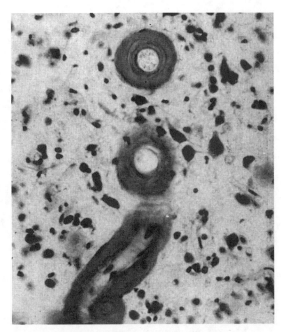

FIG 21.7 Amyloid angiopathy.

Amyloid angiopathy (Figure 21.7)

There is deposition of amyloid around the blood vessels.

Neuropathology in AD
■ cell loss
■ plaques
■ tangles
■ amyloid angiopathy

Neurochemistry

The cholinergic system is:

■ most consistently reduced in AD;
■ associated with memory functioning.

DRUG TREATMENTS FOR ALZHEIMER'S DISEASE

No drug treatments are available for dementia in the UK, although Tacrine has recently been introduced in the USA and France. Tacrine is an Acetyl Cholinesterase Inhibitor, and has been shown to be of benefit to a small number of people with AD, but it causes liver function abnormalities in a large number of recipients. New drugs of a similar nature are in the pipeline.

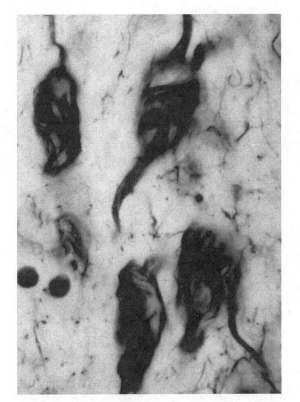

FIG 21.6 Intracellular tangles.

Other new drugs will target the deposition of amyloid, but these are still some years away.

MANAGEMENT

See the section on general management of dementia.

Vascular dementia (multi-infarct dementia)

Dementia due to vascular damage to the brain tissue can be differentiated from AD by the following features of the illness:

- sudden onset;
- 'stepwise' progression with intervening stable periods;
- episodes of confusion;
- history of stroke or cardiac ischaemia;
- risk factors for vascular disease (hypertension, diabetes, etc.);
- patchy cognitive impairment;
- neurological signs;
- carotid bruits;
- evidence of vascular disease on CT scan.

Although the above factors can differentiate between vascular dementia and AD, these features are often present in those with AD and the two conditions often coexist.

CASE 21.4

A 68-year-old man with a history of hypertension had been taken to live with his daughter after he was found to be unable to cope in his own flat. He had problems finding his way around the new house and was constantly seeking reassurance. Every few weeks he would have episodes of sleeplessness when he believed intruders were coming into his room. During these phases he urinated in inappropriate places. He never quite got back to his 'old self' after any of these episodes.

MANAGEMENT

In addition to the general management of dementia outlined above, good control of any cardiovascular risk factors is important. The role of low-dose aspirin (75 mg daily), which is useful in other cerebrovascular disorders, has not yet been clarified.

Lewy body dementia

See Chapter 6 on organic states.

Reversible causes of dementia

Reversible causes of dementia are unusual in the elderly, but you should always be on the look-out for them (see Chapter 6 on organic states).

DEPRESSION IN THE ELDERLY

Depression in elders is under-recognized, and even when it is recognized it tends to be under-treated. Community surveys have shown that 10 per cent of elders suffer from depressive illnesses of marked severity, and a further 30 per cent suffer from depressive symptoms which are not severe enough to warrant a diagnosis. If you turn to acute medical wards or nursing and residential homes the figures are even higher.

Levels of depressive illness in different settings

- 10 per cent (4 per cent severe) in the community
- 20 to 40 per cent in acute medical wards
- 30 per cent in residential/nursing care

Reasons for the under-recognition and undertreatment of depression in the elderly

These can be summarized as follows:

- social reasons;
- clinical presentation;
- pharmacological reasons.

SOCIAL REASONS

Stereotypes of the elderly suggest that it is normal to be miserable during the later years of life (see who suffer from physical illness and assume depression is normal under such circumstances (see Chapter 13 on liaison psychiatry and somatoform disorders).

CLINICAL PRESENTATION

The classic presentation of depression in the elderly

- lowered mood
- loss of interest
- loss of energy and fatigue
- feelings of guilt, worthlessness and hopelessness
- agitation and retardation
- poor concentration
- suicidal ideation or attempts
- biological symptoms
- delusions and hallucinations

CASE 21.5

A 79-year-old woman presented with a 6-week history of feeling increasingly tired and 'washed out'. She was unable to do her day-to-day activities and stopped going out. She became increasingly miserable and wished that she was dead. She ate poorly and slept badly.

Clinical presentations like the one outlined in Case 21.5 are common and vary little from those which you might expect to see at any age. These cases are relatively straightforward and are not usually difficult to diagnose. In addition, the elderly can present in different ways to a younger age group.

Complaints of physical problems

CASE 21.6

A 74-year-old man made repeated journeys to his general practitioner for minor physical ailments which could not be diagnosed. He began to call the duty doctors out of hours for reasons they could not discern. When he began to call the emergency services because of acute distress, and the family doctors were billed, a psychiatric assessment was requested. The person was found to be profoundly depressed but responded well to a combination of antidepressant treatment and social support.

Minor medical morbidity is common in the elderly. Wear and tear on the body leaves its legacy for many elders. Frequently there is a coincidental abnormality, osteoarthrosis of the knees, or diverticular disease, which is irrelevant, but which can be used to explain away the problem and so the person is dismissed ('It's your age, dear, nothing we can do').

However, the person will return again and again to the surgery with vague pains and non-specific symptoms until the depression is recognized or they give up trying this approach.

Recent onset of neurosis

'I do worry doctor, I've nothing to worry about, but I do'. 'I check things too – the doors at night, the heating, five times sometimes'. It has been said that there is only one neurosis in old age, and that is depression. This is not true, but there is some merit in thinking about a primary mood problem when people present with obsessive-compulsive symptoms or anxiety for the first time late in life.

Depressive pseudodementia

The presentation of depression as an apparently dementing illness has been dealt with elsewhere (see Chapter 6 on organic states).

Distinguishing dementia from depression

- acute, recent onset of symptoms
- no cognitive decline prior to depressive symptoms
- complaints about cognitive problems
- 'don't know' answers
- variable impairment
- inattention
- slow mental processing
- past history of depression

Behavioural disturbance

CASE 21.7

An 82-year-old woman in a rest home began to call out at night, put herself on the floor and bang on the floor with her stick during the day, demanding attention from the staff. Her problems were described as 'behavioural' and she was asked to leave when she had previously been a popular resident. A psychiatric assessment revealed her to be depressed to the point of suicide. A short course of ECT restored her to her previous ·level of functioning and she continued in the home.

Unusual behaviours which at first sight do not appear to be depressive in origin should be considered carefully. More demanding behaviour in the residential home, calling relatives when there is nothing wrong or nothing to say, and changes in the level of self-care may all point in non-specific ways to a person developing depression. Any of these could be dismissed merely as the result of the person being difficult and cantankerous.

Late-onset alcoholism

Most old age psychiatrists do not see many people with alcohol abuse as their primary problem. By the time they reach 65 years of age, most people with alcohol problems have either died as a result of their drinking or established some kind of stability which does not require input from psychiatric services.

For those who present for the first time with alcohol problems in old age, depression is the most common reason for the change in behaviour. Most are self-medicating to relieve the symptoms of anxiety and insomnia that they experience.

Sudden complaints of loneliness

Moving out of your home and into residential care is a major step, and not one to be taken lightly. Although it can provide companionship, help and a fulfilling environment, this is achieved at a huge cost, i.e. giving up your home, possibly leaving your neighbourhood, and losing independence, not to mention the financial cost. If a person talks of moving away from home for no clear reason it is advisable to look for symptoms of depression and advise that they take no decision until their mood has improved. Many other ways of reducing isolation could be tried (day centres, clubs, befrienders, etc.) before this step is taken. It is hard to get out of residential care once you are in.

Suicide attempts

In contrast to the younger age group, where episodes of deliberate self-harm may be associated with specific situations and there is no intent to kill, this is rarely the case in the elderly. Until recently, the elderly were over-represented in terms of the numbers of those committing suicide,

although there is now a trend for younger men to commit suicide more frequently than before.

Risk factors for suicide in the elderly

- *social factors* living alone, male sex, failure to adjust to retirement
- *physical factors* chronic physical problems, especially pain
- *psychological factors* depressive illness; bereavement, previous suicide attempt, threats of self-harm, putting affairs in order

The presentation of depression in old age

- 'classical'
- with physical symptoms
- neurotic symptoms
- depressive pseudodementia
- behavioural disturbance
- late-onset alcohol abuse
- complaints of loneliness
- suicide attempts

Causes of depression in the elderly

BIOLOGICAL FACTORS

Depression in the elderly is said to be more 'organic' than depression in the younger adult. The elderly person suffering from depression is less likely to have a family history than their younger counterpart. Neuro-imaging studies have not yet convincingly demonstrated a difference between the normal elder and the depressed elder, or between the young and the old person with depression.

The association with physical illness has already been noted.

SOCIAL FACTORS

Loneliness is one of the commonest complaints of those who suffer from depression in old age. As families disperse, the potential for social isolation has increased. Public transport is more difficult to use and the elderly person no longer has a place in society. Lack of a close confidant has been identified as a major factor in the development of depression in the elderly.

PHARMACOLOGICAL FACTORS

The elderly tend to be more prone to the side-effects of medication. This has two consequences:

- attempts to administer medication within a therapeutic range can be limited by its side-effects;
- doctors tend to be very cautious and to under-treat depression.

Attempts must always be made to set medication into a dose range that is likely to effect a clinical improvement within the limits of side-effects. This applies to the elderly as much as to any other group.

If a person is not responding to a given dose of an antidepressant, after checking the diagnosis and compliance the next step is to increase the dose if the person can tolerate it. This might be done more slowly in the elderly, particularly if they are frail, than in more robust people.

CASE 21.8

A 74-year-old man experienced a moderate depressive episode with marked symptoms of anxiety. He was treated by his family doctor with 75 mg imipramine daily, to which he had responded during a previous episode 20 years previously. He made some progress, but did not become symptom-free. It was not until he had received a dose of 200 mg daily that he responded fully. The dose had been increased in 25-mg steps with monitoring of his blood pressure (when lying and standing) and his ECG.

Until recently, the standard treatments for depression in the elderly were tricyclic antidepressants and monoamine oxidase inhibitors (MAOIs).

Tricyclic antidepressants

Although they are highly effective in the elderly, there are problems with these drugs (outlined in Chapter 8 on mood disorders). The elderly are more likely to have problems with drug interactions and difficulties with the antimuscarinic side-effects which include:

- glaucoma;

- urinary retention;
- delirium;
- constipation.

Postural hypotension may not be a great problem in a young adult, but for an elder a fall can mean a fractured hip and loss of independence. Rehabilitation in the presence of depression is always more difficult.

The elderly also have a greater incidence of cardiac problems, which limits the use of this group of drugs.

Problems with the use of tricyclics in the elderly

- antimuscarinic problems
- cardiac dysrhythmias
- postural hypotension

Monoamine oxidase inhibitors (MAOIs)

The traditional MAOIs are now little used in the elderly, although the introduction of moclobemide (Manerix), a reversible inhibitor of MAO (RIMA), with a much improved side-effect profile, has rejuvenated interest in this class of drugs.

Selective serotonin reuptake inhibitors (SSRIs) (e.g. paroxetine, fluoxetine)

The introduction of this class of antidepressants has been important for the treatment of depression in the elderly. The improved side-effect profile (no cardiac or anticholinergic problems) and the possibility of once-a-day dosing gives them major advantages over the tricyclics. For many old age psychiatrists they have become the first-line treatment.

There are problems, particularly with gastrointestinal side-effects which can be difficult if the person is not eating or drinking well. The SSRIs may also cause agitation and restlessness.

Neuroleptics

In the presence of marked anxiety or agitation, neuroleptics may be added to the regime and gradually withdrawn as the person settles.

For people who also have psychotic symptoms, the addition of a neuroleptic to their regime speeds their recovery.

Augmentors

For those people who do not respond to standard antidepressant regimes, augmenting the regime is the next step.

Lithium

Lithium is commonly used, but the increased prevalence of low-grade renal failure and the concurrent use of diuretics and non-steroidal anti-inflammatory drugs means that it must be monitored very closely. Toxicity may occur within the therapeutic range.

Carbamazepine

Carbamazepine has been used and is effective. However, falls are a problem.

ELECTROCONVULSIVE THERAPY (ECT)

Indications for ECT in the elderly

- severe depression
- psychotic symptoms
- not eating or drinking
- severe suicide risk
- medication failure
- previous response

Age is no barrier to ECT. It remains a highly effective treatment, even for the oldest old. The major contraindication is a recent cerebrovascular accident.

The rate of complications increases with age, confusion being the most obvious of these. Some promote the use of unilateral ECT to reduce this complication, but with a lengthening of the course. My own practice is to start with bilateral ECT, which can be changed if confusion does arise.

PSYCHOLOGICAL THERAPIES

The elderly have been relatively neglected by psychotherapists for many years. More recently, increasing interest has been shown in psychological interventions, and they play an important part in the management of any depressed person.

SOCIAL INTERVENTIONS

The importance of social interventions can be deduced from what has been said before. Strategies to relieve loneliness and to develop a meaningful role in society (e.g. encouraging mutually enjoyable relationships with grandchildren) are vital elements of recovery from depression.

Outcome

Early studies suggested that the outcome for depression in the elderly is very poor. Naturalistic studies found very high relapse rates, high levels of chronicity and mortality levels in excess of those expected.

Predictors of a poor outcome for depression in the elderly

- the presence of physical illness
- the development of physical illness
- length of the episode prior to treatment
- the presence of brain pathology

Most people recover from the initial episode, but many relapse during the next 2 years. These numbers can be reduced by keeping people on medication for this 2-year period, after which many people have a smoother course.

PSYCHOTIC DISORDERS IN LATE LIFE

CASE 21.9

A 68-year-old woman presented to the police reporting that there were men in her loft. She had heard them talking to each other about her and she believed that they were connected to a home for people with learning difficulties who wanted to take over her house for themselves. She was referred to social services, who requested a mental health assessment.

Elderly people who present with psychotic illnesses have been characterized in the following way:

- women are more commonly affected than men;
- they are frequently isolated;
- they have some kind of sensory impairment.

Presentation

Members of this group often do not come to the attention of psychiatrists directly (see Case 21.9). They go to the police, housing authorities and other statutory agencies, driven by their persecutory beliefs.

They experience delusions and hallucinations in all modalities.

CASE 21.10

A 73-year-old woman saw people on the roofs opposite her house, who spied on her and could see what she was doing even when the curtains were closed. She called them 'chimney hoppers'.

Such people frequently believe that neighbours are trying to oust them from their homes, trying to poison them or attempting to harm them in some other way.

CASE 21.11

A 90-year-old deaf woman became very distressed by the behaviour of her neighbours, who she believed were passing gas into her house in order to poison her so that they could move their family into the house.

There are two categories of patient with late-onset psychotic disorder.

Functional

People in the first category are a 'functional' group who resemble those with schizophrenia (i.e. there are more first-rank symptoms and auditory hallucinations) of early onset and are more likely to have a family history of psychotic disorder. They respond well to medication, perform well in cognitive tests and have relatively normal CT scans.

Organic

People in the second category are more 'organic'. They are less likely to have a family history, they have subtle cognitive problems on presentation, and go on to develop dementia. They do not respond so well to treatment, have more changes on CT scan, and do not live as long as those in the 'functional' group.

CLASSIFICATION

This remains difficult. Some argue that these disorders represent schizophrenia that starts late in life, while others suggest that it is a separate disorder (paraphrenia) which is specific to late life. ICD-10 and DSM-IV have a category, 'persistent delusional disorder', into which many of these people fit.

MANAGEMENT

This group is difficult to engage, often demanding a move away from their accommodation rather than treatment of any kind.

Medical treatment

Treatment is with conventional neuroleptic medications. Depot medication will aid compliance.

Social management

Merely moving the person is unlikely to produce a lasting change in their mental state. A different environment can, however, break down the isolation experienced and improve the person's quality of life.

OUTCOME

- 33 per cent do well and become symptom-free on medication.
- 33 per cent improve but do not become symptom-free.
- 33 per cent do not improve.

CASE 21.12

A 74-year-old man continued to take neuroleptic medication on the basis that he felt much more able to deal with the foreign power that controlled his life when taking the medication than when he was without it. He never developed the view that the medication was reducing the symptoms themselves.

Relocation may cause a temporary reduction in symptoms, but the ideas will soon recur in the new setting.

OTHER DISORDERS

Anxiety disorders

Anxiety disorders are common in late life, although little recognized and rarely treated. As mentioned above, depression may be the main problem underlying the anxiety.

Fears about going out, falling and being mugged are increasingly common. They may be dismissed as a natural part of being elderly and no therapy introduced.

TREATMENT

Little is known about therapy for this group. They have received little attention, but social, psychological and pharmacological strategies may be effective.

Sleep disorders in the elderly

INSOMNIA

Insomnia is a subjective complaint about the quantity and quality of sleep. The incidence of insomnia is about 35 per cent in the elderly, and it is frequently reported to have been of long duration.

Causes of insomnia in the elderly
Physical causes
■ pain
■ cough
■ dyspnoea
■ bladder problems
Drugs
■ caffeine (tea, coffee)
■ alcohol
■ beta blockers
■ amphetamines
Psychological causes
■ bereavement
■ depression
■ dementia
■ mania
Disorders of sleep
■ obstructive sleep apnoea
■ restless legs

The pattern of sleep changes with increasing age, with less time spent asleep at night, but more time spent sleeping during the day. At the same time, people with less to do spend more time in bed, and so seem to have spent more time awake when they feel that they should have been asleep.

Causes of insomnia

A very wide range of problems may cause insomnia in the elderly. Many of these are physical, and more rarely they may be psychiatric.

Management

First make a diagnosis (diary-keeping and a careful history are important here), and then treat the underlying cause. If the diagnosis is primary insomnia then 'sleep hygiene' measures should be taken (see Chapter 6 on organic states). If this fails, then medication can be used, but this should only be for a short period. Hypnotic medication is associated with a wide range of difficulties in the elderly, of which falls are perhaps the most important.

Bereavement

Bereavements are common among the elderly. The process and problems of grieving are outlined in Chapter 22 on loss and bereavement.

CONCLUSIONS

For psychiatrists and general practitioners the elderly present particular challenges which can only be met by working within the context of a multidisciplinary team. Without this structure it is unlikely that the doctor alone will make much impact upon the suffering they encounter. Inter-agency working is essential to meet the complex and varied needs of this group.

Further reading

Burns, A. and Levy, R. 1994: *Dementia*. London: Chapman and Hall.

Burns, A., Howard, R. and Petit, W. 1995: *Alzheimer's disease: a medical companion*. Oxford: Blackwell Science.

Jacoby, R. and Oppenheimer, C. 1992: *Old age psychiatry*. Oxford: Oxford University Press.

22 LOSS AND BEREAVEMENT

A 72-year-old woman had been married for 49 years. Her husband developed a chest infection which was treated with antibiotics at home. His condition worsened and he developed heart failure. He was admitted to hospital but died 2 days after admission. His wife was with him when he died, but seemed to show little emotion and arranged the funeral without major difficulties. She cried at the funeral, but continued to cope well until a week later when she found herself unable to sleep, frequently crying, eating poorly and starting at each noise in the house, thinking that it might be her husband. She felt that she had done wrong in letting him go to hospital, and if only she had taken care of him all would have been well. Over the next 2 months the feeling of sadness and guilt receded. Although she still thought of him often, it was with less pain. She took up many of her social activities again and began to feel her normal self once more.

Case 22.1 shows the normal reaction to the death of a loved one (as this is normal it can hardly be called a case at all). There are three phases, which usually evolve over a 6-month period: numbness, sadness and acceptance.

NORMAL PHASES OF MOURNING

Numbness

The bereaved individual feels unreal and bereft of emotion, finding it difficult to accept the loss fully.

Sadness

In this phase of grief the person feels distressed, is often tearful, and loses all sense of enjoyment. They have difficulty concentrating, lose their appetite and sleep badly. They can become irritable and socially withdrawn. The organization of day-to-day activities can be difficult. Feelings of irrational guilt, responsibility and self-reproach affect one third of mourners. A smaller number of people turn this anger outward, often blaming doctors or nurses for the death of their loved one. There is preoccupation with the image of the deceased. Hallucinations are not uncommon and may be alarming, but for some people they are a source of comfort. The sensations range from a sense of the deceased person's presence to auditory or visual perceptions of them.

The bereaved can experience the aches and pains of the last illness of the deceased, and they may feel a generalized fear and sense of impending catastrophe or insanity. Survivors bitterly regret the loss of opportunity for reconciliation and for making reparation for normal family quarrels or disagreements.

Features which distinguish this phase of sadness from a typical depressive disorder are the rarity of thoughts about suicide, the absence of retardation, and the absence of guilt about real or imaginary misdeeds or moral failings, as opposed to self-reproach for letting the deceased die.

Acceptance

The symptoms gradually recede and the bereaved person accepts the loss and returns to a more normal level of functioning.

These phases are seen not only after death of a loved one, but also after loss of almost any kind, e.g. loss of a pet, amputation and job loss.

> The following features distinguish normal bereavement from depressive disorder:
>
> - suicidal thoughts are rare
> - no retardation
> - self-reproach for letting the deceased die
> - no guilt about past misdeeds or moral failings

PROLONGED OR ATYPICAL GRIEF

DEFINITION

This is arbitrarily defined as the persistence of the sadness phase at a high level of intensity beyond a 6-month period. The duration and intensity of the grief appear to be proportional to the bereaved person's perception of the preventability of the loss.

In addition to the components of the sadness phase, the following additional signs of abnormal grief can be seen:

- panic attacks;
- apathy;
- self-destructive behaviour;
- agitation or retardation;
- avoidance of places, people and objects related to the deceased;
- lack of specific grieving;
- anger about the final illness or mode of death;
- over-idealization of the dead person.

Protracted or unresolved grief is more likely under the following circumstances:

- sudden unexpected death (e.g. road traffic accident or industrial accident);
- when the death is 'untimely' (e.g. death of a child as opposed the anticipated death of an elder);
- when the relationship to the deceased was ambivalent (e.g. an unhappy marriage or strained relationship between parent and adolescent);
- when the bereaved has difficulty in expressing his or her feelings;
- when there are additional negative life events;
- when the survivor lacks social support.

PHYSICAL MORBIDITY AND MORTALITY IN SURVIVORS

Widowers are at risk of fatal myocardial infarction in the first year after the death of their wives; the widower literally dies of a broken heart. Attendance at the general practitioner's surgery is more frequent following a bereavement.

ANNIVERSARY REACTIONS

These are potent precipitants of delayed and unresolved grief. They are not only triggered by the anniversary of the death, but might coincide with a significant date in the course of the dead person's terminal illness, such as an operation, a move to a hospice, or the birthday of the deceased.

CASE 22.2

A 24-year-old woman with a history of alcohol abuse was brought into the emergency department having been found in the local cemetery. She had drunk a bottle of vodka and then lacerated her wrist on the gravestone of her father. She was depressed and wanted to die. Her relationship with her father had at times been brutal, as he would drink and beat both his daughter and her mother. At other times he was 'the most wonderful man alive'. He died of complications of his alcoholism. The day of her admission was his birthday.

Treatment of prolonged and atypical grief

CASE 22.3

An 18-year-old woman became pregnant by her boyfriend who then left her. She was isolated in a high-rise flat with little social contact. The baby was born prematurely and subsequently died. She attended the funeral but showed little emotion. She had not returned to the grave when seen 8 months later in the clinic. She was miserable, apathetic and had lost weight. It was difficult for her to talk about the child, but over a period of several months, she slowly began to talk of her high hopes for the child, what kind of a mother she would have been, and her anger at her boyfriend's desertion of her. She brought in photographs of the child, and eventually managed to pack away the cot and the toys she had bought. Later she began to take up her social life again and look for work.

The basic principle of the treatment is a recapitulation of the grieving process, aiming to help the patient to move through the different phases of grief until they are eventually able to accept the loss. The bereaved person is encouraged to talk about their feelings of sadness, anger or guilt which they had previously repressed. This may also include a behavioural element (e.g. bringing in photographs of the deceased, clearing out their clothes, or visiting their grave) coupled with discussion of the feelings that these activities invoke.

It can be useful to talk about such feelings very soon after any loss, as this can help to prevent the development of abnormal grief.

Further reading

The following are classic texts on the subject and well worth reading, despite their age.

Kubler-Ross, E. 1970: *On death and dying*. London: Tavistock.

Murray Parkes, C. 1970: *Bereavement*. Harmondsworth: Pelican.

New developments in the science of genetics have begun to transform thinking in many areas of medicine, including psychiatry. Whilst the genetics of individual disorders are addressed in the relevant chapters, the basic principles underlying the discipline are investigated here.

DEFINITIONS

DNA

DNA (deoxyribonucleic acid) is a polymer composed of four bases, namely adenine (A),

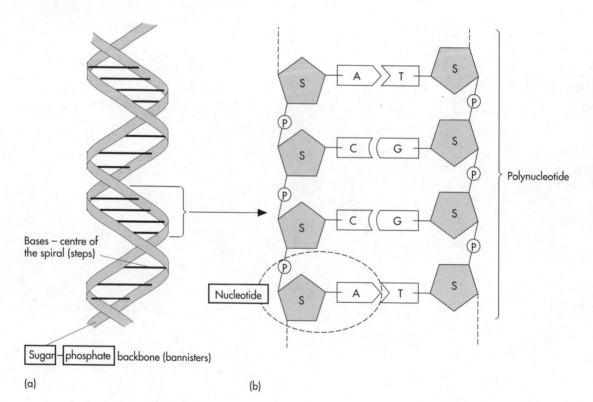

Bases – centre of the spiral (steps)

Sugar – phosphate backbone (bannisters)

Nucleotide

S A T S

P

S C G S

P

S C G S

P

S A T S

Polynucleotide

(a)

(b)

FIG 23.1 (a) The double helical structure of DNA. (b) Magnified view of DNA components; S, pentose sugar; P, phosphate; C, cytosine; T, thymine; A, adenine; G, guanine.

guanine (G), thymine (T) and cytosine (C), attached to deoxyribose sugar molecules linked by a phosphate backbone. DNA forms itself into a double helix like a spiral staircase, with bases from each strand forming the 'steps' (Figure 23.1).

The genetic code

The sequence of bases represents the 'genetic code'. This code is deciphered, and via intermediaries in the form of messenger RNA it determines the proteins produced by the cell.

The genome

The genetic material of a cell is called the genome. The human genome has the following features:

■ 3×10^9 base pairs (i.e. 3000 Mb);
■ three to four times the size of the genome of a bacterium;
■ it is over 1 m in length in each cell;
■ it is divided into 46 chromosomes (22 pairs plus a pair of sex chromosomes);
■ it is diploid (i.e. each cell contains two copies).

Genes

Genes are the part of the DNA which codes for protein. Most DNA is non-coding. The human has about 75 000 genes.

Cell division

MITOSIS

The 46 chromosomes are replicated and passed on to two diploid daughter cells (Figure 23.2).

MEIOSIS

Each chromosome becomes associated with its pair and the DNA is shuffled between them (this is known as crossing-over or recombination). After replication of the chromosomes the cell then divides to give four haploid cells (gametes) (Figure 23.2).

Genetic variation

POLYMORPHISM

Natural variation in characteristics such as eye colour is called polymorphism. It results from inheriting variations in the DNA.

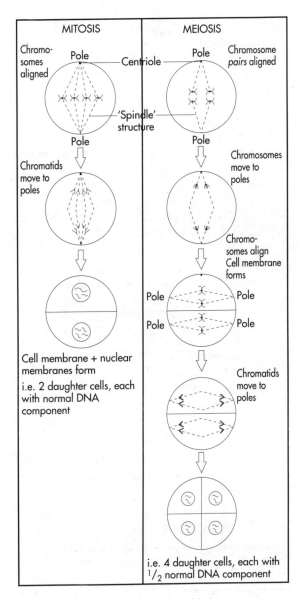

FIG 23.2 Comparison of chromosomal behaviour in mitosis and meiosis.

ALLELE

An allele is one of two or more alternative forms of a given gene.

MUTATION

A rare variation in the normal DNA sequence is known as a mutation. Mutations can range from a single base-pair change to gross abnormalities of the chromosome structure.

METHODS OF HUMAN GENETIC RESEARCH

Cytogenetics

The chromosomes of a cell are visible under the light microscope just prior to cell division. They can be identified by the size of their arms and by their characteristic 'banding pattern' after they have been stained.

THE CLASSIFICATION OF CHROMOSOMAL ABNORMALITIES

Numerical

Too many, e.g. Down's syndrome, trisomy 21, Kleinfelter's syndrome XXY.
Too few, e.g. Turner's syndrome X0.

Structural

Deletions; pieces missing.
Duplications; extra pieces.
Rearrangements between or within the chromosome.

Genetic epidemiology

Genetic epidemiology seeks to find the relative contributions of genetic components to a given trait and that ascribable to the environment.

Family studies

Within families members share different proportions of their genes. The parents siblings and children share half the genes. Second degree relatives share only a quarter.

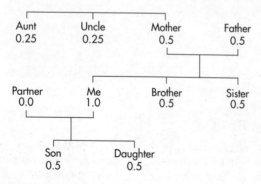

FIG 23.3 Family studies.

If a disease has a genetic component, then the relatives of the sufferer will be affected more often than members of the general population (Figure 23.3). An increased risk within a family does not prove a genetic component, but makes it likely. The family may be exposed to the same environmental risk factor (e.g. exposure to lead).

Twin studies

Monozygotic twins share the same genetic material. Any differences between them are the result of environmental influences. Dizygotic twins share 50 per cent of their genetic material.

Concordance

If two people share the same trait they are said to be concordant. If DZ twins have a lower concordance for a particular trait than MZ twins, then it is likely that genetic factors are playing a role.

Adoption studies

An adoptee is brought up by genetically unrelated parents. Resemblance to genetic parents is caused by genes, whereas resemblance to adopted parents is caused by environmental factors.
Two types of adoption study can be done:

- investigation of the incidence of illness in the adopted-away offspring of an affected individual compared to the incidence of that illness in the adopted-away offspring of an unaffected individual;
- investigation of the incidence of illness in the biological parents compared to that in the adopted parents of an affected individual.

GENETIC MODELS

Mendelian models

These are simple models, usually of a single gene influencing a single trait.

Autosomal dominant

Only one copy of the gene is required to express the disease (e.g. Huntington's chorea).

Autosomal recessive

Two copies of the gene are required to express the disease. Individuals with one copy of the gene are carriers.

X-linked recessive

All males will be affected, and females are unaffected carriers. Male-to-male transmission is never seen, as only the Y-chromosome is passed on.

X-linked dominant

Both males and females can be affected, but the disease may be less severe in females with a normal X-chromosome in addition to the damaged one.

MODIFYING FACTORS

Single-gene mutations may not produce the patterns of disease predicted by the 'Mendelian model' if they are subject to modifying factors.

Expressivity

All individuals have the disease, but to greater or lesser degrees.

Penetrance

Not all carriers of the gene become ill. Penetrance represents the number of individuals who carry the gene who actually become ill.

Imprinting

Expression of the damaged gene depends upon the parent of origin.

Anticipation

The disease gets worse in each successive generation.

Quantitative and complex traits

If the inheritance of a disease does not fit a simple (Mendelian) model, even after modifying factors have been taken into account, then less specific models are proposed.

Single major locus (SML) model

The disease is caused by one major defective gene, the effect of which is modulated by random environmental influences.

Polygenic-multifactorial inheritance

The disease is caused by a number of genes (polygenic) in combination with many environmental factors, the effects of which are small, independent and additive.

This model has been proposed for many disorders, e.g. diabetes, heart disease, Alzheimer's disease, schizophrenia and affective psychosis.

These disorders are probably genetically heterogeneous, i.e. one disorder may be caused by a variety of different gene combinations. Mild to moderate learning difficulties are probably the result of several genes interacting, whereas severe problems are less heritable and more likely to result from biological factors (e.g. trauma, infection or chromosome aberrations).

Molecular genetics

Molecular genetics involves searching for mutations which are responsible for a disorder, or which influence its course. Using experimental techniques to establish the order of bases in a particular fragment of DNA, it is possible to identify the position of mutations.

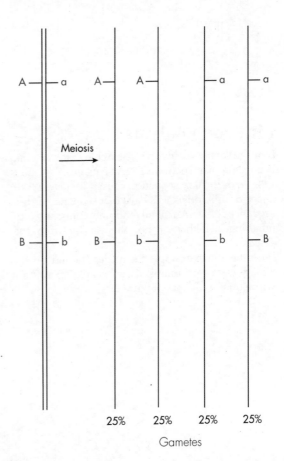

FIG 23.4 Linkage analysis.

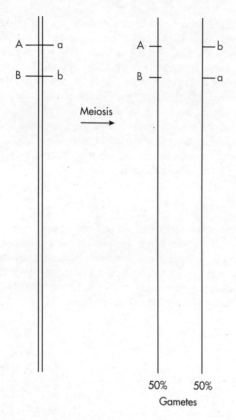

Meiosis

50%   50%
Gametes

FIG 23.5 Linkage analysis

Linkage analysis

Linkage analysis involves searching for a link between a disease and a DNA sequence.

If a particular sequence causes a disease, all affected individuals will have that sequence. Other sequences of DNA will be randomly transmitted to offspring, whether or not they suffer from the disease.

In the above example the alleles Aa and Bb are a long way apart (unlinked), and haplotypes occur with equal frequency (Figure 23.4).

In the second example (Figure 23.5) the alleles are closer together and do not segregate randomly to the gametes but are passed on unchanged.

LOD SCORE

This genetic distance is measured by the LOD (logarithm of odds) score. A LOD score of 3 is regarded as evidence of linkage, a score of zero is non-informative and a score of –2 is evidence of non-linkage.

Allelic association analysis

This involves comparing the frequency of an allele in a diseased population with its frequency in a normal control population. Allelic association assumes that the mutation has only arisen a few times and that alleles close to it will be inherited with it. Individuals with the disease will have a greater frequency of these alleles closely associated with the mutation.

CONCLUSIONS

Psychiatric disorders result from a complex inter-action between environmental and genetic factors. Mutations which cause disorders directly may be identified using molecular genetic techniques. These techniques allow the identification of the responsible gene in the absence of any biochemical clues to the aetiology of the disease. As increasing numbers of genes and susceptibility factors are identified, the treatment for psychiatric disorders will be revolutionized.

Further reading

Guffin, P., Owen, M.J., O'Donovan, M.C., Thapar, A. and Gottesman, I. 1994: *Seminars in psychiatric genetics.* London: Gaskell.

INTRODUCTION

Throughout this book you will have encountered references to people who have been admitted to hospital when they do not consider themselves ill or in need of treatment. To remove a person from their home and detain them against their will could be a major infringement of their civil liberties, whatever the benign and paternalistic intentions of those who make the decision to remove them. The Mental Health Act 1983 is the body of legislation which deals with the compulsory detention and treatment of people suffering from mental disorder.

Conditions included in the term 'mental disorder'

- mental illness (e.g. mania)
- arrested or incomplete development of mind (i.e. severe mental disability)
- psychopathic disorder (see Chapter 19 on personality and its disorders) psychopathic disorder is not included in the Mental Health legislation covering Scotland and Northern Ireland. The compulsory admission procedures referred to in this chapter deal with legislation which covers England and Wales)

Promiscuity, sexual deviancy and dependence on drugs or alcohol are not included in the category of mental disorder. However, a drug- or alcohol-induced psychosis (e.g. paranoia or hallucinosis) is covered by the term 'mental illness'.

All doctors should be familiar with the procedures for compulsory admission because they will be involved either as general practitioners or as medical staff in an Accident and Emergency department.

- Compulsory admission and detention involve Sections 4, 5 and 136.
- Compulsory longer term admissions involve Sections 2 and 3.

Sections 2, 3 and 4 require the carefully considered completion of two standard forms:

- the medical recommendation;
- the approved social worker's (or relative's) application.

The medical recommendation must include those symptoms and aspects of behaviour which satisfy the criteria set out below.

SECTION 2

From the general practitioner's point of view, Section 2 (Figure 24.1) is the most commonly used section.

Medical recommendation for admission for assessment

Mental Health Act 1983
Section 2

Form 4

(full name and address of medical practitioner)

I _____

_____

a registered medical practitioner, recommend that

(full name and address of patient)

_____

_____

be admitted to a hospital for assessment in accordance with Part II of the Mental Health Act 1983

I last examined this patient on

(date) _____

*Delete if not applicable

* I had previous acquaintance with the patient before I conducted that examination.

* I have been approved by the Secretary of State under section 12 of the Act as having special experience in the diagnosis or treatment of mental disorder.

I am of the opinion

(a) that this patient is suffering from mental disorder of a nature or degree which warrants detention of the patient in a hospital for assessment

AND

(b) that this patient ought to be so detained

Delete the indents not applicable

    (i)   in the interests of the patient's own health

    (ii) in the interests of patient's own safety

    (iii) with a view to the protection of other persons

AND

(c) that informal admission is not appropriate in the circumstances of this case for the following reasons:–

(The full reasons why informal admission is not appropriate must be given)

_____

_____

_____

_____

_____

_____

Signed _____ Date _____

FIG 24.1 Section 2. Reproduced with the permission of HMSO, London.

This section allows compulsory admission for assessment or for assessment followed by medical treatment for up to 28 days. The recommendation is made by two medical practitioners, one of whom is preferably the person's own general practitioner, and the other an 'approved doctor', i.e. one who is recognized as having special training in psychiatry. The medical examination requires direct personal examination of the person's mental state and consideration of all the available medical information, e.g. the general practitioner's records. The views of the community psychiatric nurse should also be taken into account.

The application is made by an approved social worker or nearest relative, preferably the former.

Points that the doctors must agree on

- the person is suffering from a mental disorder (i.e. mental illness, arrested or incomplete development of mind, or psychopathic disorder) which is so severe that they should be detained in hospital for assessment followed by treatment
- the person should be detained in the interest of either preventing a deterioration in their own mental health or safety, or for the protection of other people

Assessment of the person should be carried out jointly by the doctors and the approved social worker, who must consider whether to request assistance from the police if there is a significant risk of violence.

Two doctors must discuss their views with the applicant and with each other, and they must consider realistic alternative forms of care, including informal admission, out-patient or domiciliary treatment, or arranging for willing and capable friends or relatives to stay with the person. When considering alternatives to hospital admission, the burden on the 'carers' and any risk to their safety and physical and psychological well-being must be taken into account. The safety of the community must also be taken into consideration.

Doctors and social workers must beware of making false assumptions based on gender, social and cultural background. Certain religious practices, such as prolonged fasting or praying, must be evaluated with the assistance of a religious authority from the person's community. In addition, in those cases where the person and the doctors do not have fluent knowledge of each other's language, the services of a trained interpreter with some basic knowledge of psychiatry and its terminology and of the person's cultural background should be enlisted. Interpreters are generally available through Social Services

Points to consider when recommending a section

- alternative forms of care
- carer burden
- gender, and religious, social and cultural background
- communication problems due to language differences
- communications due to intercurrent illness or disability (deafness, dysphasia, etc.)

Departments or through a hospital's 'ethnic switchboard'. Consideration should also be given to the possibility of misunderstandings due to intercurrent health problems such as deafness or dysphasia.

The doctors are responsible for ensuring that a hospital bed will be available. If direct access to the person is not immediately possible, and there is reason to believe that the situation is urgent, Section 135 may be invoked (see below), or the police may be called to gain entry in a case of extreme emergency.

Section 2 authorizes detention for a maximum period of 28 days.

SECTION 3

This compulsory admission (Figure 24.2) is for treatment, and requires the medical recommendation of two doctors (one of whom is 'approved', while the other is preferably the person's own general practitioner). The maximum period of detention under Section 3 is 6 months, but it is renewable for a further 6 months.

Medical recommendation for admission for treatment

Form 11

Mental Health Act 1983
Section 3

(full name and address of practitioner)

I ⬚

⬚

a registered medical practitioner, recommend that

(full name and address of patient)

⬚

⬚

be admitted to hospital for treatment in accordance with Part II of the Mental Health Act 1983

(date)   I last examined this patient on ⬚

*Delete if not applicable

*(a) I had previous acquaintance with the patient before I conducted that examination.

*(b) I have been approved by the Secretary of State under section 12 of the Act as having special experience in the diagnosis or treatment of mental disorder.

In my opinion this patient is suffering from —

(complete (a) or (b))

**The phrase which does not apply <u>must</u> be deleted

(a) mental illness/severe mental impairment **and his mental disorder is of a nature or degree which makes it appropriate for him to receive medical treatment in a hospital;

(b) psychopathic disorder/mental impairment **and his mental disorder is of a nature or degree which makes it appropriate for him to receive medical treatment in a hospital and such treatment is likely to alleviate or prevent a deterioration of his condition.

This opinion is founded on the following grounds:-
[Give clinical description of the patient's mental condition]

_____

_____

_____

_____

_____

_____

Delete the indents not applicable

I am of the opinion that it is necessary
(i)   in the interest of the patient's own health
(ii)   in the interest of patient's own safety
(iii)   with a view to the protection of other persons

that this patient should receive treatment and it cannot be provided unless he is detained under section 3 of the Act, for the following reasons:–

[Reasons should indicate whether other methods of care or treatment (eg out-patient treatment or local social services authority services) are available and if so why they are not appropriate, and why informal admission is not appropriate.]

_____

_____

_____

_____

_____

_____

Signed _____ Date _____

FIG 24.2 Section 3. Reproduced with the permission of HMSO, London.

Medical recommendation for emergency admission for assessment

Form 7

Mental Health Act 1983
Section 4

THIS FORM IS TO BE USED ONLY FOR AN EMERGENCY APPLICATION

(name and address of medical practitioner)

I

a registered medical practitioner, recommend that

(full name and address of patient)

be admitted to a hospital for assessment in accordance with Part II of the Mental Health Act 1983

(date)   I last examined this patient on

(time)   at

*Delete if not applicable

* I had previous acquaintance with the patient before I conducted that examination.

* I have been approved by the Secretary of State under section 12 of the Act as having special experience in the diagnosis or treatment of mental disorder.

I am of the opinion —

(a) that this patient is suffering from mental disorder of a nature or degree which warrants the patient's detention in a hospital for assessment for at least a limited period

AND

(b) that this patient ought to be so detained

Delete the indents not applicable

    (i)   in the interests of the patient's own health
    (ii) in the interests of the patient's own safety
    (iii) with a view to the protection of other persons

AND

(c) that informal admission is not appropriate in the circumstances of this case.

In my opinion it is of urgent necessity for the patient to be admitted and detained under section 2 of the Act. Compliance with the provisions of Part II of the Act relating to applications under that section would involve undesirable delay.

In my opinion an emergency exists, because I estimate that compliance with those provisions would cause about ☐ hours' delay, and I consider such a delay might result in harm as follows

(state reasons)

_____

_____

_____

_____

_____

to

*(a) the patient
*(b) those now caring for him
*(c) other persons.

I understand that the managers of the hospital to which the patient is admitted may ask me for further information relevant to this recommendation.

I was first made aware that his condition was causing anxiety, such that it might warrant immediate admission to hospital—

†Delete whichever
do not apply

†(a) Today at (time) ☐
†(b) Yesterday
†(c) On (date if within one week) ☐
†(d) more than a week ago

Signed _____   Date _____

                                            Time _____

FIG 24.3 Section 4. Reproduced with the permission of HMSO, London.

Report on hospital in-patient

Form 12

Mental Health Act 1983
Section 5 (2)

(name of hospital or
mental nursing home
in which the patient is)

To the Managers of

I   am

delete the phrase
which does not
apply

the registered medical practitioner

the nominee of the registered medical practitioner

in charge of the treatment of

(full name of patient)

who is an in-patient in this hospital and not at present liable to be detained under the Mental
Health Act 1983. I hereby report, for the purposes of section 5(2) of the Act, that it appears
to me that an application ought to be made under Part II of the Act for this patient's
admission to hospital for the following reasons:–

(Reasons should indicate why informal treatment is no longer appropriate)

Signed _____   Date _____

Time _____

FIG 24.4 Section 5(2). Reproduced with the permission of HMSO, London.

COMPULSORY EMERGENCY ADMISSIONS AND DETENTION UNDER THE MENTAL HEALTH ACT

Section 4

This section (Figure 24.3) is only to be used in genuine emergencies when admission is an urgent necessity and in cases where there is a significant danger of mental or physical harm to others and/or the danger of serious harm to property and/or the need for physical restraint. It is only to be implemented when there is not enough time to get a second medical recommendation. A Section 2 is preferable because of the greater safeguard of civil liberties that it offers. The assessment criteria are the same as for a Section 2.

Section 5(2) – the doctor's holding power

This section (Figure 24.4) only applies to people who are already in-patients, whether in psychiatric, medical or surgical wards. It does not apply to out-patients or to people in the Accident and Emergency department, i.e. it is not an admission Section. The Section must be implemented immediately after examination of the person and it must not be left on the ward for nurses to submit if and when they fear that the person is about to leave. The person can be detained on a Section 5(2) for up to 72 hours when the person's consultant or their deputy concludes that an application for formal admission (Sections 2 or 3) is indicated. The Section 5(2) cannot be renewed.

Section 5(4) – the nurse's holding power

When a psychiatric emergency (e.g. risk of suicide or violence) arises which involves an informal psychiatric patient, and a doctor is not immediately available, a registered mental nurse can lawfully prevent a person from leaving the ward for 6 hours or until the arrival of a doctor who is empowered to use Section 5(2).

Section 136 – police power to remove to a place of safety

DEFINITION

A 'place of safety' is a hospital or police station where a person can be detained for assessment by a (preferably approved) doctor and an approved social worker, and assessments can be made for treatment and care. People detained under Section 136 cannot have their detention prolonged by a Section 5(2) or Section 5(4). If compulsory admission is indicated, this should be under Section 2 or Section 3. Under exceptional circumstances a person may be admitted from a police station under Section 4.

Section 135

An approved social worker who believes that a person is suffering from a mental disorder and is unable to care for himself or herself or who is being ill-treated or neglected can apply to a magistrate for a warrant to remove that person to a place of safety.

Further reading

Department of Health and Welsh Office 1993: *Code of practice: Mental Health Act 1983*. London: HMSO.
Lipsedge, M. 1989: Choices in psychiatry. In Dunstan, G.R. and Shinebourne, E.A. (eds), *Doctor's decisions. Ethical conflicts in medical practice*. Oxford: Oxford University Press.

INDEX